HEALTH PROMOTION IN NURSING PRACTICE

Eighth Edition

Health Promotion in Nursing Practice

Carolyn L. Murdaugh, PhD, RN, FAAN
Professor Emerita and Adjunct Professor
University of Arizona
College of Nursing
Tucson, Arizona

Mary Ann Parsons, PhD, RN, FAAN
Professor Emerita and Dean Emerita
University of South Carolina
College of Nursing
Columbia, South Carolina

Nola J. Pender, PhD, RN, FAAN
Professor Emerita
University of Michigan
School of Nursing
Ann Arbor, Michigan

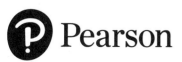 Pearson

330 Hudson Street, NY, NY 10013

Vice President, Health Science and TED: Julie Levin Alexander
Director, Portfolio Management and Portfolio Manager: Katrin Beacom
Editor in Chief: Ashley Dodge
Portfolio Management Assistant: Erin Sullivan
Associate Sponsoring Editor: Zoya Zaman
Product Marketing Manager: Christopher Barry
Field Marketing Manager: Brittany Hammond
Vice President, Digital Studio and Content Production: Paul DeLuca
Director, Digital Studio and Content Production: Brian Hyland

Managing Producer: Jennifer Sargunar
Content Producer (Team Lead): Faraz Sharique Ali
Content Producer: Neha Sharma
Manager, Rights Management: Gina Cheselka
Operations Specialist: Maura Zaldivar-Garcia
Cover Design: Cenveo Publisher Services
Cover Art: dharshani Gk-arts/123RF
Full-Service Management and Composition: iEnergizer Aptara®, Ltd.
Printer/Binder: LSC Communications
Cover Printer: LSC Communications
Text Font: Palatino LT Pro 10/12

Library of Congress Cataloging-in-Publication Data
Names: Murdaugh, Carolyn L., author. | Parsons, Mary Ann, author. | Pender, Nola J., 1941– author.
Title: Health promotion in nursing practice / Carolyn L. Murdaugh, PhD, RN, FAAN, Professor Emerita and Adjunct Professor, University of Arizona, College of Nursing, Tucson, Arizona, Mary Ann Parsons, PhD, RN, FAAN, Professor Emerita and Dean Emerita, University of South Carolina, College of Nursing, Columbia, South Carolina, Nola J. Pender, PhD, RN, FAAN, Professor Emerita, University of Michigan, School of Nursing, Ann Arbor, Michigan.
Description: Eighth edition. | Boston : Pearson, [2019] | Revised edition of: Health promotion in nursing practice / Nola J. Pender, Carolyn L. Murdaugh, Mary Ann Parsons. Seventh edition. [2015]. | Includes bibliographical references and index.
Identifiers: LCCN 2017061583 | ISBN 9780134754086 | ISBN 0134754085
Subjects: LCSH: Health promotion. | Preventive health services. | Nursing.
Classification: LCC RT67 .P56 2019 | DDC 613--dc23 LC record available at https://lccn.loc.gov/2017061583

1 18

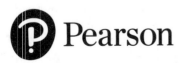

ISBN 13: 978-0-13-475408-6
ISBN 10:   0-13-475408-5

Dedication

To nurse educators and practicing nurses who teach and role model health promotion. I bid you success as you face the challenges of promoting a culture of health for all.

— C. L. Murdaugh

To my family and friends for their support during the preparation of this edition; I wish all of you happy and healthy lives.

—M. A. Parsons

CONTENTS

FOREWORD

I am pleased to write the foreword for the eighth edition of *Health Promotion in Nursing Practice*. The promotion of health is recognized globally as essential to the well-being of the world population and to the achievement of health equity across diverse racial, ethnic, and economic groups. Many organizations speak of the need to develop a "culture of health" worldwide. Increasingly, health policies are being designed and implemented to move toward the goal of high-level health and wellness for all. Widespread adoption of this goal by health care providers would result in new models of care, decreased monies spent on acute illness, and a lower incidence of devastating chronic diseases. Access to innovative health promotion programs for all populations, particularly those most vulnerable, is a major focus of this eighth edition.

This book helps the nurse link health promotion practices with national health goals such as those articulated in *Healthy People 2020*. Nurses must lead positive change in health promotion and prevention policies and design health promotion programs as a multisectoral endeavor. Healthy environments, schools, and worksites with adequate air quality, water supply, housing, vector control, and shelter from the devastating effects of natural disasters are essential to quality living. Community-based health promotion strategies are the first lines of support for the health of all people. This new edition provides strategies that nurses can use to help communities activate their power to engage in competent individual, family, and community self-care. These strategies address the social and physical environments critical for healthy longevity. Approaches to evaluating the effectiveness of behavior change programs in communities and in primary care are also described.

New communication, tracking, and linking technologies are developing at a rapid pace, thus enabling widespread dissemination of health promotion information and innovative support of individuals and families who want to make positive lifestyle and environmental changes. Sporadic programs do not result in the continuity of care needed for real health behavior change at the family and community levels. In this edition, the authors speak to the importance of social media, mobile applications (apps), and other digital technologies to support better continuity of care and follow-up essential to effective long-term behavior change.

Cultural sensitivity to the health promotion needs of diverse populations is important as many communities are experiencing a wider array of languages, cultural practices, and lifestyles. Fitting health promotion services to individuals, families, and communities from diverse backgrounds requires listening to their priorities, respecting them as persons with dignity and worth, and adapting health promotion strategies and technologies to differing cultural values, levels of education, and life stages.

It is important that health promotion services be provided by nurses and other health care workers who maintain healthy lifestyles and healthy work environments. The American Nurses' Association declared 2017 as the year of the *Healthy Nurse*. Educational programs for nurses and other health professionals must provide healthy learning environments and preparation for healthy lifestyles to be consistent with valuing health promotion as an important aspect of nursing practice.

Knowledge about health promotion and effective interventions continues to emerge. This eighth edition integrates the results of the latest research and theoretical advances into useful, evidence-based information to help nurses provide scientifically sound health promotion and prevention services. Dr. Carolyn L. Murdaugh and Dr. Mary Ann Parsons, nurse experts in health promotion, will inspire you to incorporate new health promotion strategies into your organizational policies, create scientifically sound nursing protocols, and provide leadership in the development of a culture of health.

Nola J. Pender, PhD, RN, FAAN
Distinguished Professor
Marcella Niehoff School of Nursing
Loyola University Chicago
Professor Emerita
School of Nursing
University of Michigan

PREFACE

The overall goal of the eighth edition is to provide nurses and other health promotion practitioners practical, evidence-based information to promote the health of racially, ethnically, and culturally diverse individuals, families, and communities. The book aims to (1) present a comprehensive approach to health promotion that is based on the most recent research and federal guidelines; (2) describe the role that digital technologies are playing in health promotion in all ages and populations; (3) integrate factors in the social and physical environments that influence health and health inequities; and (4) offer strategies to implement and evaluate programs to promote health in individuals across the life span, and in schools, worksites, and communities. We believe information in the book provides the foundation on which to build the practice of health promotion.

ORGANIZATION OF THIS BOOK

- *Part I, The Human Quest for Health:* Multiple conceptions of health are reviewed, and both individual and community models are described to guide the development of health promotion programs.
- *Part II, Planning for Health Promotion and Prevention:* Strategies are presented to assess health, health beliefs, and health behaviors, and develop a health promotion plan.
- *Part III, Interventions for Health Promotion and Prevention:* Four core health-promoting behaviors are addressed: physical activity, nutrition, stress management, and social support.
- *Part IV, Evaluating the Effectiveness of Health Promotion:* Practical methods for evaluating health promotion programs are described.
- *Part V, Approaches for Promoting a Healthy Society:* Four areas are included: empowering individuals for self-care; promoting health and health literacy and decreasing health inequities in diverse populations with culturally sensitive approaches; promoting health in schools, worksites, and communities; and building a healthy society through social and environmental change.

NEW TO THIS EDITION

- An overview of several theories and models that currently guide the development of digital health promotion applications.
- The role of technology in health assessment and health planning.
- The application of social media, mobile health, and other digital technologies in promoting healthy behaviors for physical activity, healthy eating, and stress reduction.
- The use of online communities to provide support.
- Strategies to empower individuals and communities for self-care.
- Federal plain language guidelines to promote health literacy.

- Updated information on environmental contaminants, including herbicides, lead, and shale gas extraction.
- Information about the Robert Wood Foundation goal to create a national movement to promote a culture of health which promotes health equity.
- Incorporation of *Healthy People 2020* midcourse evaluations and *Healthy People 2030*.
- Updated chapter content, tables, and figures based on the most recent literature.

For the learner, each chapter contains learning objectives, figures, tables, and displays to highlight and reinforce material covered in each chapter; suggestions for applying the information to practice; recommended avenues for research; and learning activities to provide experiences in health promotion activities and challenge the student to critically think about the chapter content. Last, an extensive reference list is available at the end of each chapter, and relevant websites are included throughout the book.

The book is ideally suited for undergraduate students in nursing and health promotion, graduate students in advanced practice programs, including the DNP, and nurses and other health care professionals who practice in health promotion settings.

ACKNOWLEDGMENTS

We are deeply indebted to Alice Pasvogel, PhD, Assistant Research Scientist, College of Nursing, University of Arizona, who spent countless hours editing, formatting, and preparing the tables and figures. Her patience, attention to detail, and expert editorial assistance enabled us to finish the book in a timely manner.

Our sincere appreciation is also extended to many persons at Pearson who have supported us in completing this revision. We are especially appreciative of Ashley Dodge, who guided the revision of the eighth edition, and Neha Sharma and Cheena Chopra at Noida, India, who worked closely with us during the final preparation and production stages. Neha's sensitivity to the stressors of writing and deadlines, and both Neha's and Cheena's expertise and attention to detail are sincerely appreciated. Last, we acknowledge the reviewers who provided valuable feedback on several chapters for this edition.

Carolyn L. Murdaugh
Mary Ann Parsons

Reviewers

Sharrica Miller, PhD, CPNP-PC, RN
Assistant Professor
College of Health & Human Development
School of Nursing
California State University
Fullerton, California

Judith Peters, Ed.D. RNC
Associate Professor
School of Nursing
Loma Linda University
Loma Linda, California

Ira Scott-Sewell, PhD, RN
Associate Professor
Associate of Science in Nursing Department
Alcorn State University
Natchez, Mississippi

Jutara Srivali Teal, DNP, MTOM, RN, L.Ac.
Assistant Professor
College of Health & Human Development
School of Nursing
California State University
Fullerton, California

Health Promotion in a Changing Social and Digital Environment

The rapid expansion of digital technologies, along with rising health care costs, increasing population diversity, and persistent health inequities, has moved the need for health care reform and health promotion to center stage. Dramatic advances have occurred in health and health care over the past century, mainly due to public health efforts and new medical technologies. However, the health care system in the United States is no longer the best in the world, and persistent health care inequities have resulted in declining health for many Americans. The need to promote health brings both opportunities and challenges, as culturally diverse individuals and their social and physical environments must be addressed.

HEALTH EXPENDITURES AND HEALTH IN THE UNITED STATES

Expenditures for health care in the United States are higher than any other high-income country in the world, and were before the Affordable Care Act (Dieleman et al., 2016). In spite of the amount of money spent on health care, of 35 industrialized countries, the United States reports the highest child and maternal mortality rates, homicides, body mass index, sexually transmitted diseases, and major chronic diseases, including diabetes, ischemic heart disease, and chronic lung disease. Although the projected life expectancy is predicted to increase in most countries by 2030, life expectancy gains for the United States are projected to be one of the lowest. In addition, the United States is the first country to experience a reversal of height in adulthood, which is associated with greater longevity (Kontis et al., 2017). These findings have been described as the American "health care paradox," as the large number of dollars spent on health care in this country has not resulted in better health and longevity, compared to other countries (Bradley, Sipsma, & Taylor, 2017).

How health care dollars are spent matters. Countries projected to have greater longevity have higher ratios of social service to health care spending to address the social determinants of health. The ratio of social service to health care spending in the United States is the lowest of all 13 high-income countries, and the United States is the only one of the 13 countries without universal health coverage. In 2013, the second highest health care spending in the United States was for chronic illnesses, such as diabetes, ischemic heart disease, chronic lung disease, and cerebrovascular disease, all conditions with modifiable lifestyle factors. Pharmaceutical costs were highest for hyperlipidemia and hypertension, two risk factors that can frequently be reduced with lifestyle change. Most of public health spending went to manage communicable diseases, with little allocation to the promotion of healthy lifestyles (Dieleman et al., 2016).

HEALTH AND THE SOCIAL ENVIRONMENT

Where people live also determines their health. The contributions of the social, economic, and environmental conditions of communities to health and longevity are no longer questioned. Longevity increases with income. In research reported in 2016, a longevity difference of 15 years for men and 10 years for women was observed in persons who were in the top 1% income bracket compared to persons in the bottom 1%, and this inequality has increased over the past 12 years (Chetty et al., 2016). Geographic differences in longevity in low-income persons were observed; low-income persons who live in affluent cities have greater life expectancies that those who live in less affluent cities. Affluent cities are more likely to provide public services for all its citizens than poorer cities.

The role of social determinants in health was recognized in the *Healthy People 2020* goals; two overarching goals in the proposed *Healthy People 2030* framework are to achieve health equity for all and eliminate disparities, and to create social and physical environments that promote attainment of health and well-being for all (Office of Disease Prevention and Health Promotion, 2017).

THE SOCIAL ENVIRONMENT AND A CULTURE OF HEALTH

In 2010, the Robert Wood Johnson Foundation (RWJF) developed a long-term vision for a culture of health in all communities (Robert Wood Johnson Foundation & RAND Corporation, 2015). The major outcome of the culture of health action framework is improved population health, well-being, and equity. Priority areas include interventions to develop healthy children, increase access to affordable care, and address components of social and built environments that promote health.

Creating a culture of health presents opportunities for nurses who incorporate health promotion in their practice. Expanded skills, knowledge, and innovative practice models are required to integrate the social determinants of health into health promotion (Denham, 2017). Knowledge that promotes communication, collaboration, and leadership to foster community engagement, partnerships, and empowerment will enable nurses to improve the health of individuals in diverse communities. Becoming culturally competent and gaining skills to promote health literacy are also necessary. Interdisciplinary teams are essential to building a culture of health in a community, so nurses should also possess skills needed to work as a team member in a community and be able to provide team leadership.

DIGITAL TECHNOLOGIES, HEALTH PROMOTION, AND HEALTH EQUITY

The high costs of health care and limited funds spent on social services to decrease health inequities place the burden on the federal government to eliminate unnecessary spending and invest in upstream determinants of health (Shortell & Rittenhouse, 2016). Investment in health promotion programs and services that address lifestyle risk factors instead of secondary and tertiary prevention can reduce costs and promote health. Incorporating digital technologies is a potentially powerful strategy to promote health and decrease health inequities for hard-to-reach, low-income, racially and ethnically diverse populations.

Digital technologies are widespread and found in all aspects of people's lives. Information and communication technologies are constantly expanding and influencing lives around the world. According to a Pew Research Center report, in 2016 the median for adults owning either a cellphone or a smartphone was 88% globally. Over 95% of adults in the United States had a cellphone in 2016, compared to 53% in 2000. Of the 95% having a cellphone, 77% owned a smartphone (Pew Research Center, 2017a). Mobile smartphones offer sophisticated technology and connection to the Internet. They enable users to browse the Internet to access information, run applications (apps), send and receive e-mail, and communicate health data to health care professionals (Singh & Landman, 2017). Smartphones may include video cameras, accelerometers, pedometers, and global positioning systems (GPS).

Traditionally, health promotion has been a low-tech area compared to innovations in medical technologies used in acute health care settings. However, health information technologies are one of the fastest trends in the health care system. The expansion of mobile wireless computer technologies, social media applications, telemedicine, and telehealth is having a significant influence on health promotion and prevention, unlike any in recent history. Mobile health (mHealth) applications, a subset of electronic health (eHealth), offer mobile computing for health care and represent a significant change in health promotion strategies. These apps enable clients to track health information, receive prompts, record, visualize, and communicate information, and interact in peer support groups. Internet coaches (eCoach) are also used in many health and wellness apps. Social media and social networking sites are also avenues for sharing health information.

In spite of the growth of Internet access and mobile phones, the economic, access, and literacy barriers have not been addressed, as they have been slow to spread to disadvantaged social groups, including persons with low income, low education, low health literacy, or limited English language skills; racial/ethnic minorities; the elderly; and persons living in rural areas (Pew Research Center, 2017b). The differences in access are described as the digital divide or digital inequality between disadvantaged and advantaged groups worldwide due to lack of Internet access and personal computer ownership. Digital inequalities are seen across the life span in socioeconomically disadvantaged children and adolescents, adults, and older persons. Internet access should be a priority for all citizens in all communities (Hicks, 2017).

mHEALTH, HEALTH LITERACY, AND HEALTH PROMOTION

Internet and mHealth applications are seen as potentially significant strategies to decrease health inequities and promote health, as they increase access to health professionals, health information, and health promotion apps, and empower clients to engage in healthy self-care behaviors (Robinson et al., 2015). However, persons with low health literacy do not possess the skills needed to interact with technology-based apps. Poor health literacy is a health risk as persons with inadequate literacy skills have limited understanding of their health problems and treatments. Health inequities are decreased when individuals have access to the Internet and digital technologies and the necessary literacy and computer skills to interact with the health apps. Nurses play a role in making sure that mHealth apps address culturally appropriate health information and the literacy levels of their clients; designing and teaching health literacy programs that are sensitive to culturally diverse populations; and engaging community organizations to find solutions to address access and cost issues.

Some eHealth advocates view empowerment as a positive outcome of mHealth as clients take an active role in managing their health and lifestyle. Unfortunately, there is limited evidence that all clients are willing or capable of assuming responsibility for their health. Other critics warn about focusing solely on individual responsibility without attending to the social determinants of health. Information and quality remain a concern in social media platforms. Potential ethical and privacy issues signal caution and demand constant monitoring by health care professionals. Evidence clearly shows that mobile technologies, including mHealth and social media, have the potential to bridge the digital divide and play a significant role in promoting the health of all individuals and communities.

HEALTH PROMOTION: GOING FORWARD

The changing social and digital environment and persistent inequities in health and health care, along with the increasing burden of noncommunicable diseases, create tremendous health challenges for nurses and all health professionals. Individual lifestyle factors play a role in noncommunicable diseases, and persons with inequities in income, education, housing, employment, and safe communities are less likely to practice health behaviors (Davies et al., 2014). The need to address both individual and community level health has resulted in a call for a new wave in public health. The "fifth" wave is described as a shift to a culture of health to promote the health of all (Davies et al., 2014). In this wave, individuals and communities are interdependent and engaged to promote health equity. A culture of health has also been envisioned and supported by the RWJF in this country as described earlier.

Practicing nurses and nurse educators are challenged to envision a new wave in practice and education that promotes both individual behavioral change and healthy communities where healthy lifestyles can be practiced. Denham (2017) calls for "disruptive" changes in nursing education and practice to place an emphasis on societal concerns. In a new wave of health promotion practice, collaborative partnerships offer a powerful strategy to bring stakeholders together to address the many individual and social issues; they might include local and state organizations and governments and private and public agencies. Digital technologies also offer venues to promote communication and facilitate change at all levels. The pace of change in health care and the social and digital environments present many challenges; they also bring many new opportunities for nurses who have a desire to promote health for all.

References

Bradley, E., Sipsma, H., & Taylor, L. (2017). American health care paradox—High spending on health and poor health. *QJM: An International Journal of Medicine, 110*(2), 61–65. doi:10.1093/qjmed.hcw187

Chetty, R., Stepner, M., Abraham, S., Lin, S., Scuderi, B., Turner, N., . . . Cutler, D. (2016). The association between income and life expectancy in the United States, 2001–2014. *JAMA, 315*(16), 1750–1766. doi:10.1001/jama.2016.4226

Davies, S., Winpenny, E., Ball, S., Fowler, T., Rubin, J., & Nolte, E. (2014). For debate: A new wave in public health improvement. *The Lancet, 384*(9971), 1889–1895. doi:10.1016/S0140-6736(13)62341-7

Denham, S. (2017). Moving to a culture of health. *Journal of Professional Nursing, 33*(5), 356–362. doi:10.1016/j.profnurs.2017.07.010

Dieleman, J., Baral, R., Birger, M., Bui, A., Bulchis, A., Chapin, A., . . . Murray, C. (2016). US spending on personal health care and public health, 1996–2013. *JAMA, 316*(24), 2627–2646. doi:10.1001/jama.2016.16885

Hicks, E. (2017). Digital citizenship and health promotion programs: The power of knowing. *Health Promotion Practice, 18*(1), 8–10. doi:10.1177/1524839916676263

Kontis, V., Bennett, J., Mathers, C., Li, G., Foreman, K., & Ezzati, M. (2017). Future life expectancy in 35 industrialized countries: Projections with a Bayesian model ensemble. *The Lancet, 389*(10076), 1323–1335. doi: 10.1016/S0140-6736(16)32381-9.

Office of Disease Prevention and Health Promotion. (2017). *Healthy People 2030.* Retrieved from https://healthypeople.gov

Pew Research Center. (2017a). *Mobile fact sheet. Who owns cellphones and smartphones.* Retrieved October 1, 2017, from www.perinternet.org/fact-sheet/mobile/

Pew Research Center. (2017b). *Digital divide persists even as lower-income Americans make gains in tech adoption.* Retrieved October 1, 2017, from http://www.pewresearch.org/fact-tank/2017/03/22/digital-divide-persists-even-as-lower-income-americans-make-gains-in-tech-adoption/

Robert Wood Johnson Foundation & RAND Corporation. (2015). *From vision to action: A framework and measures to mobilize a culture of health.* Robert Wood Johnson Foundation. Retrieved October 1, 2017, from https://www.cultureofhealth.org/content/dam/COH/RWJ000_COH-Update_CoH_Report_1b.pdf

Robinson, L., Cotten, S., Ono, H., Quan-Haase, A., Mesch, G., Chen, W., . . . Stern, M. (2015). Digital inequities and why they matter. *Information, Communication, & Society, 18*(5), 569–582. doi:10.1080/1369118X.2015.1012532

Shortell, S., & Rittenhouse, D. (2016). The most critical health care issues for the next president to address. *Annals of Internal Medicine, 165*(11), 816–818. doi:10.7326/M16-2471

Singh, K., & Landman, A. (2017). Mobile health. In A. Sheikh, K. Cresswell, A. Wright, & D. Bates (Eds.), *Key Advances in clinical informatics: Transforming health care through health information technology* (pp. 183–196). San Diego, CA: Elsevier.

PART 1

The Human Quest for Health

CHAPTER 1

Toward a Definition of Health

OBJECTIVES

This chapter will enable the reader to:

1. Compare traditional and holistic beliefs about health.
2. Contrast stability and actualization concepts of individual health.
3. Discuss viewpoints of health by nurse theorists.
4. Summarize family and community definitions of health.
5. Describe the social determinants of health.
6. Discuss strategies to build a culture of health.
7. Justify the significance of global health.
8. Discuss the changing perspectives of health promotion to promote health.

Although health is one of the four concepts expressed in the nursing metaparadigm and a stated goal of nursing, different views about the meaning of health are common (American Nurses Association, 2010; Fawcett & Desanto-Madeya, 2013). These differences result from a greater understanding of determinants of health and the diverse social values and norms in our multiple ethnic, religious, and cultural groups. What many health professionals once accepted as the definition of health—the absence of diagnosable disease—is only one of many views of health held today. All people who are free of disease are not equally healthy. Furthermore, health can exist without illness, but illness does not exist without health as its context.

Health promotion, the central strategy for improving health, has shifted the paradigm from defining health as a dichotomy (presence or absence of illness or disease) to a multidimensional definition of health with social, economic, cultural, and environmental dimensions. In a multidimensional model, health benefits can potentially be achieved from positive changes in any one of the health dimensions. This expanded health perspective encompasses multiple options for improving health and no longer places the responsibility for poor health entirely on the individual.

Definitions of health change over the life span. As children mature and move into adolescence, their explanation of health becomes more inclusive and more abstract. Health definitions of adolescents begin to expand to include physical, mental, social, and emotional health and not just the idea of absence of illness. Young adults ages 16 to 24 years report less priority on health and less engagement in health behaviors than adolescents ages 12 to 15 years and adults 25 years and older (Goddings, James, & Hargreaves, 2012). Older adults hold a more holistic definition of health, placing emphasis on physical, mental, social, and spiritual dimensions (Song & Kong, 2015).

Gender is also an important sociocultural determinant of health throughout the life span (Diaz-Morales, 2017). Many factors contribute to gender differences in health, including genetic, biological, social, and behavioral factors such as risk-taking behaviors, health-seeking behaviors, and coping styles (Caroli & Weber-Baghdiguian, 2016; Diaz-Morales, 2017). The social context of men and women is also a major determinant of gender differences. Gender equality is considered a major social determinant of health and crucial to improving the health of women and transgender individuals. In addition, a greater understanding is needed of the influence of gender on health behaviors.

A positive model of health emphasizes strengths, resiliencies, resources, potentials, and capabilities. The nature of health as a positive life process is less commonly discussed; attention still focuses on forces that undermine health, rather than factors that lead to health. Morbidity (prevalence of illness) and mortality (death) continue to be used to define the health of a population. Although these indicators are essential, they do not provide a complete picture, as they reflect disease burden and the need for health care, not health. Complex interwoven forces within the social and physical environmental context of people's lives also determine health. Health cannot be separated from one's life conditions, as neighborhood, social relationships, work, and leisure, which lie outside the realm of health practices, positively or negatively influence health long before morbid states are evident.

HEALTH AS AN EVOLVING CONCEPT

The historical development of the concept of health provides the background for examining definitions of health found in the professional literature. The Greeks were the first to write that health could not be separated from the physical and social environments and human behavior (Tountas, 2009). Their philosophy maintained that harmony, equilibrium, and balance were the key elements to health, and illness resulted when this balance was upset. Plato considered health to be a state of being in complete harmony with the universe. Hippocrates went on to define health as a balance between environmental forces and individual habits. Illness was considered an upset of this equilibrium (Tountas, 2009).

The word *health* as it is commonly used did not appear in writing until approximately AD 1000. It is derived from the Old English word *health*, meaning being safe or sound and whole of body (Sorochan, 1970). Historically, physical wholeness was important to be accepted in social groups. Persons suffering from disfiguring diseases, like leprosy, or congenital malformations were ostracized from society. This was due to others' fear of contracting contagious diseases as well as discrimination against those whose appearance was altered due to disease or deformity. Being healthy was considered natural or in harmony with nature, while being unhealthy was thought of as unnatural or contrary to nature.

Society became concerned about helping individuals escape the catastrophic effects of illness beginning with the scientific era that produced new medical discoveries and treatments. *Health* was described as "freedom from disease." Because disease could be traced to a specific cause, often microbial, it could be diagnosed. The notion of health as a disease-free state was extremely popular into the first half of the 20th century. Health and illness were viewed as extremes on a continuum; the absence of one indicated the presence of the other. This gave rise to "ruling out disease" to assess health, an approach still prevalent today. The underlying erroneous assumption is that a disease-free population is a healthy population.

The concept of mental health did not exist until the latter part of the 19th century. Individuals who exhibited unpredictable or hostile behavior were labeled "lunatics" and ostracized in much the same way as those with disfiguring physical ailments. Being put away with little or no human care was considered their "just due," because mental illness was often ascribed to evil spirits or satanic powers. The visibility of the ill only served as a reminder of personal vulnerability and mortality, aspects of human existence that society wished to ignore.

The psychological trauma resulting from the high-stress situations of combat during World War II expanded the scope of health to include the mental status of individuals. Mental health was seen as the ability of an individual to withstand stresses imposed by the environment. When individuals succumbed to the rigors of life around them and no longer were able to carry out the functions of daily living, they were declared to be mentally ill. Despite efforts to develop a more holistic definition of health, the dichotomy between individuals suffering from physical or mental illness persisted for many years. In 2011, the World Health Organization (WHO) published an expanded view of mental health as a state of well-being in which individuals realize their potential, can cope with normal life stresses, work productively, and are able to make a contribution to their community (World Health Organization, 2014).

In 1946, the WHO proposed a landmark definition of health that emphasized "wholeness" and the positive qualities of health: "Health is a state of complete physical, mental, and social well-being and not merely the absence of disease and infirmity" (World Health Organization, 2005). The definition was revolutionary in that it

1. Reflected concern for the individual as a total person
2. Placed health in the context of the social environment
3. Overcame the reductionist definition of health as the absence of disease.

The breadth of this historical definition mandated a comprehensive approach to health promotion, and inherently created an imperative for health equity (Friel & Marmot, 2011).

Many continue to think that the WHO definition is utopian, too broad, and the absoluteness of the term "complete" renders health impossible to achieve (Bok, 2017; Huber & Bok, 2015). The definition was formulated when acute infectious illnesses were the major health burden. However, chronic diseases have replaced acute illnesses as the major cause of disability and death, and people are living with chronic diseases for decades. This change is not accounted for in the definition. In addition, the influence of the genome in disease, the inability to separate individuals from their environment, and the relationship of the earth's climate and human health cannot be ignored. Despite multiple acknowledged influences on health, the WHO definition of health continues to be the most popular and comprehensive definition of health worldwide and was reaffirmed at the 2005 assembly (World Health Organization, 2005). It is now accepted that individual health cannot be separated from the health of society. Moreover, the relationship of human health to the health of the earth's ecosystem is also recognized as an important dimension. In other words, one cannot be healthy in an unhealthy society or world. Within these dimensions, health has more recently been defined as "the ability to adapt and to self-manage in the face of social, physical and emotional challenges" (Bok, 2017). Health is not a fixed state, as it varies depending on an individual's life circumstances.

In the following sections, health definitions are discussed that focus on the individual and the community. Although health care professionals cannot ignore individual health, the health of the individual's larger community is also critical, as the health of the community influences the overall health status of its members.

DEFINITIONS OF HEALTH THAT FOCUS ON INDIVIDUALS

Health as Stability

Stability-based definitions of health are based on the physiological concepts of homeostasis (internal stability) and adaptation. Dubos (1965), an early advocate of the stability position, defines health as a state that enables the individual to adapt to the environment. The degree of health experienced is dependent on one's ability to adapt to the various internal and external tensions that one faces. Dubos considered optimum health to be a mirage because in the real world individuals must face physical and social forces that are forever changing, frequently unpredictable, and often unsafe. An early scientist who viewed the environment as a major influence on health, Dubos considered the closest approach to optimum or high-level health to be a physical and mental state that permits one to function effectively within the environment (Flannery, 2009).

Definitions of health based on normality can be considered stability oriented. Norms represent average states rather than excellence in human functioning (Ereshefsky, 2009). Health is considered a normal function and disease represents an impairment of normal function. A major issue with normative definitions of health is that they leave little room for incorporating growth, maturation, and evolutionary emergence into a definition of health.

Environmentally focused models of health can also be considered stability oriented, as these models are based on adaptation to one's environment. Health is considered an individual's ability to maintain a balance with the environment. Health exists when one is able to adapt to the environment successfully and is able to grow, function, and thrive. In contrast, lack of adaptation is seen as a gap between one's ability to adapt and the demands of the environment.

Parsons' conceptualization of health is compatible with a stability-oriented environmental model. More than 50 years ago, Parsons defined health in terms of social norms rather than physiological norms, describing health as individuals' effective performance of roles and tasks for which they have been socialized (Parsons, 1958).

A number of nurse theorists have proposed definitions of health emphasizing stability beginning with Florence Nightingale. Nightingale viewed health as being the best that one could be at any point in time (Selanders, 2010). Levine, an early nurse theorist, defines health as a state in which there is balance between input and output of energy and in which functional, personal, and social integrity exists (Schaefer, 2014). Johnson, in her behavioral system model, does not explicitly define health. However, a view of health that focuses on stability can be inferred from her conceptualization of internal homeostasis (Holaday, 2014). Behavioral system stability is demonstrated by efficient and effective behavior that is purposeful, goal directed, orderly, and predictable.

Roy also subscribes to a stability definition of health. The central concept in Roy's model is adaptation. Health is a state and process of successful adaptation that promotes being and becoming an integrated whole person. The four adaptive modes through which coping energies are expressed are physiological, self-concept, role performance, and interdependence. Adaptation promotes integrity, which implies soundness or an unimpaired condition that can lead to completeness and unity. In an adapted state, one is freed from ineffective coping attempts that deplete energy. Available energy can be used to enhance health (Doucet & Merlin, 2014).

Health as Actualization

When individual health is defined more broadly as actualization of human potential, some prefer to use the term *wellness*, as it is considered less restrictive than the concept of health. Halbert Dunn, the creator of the modern-day definition of wellness, was an early advocate for emphasizing actualization in a definition of health. Dunn coined the term *high-level wellness*, which he described as integrated human functioning that is oriented toward maximizing an individual's potential. This requires that individuals maintain balance and purpose within the environment where they are functioning (Dunn, 1959, 1980). Although the definition identifies balance as a dimension of wellness, major emphasis is on the realization of human potential as individuals move toward their personal optimum level based on their capabilities and potential.

Definitions of wellness have evolved since Dunn initially defined the concept and launched the wellness movement. The dominant view is that wellness is holistic and includes multiple positive dimensions of health. These dimensions include social, emotional, physical, spiritual, and intellectual wellness. The wellness definition includes building on one's strengths and optimizing one's potential. The terms health, well-being, and wellness are used interchangeably in the literature, although each concept is thought to have distinguishing features. Consistencies across the definitions of health and wellness include the following:

1. Health and wellness are not merely the absence of disease.
2. Health and wellness consist of multiple dimensions that are holistic and interrelated.
3. There is a dynamic balance among the dimensions of health and wellness.
4. Health and wellness represent optimal functioning.

The WHO Regional Office in Europe convened an expert group to define well-being and develop objective and subjective measures of the domains of well-being. The first meeting was held in 2012 (World Health Organization, 2013a). The definition that was developed is considered to support the original WHO definition of health. They defined well-being as comprising individuals' experiences of their lives as well as a comparison of life circumstances with social norms and values (World Health Organization, 2013a). Wellness contains both subjective and objective dimensions. Health is considered a separate concept that influences subjective well-being, and well-being is linked to health (World Health Organization, 2013b).

Orem uses *health* and *well-being* to refer to two different but related human states in her self-care theory (Orem & Taylor, 2011; Shah, 2015). She defines *health* as a state characterized by soundness or wholeness of human structures and bodily and mental functions. *Well-being* is considered an ideal state characterized by experiences of contentment, pleasure, and happiness; by spiritual experiences; and by continuing personalization. Personalization refers to movement toward maturation and achievement of human potential (self-actualization). Engaging in responsible self-care and continuing development of self-care competency are qualities of personalization. Individuals can experience well-being even under conditions of adversity, including disease. In describing her man-living-health theory of nursing, Parse defines health as an open process of becoming (Doucet & Merlin, 2014; Parse, 2011), which is consistent with health as actualization.

Newman, building on the grand theory of Martha Rogers, defines health as the totality of the life process, which is evolving toward expanded consciousness (Bateman & Merryfeather, 2014; Neuman & Fawcett, 2012). This definition emphasizes the actualizing properties of individuals throughout the life span. Health encompasses the entire life process, which evolves toward a higher and greater frequency of energy exchange. Newman's model of health addresses holistic characteristics of human beings. However, similar to Roy's theory, there is no intent to create strategies to measure many of the terms, limiting potential testing and clinical applicability of her definition.

Both Newman and Parse build on Martha Rogers' theory of unitary person. Both represent attempts to define health in terms of holism as opposed to defining health in components or parts. The emergent nature or actualization potential of the healthy individual and the capacity for open energy exchange with the environment are characteristics of both Newman's and Parse's definitions of health.

Actualization or wellness models have been criticized because of the difficulties in measuring subjective perceptions. In addition, perceptions of health and wellness vary according to age and sociocultural context. Some believe that the expanded definitions of health in some of the wellness models do not differentiate health from happiness, quality of life, and other global concepts. In spite of these limitations, the wellness definitions provide a holistic focus and promote the positive aspects of health.

Health as Actualization and Stability

Models of individual health also incorporate both stability and actualization. In these models, health is defined as a feeling of well-being, a capacity to perform to the best of one's ability, and the flexibility to adapt and adjust to stressful situations created by one's environment. King, an early nurse theorist, proposes a definition of health that emphasizes both stabilizing and actualizing tendencies. She identifies health as the goal of nursing and defines *health* as a dynamic state in the life cycle of a person that implies

TABLE 1–1   Nurse Theorists' Conceptualizations of Health

Nurse Theorist	Health Conceptualization
Health as Stability	
Florence Nightingale	The best that one could be at any point in time
Myra Levin	A state of balance between inputs and outputs of energy in which functional and personal integrity exists
Dorothy Johnson	Internal homeostasis; balance and stability among all behavioral systems demonstrated by purposeful, goal-directed behavior
Calista Roy	Process of successful adaptation that promotes being and becoming integrated to function as a whole person
Health as Actualization	
Dorothea Orem	Wholeness of physical and mental functions as one progresses toward maturation and achievement of human potential
Margaret Newman	The totality of life processes that are evolving toward expanded consciousness (self-actualization)
Health as Stability and Actualization	
Imogene King	A dynamic state in which one is successfully adjusting to environmental stressors to achieve maximum potential for everyday living

adjustment to stressors in the environment through optimum use of resources to achieve one's maximum potential for daily living (Gunther, 2014; King, 1990, 2007). In King's model, a holistic health perspective relates to the way individuals handle stressors while functioning within the culture to which they were born. King views health as a functional state in the life cycle, while illness interferes in the life cycle. Table 1–1 summarizes the conceptualizations of health by the early nurse theorists.

A definition of health must be applicable to everyone—to the well, to those with an acute illness, and to those with chronic disease or disability. The authors of this text believe a definition of health should incorporate both actualizing and stabilizing tendencies, and define *health* as the realization of human potential through goal-directed behavior, competent self-care, and satisfying relationships with others, while adapting to meet the demands of everyday life within one's social and physical environments. The definition is based on the assumptions that health is an expression of person and environment interactional patterns that become increasingly complex throughout the life span. These interactional patterns are influenced by conditions of daily living as well as the economic, political, and sociocultural context. The authors of this book believe health and illness are qualitatively different, interrelated concepts that may coexist. In Figure 1–1, multiple levels of health are depicted in interaction with episodes of illness. Illnesses, which may have a short (acute) or long (chronic) duration, are represented as discrete events within the life span. Health can still be an aspiration to

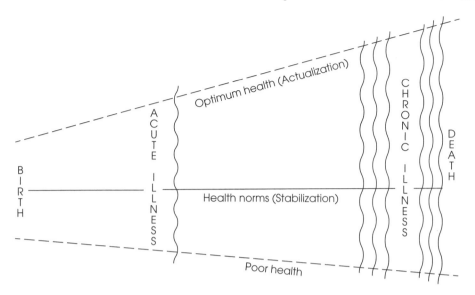

FIGURE 1–1   The Health Continuum Throughout the Life Span

those with a chronic illness or disability, and health can be achieved despite being diagnosed with a disease or living with a disability. Illness experiences can either hinder or facilitate one's continuing quest for health. Thus, good health or poor health may exist with or without overt illness.

Health as an Asset

The conceptualization of health as a resource or asset was introduced in 1986 at the First International Conference on Health Promotion (World Health Organization, 1986a), when health was defined as not an end in itself but a resource for daily living. This conception was further described as the capacity to engage in various activities, fulfill roles, and meet the demands of daily life. This definition builds on the WHO recognition of health as the strengths and capabilities inherent in individuals. Health as an asset has also been described as the internal and external attributes of the individual that mobilize positive health behaviors and optimum outcomes (Rotegard, Moore, Fagermoen, & Ruland, 2010). Health as an asset was noted in Schlotfeldt's early model of nursing. She described health as an asset and stressed focusing on individual strengths, rather than problems. Internal attributes are characteristics that are inherent within individuals, such as personality, attitude, and motivation. Internal attributes are influenced by an individual's external attributes, which include the social and cultural environments. Inclusion of external assets is consistent with the focus on the social determinants of health.

An Integrative View of Health

Although the biological model provides technological excellence and sophisticated medical care, it has led to a narrow focus on disease. An expansive view of health goes beyond disease prevention and risk reduction and emphasizes mind, body, and spirit: personal and social resources as well as physical capacities (Witt et al., 2017). When this view is integrated with traditional biomedical models (disease) and public health models (mortality, morbidity, and risks) of health, a holistic biopsychosocial view is possible. Understanding the relevance of an integrative definition of health for individuals in their everyday life experiences in different social contexts acknowledges the social determinants of health. An integrative definition of health acknowledges the need to expand traditional health promotion programs to empower individuals to improve the health of their communities.

DEFINITIONS OF HEALTH THAT FOCUS ON THE FAMILY

The complexity of the family and the diversity of family life in different ethnic, cultural, and geographic settings pose a challenge for defining and promoting family health. The traditional definition of family as two or more persons living together who are related by marriage, blood, or adoption is no longer adequate in American society. Families may be defined by biological, legal, or emotional ties, whether or not they are living together. Families may include nuclear families, single-parent families, blended families, same-sex partnerships, families without children, and sibling families. One broad definition of *family* now accepted is two or more persons who depend on one another for emotional, physical, or financial support. In this definition, family members are self-defined and may include any individuals who make a significant commitment to each other outside of marriage. Variation in family structure is essential when defining, measuring, and promoting family health.

A biopsychosocial definition of *family health* describes family health as a dynamic changing state of well-being, including biological, psychological, sociological, spiritual, and cultural factors of the family system. In this definition, an individual's health affects the functioning of the family, and in turn, family functioning affects the health of the individual. Thus, both the family system and the individual members must be part of the health assessment.

A family model of reciprocal determinism also takes into account the complexity of the family environment in promoting health (Knowlden & Sharma, 2016). In this model, health behaviors of individuals are a function of the environment that is shared with other family members and their behaviors and personal characteristics. Health information is shared and behaviors are learned, practiced, and reinforced in the daily routine, which are facilitated or hindered by family values and beliefs. In other words, the interaction of the individual with other members of the family or other units in society, including work and play, is emphasized.

Characteristics of healthy families have been described and include affirmation and support for one another, a shared sense of responsibility, shared leisure time, shared religious core, respect, trust, and family rituals and traditions. These qualities address stability of family functioning and balance in interactions among family members. Family typologies have also been developed to identify common profiles that may be linked to health in families. Typologies also suggest that health promotion interventions must be compatible with family values, beliefs, and orientations.

Many factors influence how family health is defined. Social, cultural, environmental, and religious/spiritual factors play a central role in determining how families view their health. Families' strengths, resources, and competencies are also an integral part of a positive view of health. Implementing and evaluating family models of health will assist nurses in promoting family health.

DEFINITIONS OF HEALTH THAT FOCUS ON THE COMMUNITY

Communities are usually defined within one of two frameworks: spatial/geographical area or relational/functional. Geographical definitions are based on legal or geopolitical areas such as cities, towns, or census tracts. Relational definitions are based on how people interact to achieve common goals. The WHO defines community as a social group determined by both geographical area and common values, with members who know each other and interact within a social structure (World Health Organization, 1974). Members of the community create norms, values, and social institutions for its members. The WHO definition focuses on both the spatial and relational/functional dimensions of a community.

Social ecological theories of community health emphasize the interaction and interdependence of individuals with their family, community, social structure, and physical environment (Golden, McLeroy, Green, Earp, & Lieberman, 2015). A social ecology model described in the *Ottawa Charter for Health Promotion*, a landmark health promotion policy statement, outlines the essential dimensions of community health (World Health Organization, 1986b). Fundamental to community health are peace, shelter, education, food, income, a stable ecosystem, sustainable resources, social justice, and equity. The Healthy Cities project in the United States, Europe, and Australia is based on a social ecological view that the roots of ill health lie in social and economic factors. The international project supports the premise that the responsibility for health is widely shared in the community with collaborative decision-making about health issues (de Leeuw, Tsouros, Dyakova, & Green, 2014). Cultivating healthy communities continues to be a priority for WHO, which maintains that four key ingredients are essential:

1. There must be local investment in communities.
2. Venues need to be provided for communities to learn about effective change strategies.
3. Partners need to be mobilized for change.
4. Communities need resources for local health promotion.

Informed political action and healthy public policies are also essential to a healthy community. At the 9th Global Conference on Health Promotion, in Shanghai, a continuing commitment to a Healthy Cities program was supported as a comprehensive approach for health (World Health Organization, 2016).

Community health has also been defined as meeting the collective needs of its members through identifying problems and managing interactions within the community and between the community and the larger society (Stanhope & Lancaster, 2016). Community health is more than the sum of the health states of its individual members; the characteristics of the community as a whole must be included. Individual, family, and community health are intimately related. The health of the community depends on individual health as well as the availability of social, physical, and political resources to enable individuals to live healthy lives. The relationship between social and economic conditions and the health of individuals in a community is widely documented and addressed in the *Healthy People 2020* objectives as well as the *Healthy People 2030* overarching framework (U.S. Department of Health and Human Services, 2013).

Social capital is considered to be a major determinant of health in communities. This term, which includes trust, reciprocity, and cooperation among families, neighborhoods, and entire communities, is discussed in more detail in Chapter 3. Healthy communities support healthy lifestyles. Likewise, the collective attitudes, beliefs, and behaviors of individuals who live in the community influence the health of the community. All social and physical environmental components of a community must be assessed prior to developing strategies to create healthier communities.

A body of evidence supports an expanded view of health that is inseparable from the community and larger society. Effective health promotion interventions are based on an assessment of a community's social, economic, and physical resources recommended in the *Healthy People 2020* document, as these factors affect the health of individuals, families, and communities (U.S. Department of Health and Human Services, 2013).

SOCIAL DETERMINANTS OF HEALTH

More than 100 years ago, Florence Nightingale understood that the environment in which people live was a major contributor to health and disease (Koffi & Fawcett, 2016). She also believed that environments could be altered to improve health. Her observations during the Crimean War and working in poor communities led to these observations. Of the four broad determinants of health (biological attributes, health care access, life style, and the social, economic, and physical environments), the social, economic, and physical environments in which people live are considered to be the most significant, as they influence health directly and indirectly (Mariner, 2016).

The social determinants of health are the conditions in which people are born, live, work, and age, including the health care system (Bircher & Kuruvilla, 2014). They are responsible for the differences in health seen within and between individuals, families, communities, and countries (World Health Organization, 2008). The social conditions under which people live, including poverty with its accompanying inadequate housing, poor sanitation, suboptimal food, lack of education, and social discrimination, have a dramatic impact on health. Differences in health can be attributed to socioeconomic, political, cultural, and geographic dimensions as they are driven by inequities in power, money, and resources (Friel & Marmot, 2011). The influence of these factors is evident when comparing the health of those at the top of the social ladder with those at the bottom. The *Ottawa Charter for Health Promotion* stated eight fundamental conditions and resources for health, including peace, shelter, education, food, income, a stable ecosystem, sustainable resources, social justice, and equity. The social determinants are discussed in detail in Chapter 12.

Both downstream and upstream determinants of health should be identified prior to planning and implementing interventions to promote health. Individual factors, including knowledge, beliefs, attitudes, and behaviors, are downstream factors that are shaped by upstream determinants. Upstream determinants include living and working conditions, and economic and social opportunities and resources (Braveman & Gottlieb, 2014). A conceptual framework developed for the Robert

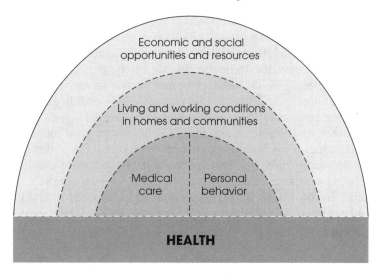

FIGURE 1–2   A Conceptual Framework for Describing Downstream and Upstream Determinants of Health

Wood Johnson Commission to Build a Healthier America depicts how downstream factors are shaped by an individual's upstream factors. This framework (see Figure 1–2) highlights a critical need to address downstream factors within an individual's socio-environmental context.

In *Healthy People 2020*, the national health agenda, one of the four major goals is to create social and physical environments that promote health (U.S. Department of Health and Human Services, 2013). The *Healthy People 2020* agenda documents the multiple determinants of health and health behaviors, including personal, social, and physical environments and the interrelationships among these different levels of health determinants. The need for multilevel (individual, family, community) interventions is emphasized to promote health and well-being.

Use of the term *social determinant* has been criticized based on the thinking that the expanded focus results in a loss of individual identity. Others state that the term *social* should not be used. Rather, determinants of health should be the focus to avoid the politicized view of health. Regardless of the terms used, it is now understood that a broader view of health that takes into account the social, cultural, and physical environments is necessary to improve the health of all. An understanding of the social determinants is important for nurses and other health care professionals to effectively intervene in neighborhoods, organizations, and communities to improve individual health. This is discussed in more detail in Chapter 14.

SOCIAL DETERMINANTS AND GLOBAL HEALTH

Global health is described as the health of the world's population resulting from worldwide interconnectedness and interdependence (Frenk, Gomez-Dantes, & Moon, 2014). Global health places a priority on improving and achieving equity for all (Koplan et al., 2009). Global health issues include the vulnerability of refugee populations, the marketing of harmful products such as tobacco, the erosion of social and environmental conditions, the exacerbation of income differences, pandemics such as the Ebola virus outbreak, the emergence of superbugs and antibiotic resistance, and global climate change.

Globalization has resulted in health threats extending across borders, bringing about health interdependence of nations to promote health and reduce health threats (U.S. Department of Health and Human Services, 2017). Global health security is more important than ever, as no country is immune to global health threats as noted with the Ebola virus outbreak in 2015. Solutions to global health security include the development of new technologies, such as vaccines; improved capacities and resources, including workforce training; new health care systems to promote population health; improved global governance and coordination; and a global identity that promotes global solutions (Horton & Das, 2015). The goal of a global health agenda is to improve the health of all people in all nations by promoting wellness and eliminating avoidable diseases, disabilities, and deaths. Although the major drivers in global health are government and nongovernment agencies, health care providers play a crucial role in assisting in identifying and addressing community and population health issues through community activism and civic engagement.

BUILDING A CULTURE OF HEALTH

In 2013, Robert Wood Johnson Foundation (RWJF) proposed a 20-year agenda to address the health of individuals and communities by building a national movement to create a national Culture of Health (Lavizzo-Mourey, 2015; Plough, 2014). A culture of health builds on the WHO definition of health that recognizes its social, cultural, economic, and political determinants. Ten core principles support the foundation for a culture of health. These principles are listed in Table 1–2. The RWJF states that a culture of

---

TABLE 1–2   Principles Underlying a Culture of Health

1. Good health flourishes across geographic, demographic, and social sectors

2. Attaining the best health possible is valued by our entire society

3. Individuals and families have the means and the opportunity to make choices that lead to the healthiest lives possible

4. Business, government, individuals, and organizations work together to build healthy communities and lifestyles

5. No one is excluded

6. Everyone has access to affordable, quality health care because it is essential to maintain or reclaim health

7. Health care is efficient and equitable

8. The economy is less burdened by excessive and unwarranted health care spending

9. Keeping everyone as healthy as possible guides public and private decision-making

10. Americans understand that we are all in this together

Source: Accessed from the Robert Wood Johnson Foundation culture of health website (http://cultureofhealth.org). Copyright 2017. Robert Wood Johnson Foundation. Used with permission from RWJF.

health is a set of ideas and practices that promote the health of individuals, families, communities, and nations (Chandra, Acosta, et al., 2016). A culture of health exists when individuals and organizations are able to:

1. Promote individual and community well-being
2. Create environments that prioritize health
3. Support access to opportunities for healthy lifestyles and high-quality health care (Chandra, Acosta, et al., 2016).

In communities where a culture of health is valued, its members work together to address the social determinants to improve the collective well-being of everyone.

Collaborating with the RAND Corporation, RWJF developed a Culture of Health Action Framework to motivate dialogue and collaboration among individuals, communities, and organizations in order to change the health of the nation by enabling everyone to lead a healthier life (Trujillo & Plough, 2016). The RWJF's goal is to mobilize a social movement to build a national culture of health. The action framework consists of four drivers that are expected to generate health, well-being, and equity for all. The drivers include:

1. Making health a shared value
2. Fostering cross-sector collaboration to improve well-being
3. Creating healthier, more equitable communities
4. Strengthening integration of health services and systems (Chandra, Miller, et al., 2016).

The framework is currently being implemented in multiple communities throughout the United States. Ongoing individual and community level evaluations will closely examine the process for building a culture of health to identify successful strategies for moving to a national culture of health (Trujillo & Plough, 2016). Changing cultures to value health will not occur overnight, as a social change that moves the emphasis from disease and illness to health will take many years. Nurses will play a major role in helping to shift the nation's values and actions to promote health through activities such as implementing health promotion programs and advocating for policies to decrease health inequities in communities.

CONCEPTIONS OF HEALTH PROMOTION

Expanding definitions of health have led to changing views of health promotion. Early health promotion efforts focused on individual responsibility for health and emphasized behavioral determinants and educational approaches. However, evidence has shown that health promotion programs must also address social and physical environments, as these also contribute to poor health. This view was expressed in the *Ottawa Charter for Health Promotion*, the first document to focus on health promotion, which was defined as a process to enable people to overcome challenges and increase control over their environments to improve their health (World Health Organization, 1986b). The Ottawa document laid the foundation for the theory and practice of health promotion and emphasized the role of social and personal resources, physical capabilities, and the need to achieve equity in health. The *Ottawa Charter* also documented the responsibility of nongovernment and government agencies in creating supportive environments and health public policy.

The *Bangkok Charter for Health Promotion* updated the *Ottawa Charter* to make health promotion central to the global development agenda and a core responsibility of all governments (World Health Organization, 2005). The *Bangkok Charter* addressed the changing context of health promotion that had occurred since the adoption of the *Ottawa Charter*. The document has been described as moving health promotion from an individual health lifestyle education model toward a socio-ecological model that addresses social determinants of health. In the *Bangkok Charter*, many challenges are recognized due to the multiple determinants of health in a globalized world; health promotion is considered a core responsibility of all governments.

The 9th Global Conference on Health Promotion resulted in the *Shanghai Declaration*, where health as a universal right was reaffirmed. The document also recognizes that health and well-being are essential to achieving the United Nations Development Agenda 2030 and sustainable development goals (SDGs). The SDGs establish a duty to invest in health (World Health Organization, 2016). Although the document is a commitment to promote universal health coverage and health equities for people of all ages, challenges are ahead to achieve the goals. The *Shanghai Declaration* is similar to the RWJF call for a culture of health, as the declaration promotes cities and communities as critical settings for health promotion and recognizes the role of governments in addressing health equity. It also recognizes the role of health literacy and the new global context for health promotion.

Health promotion and *health education* are often used interchangeably. Although the terms are closely linked, they are not the same. Health education focuses on learning activities and experiences for individuals and groups. It is a component of health promotion and is an essential part of communication between health care professionals and clients. Health education has progressed from health care professionals providing information they think the client should know to a shared decision-making process. The *Ottawa Charter* was the catalyst that moved health promotion beyond being defined as an educational activity to a broader concept that also focused on the social and political environment. The expanded definition of health promotion is evident in the principles defined to guide health promotion programs (Tremblay, Richard, Brousselle, & Beaudet, 2013). These seven principles are summarized in Table 1–3.

Health protection has also been used interchangeably with health promotion. Health protection refers to legal or fiscal controls and other regulations to enhance health and prevent disease (Tannahill, 2009). Health protection interventions emphasize worker safety to prevent disease. Disease prevention has also been used interchangeably with health promotion (Mittelmark, Kickbusch, Rootman, Scriven, & Tones, 2017). Disease prevention activities stress modifying individual or environmental factors to reduce or eliminate risk (primary prevention) for a specific disease such as cardiovascular disease or cancer, or lifestyle change to reduce risk factors present in the early stages of a disease (secondary prevention), such as dietary modifications for hypertension. Disease prevention is focused on specific diseases, while health promotion targets changing lifestyles and promoting healthy environments. Health promotion can include disease prevention when the focus is on reducing risks for healthy living.

TABLE 1–3   Core Principles of Health Promotion

Principle	Explanation
Participation	Involve the stakeholders at all stages of the project
Empowerment	Enable individuals and communities to take control over the personal, socioeconomic, and environmental factors that affect their health
Holism	Consider all health components: physical, mental, social, and spiritual
Intersectoral	Ensure collaboration from all the disciplines and areas concerned
Equity	Seek fairness in health and social justice
Sustainability	Implement changes that can be maintained after programs have ended
Multiple strategies	Rely on several approaches in combination

Source: Adapted from Rootman, I., Goodstadt, M., Hyndman, B., McQueen, D. V., Potvin, L., Springett, J., & Ziglio, E. (2001). *Evaluation in health promotion: Principles and perspectives.* WHO Regional Publication, European Series No. 92. Denmark: World Health Organization.

Health promotion has moved from being considered a goal or desired end point to a process to facilitate movement toward accomplishment of health goals. It is both the art and science of supporting people to make lifestyle changes and creating environments that are conducive to health (Mittelmark et al., 2017). A combination of health promotion strategies is needed to address the multiple determinants of health. Ecological strategies address the social, economic, and physical environments that influence health. Health promotion spans from the prevention of disease to empowering individuals, to promoting environmental and policy change. Settings for health promotion include the workplace, schools, hospitals, prisons, and communities—where individuals spend their everyday lives.

Multiple factors in society influence how the delivery of health promotion is changing and will continue to do so in the 21st century (Edington, Schultz, Pitts, & Camilleri, 2016). Evolving lifestyles and relationships occur with each new generation. These are influenced by where individuals choose to work and live. New discoveries in the neurosciences about the mind–body connection and brain plasticity and epigenetics offer new insights into the interplay of lifestyle, environment, and health. Technology continues to expand at an accelerated rate, including wearable technology, mobile health (mHealth), health monitors with wireless modules to track fitness and monitor and analyze behaviors and send alarms, and many applications to facilitate healthy behaviors.

Information and communication technologies are changing the way health information is shared and health promotion programs are being delivered. The increase in use of the Internet has resulted in social network communities that are providing instant information and health promoting programs (Ortega-Navas, 2017). The technologies offer many benefits for health promotion, including easier access to information and support for healthy behaviors. The technologies are also changing the nurse–client relationship, including the degree of engagement in the health promotion process. In addition, information accessed may not have a scientific background and should be followed up with a health care professional (Ortega-Navas, 2017).

Currently, the research base documenting the role of technology in improving health is limited so it should be considered a tool or adjunct to health promotion efforts until there is more evidence of its role in lifestyle change (Patrick et al., 2016). In spite of the limitations of the research designs (no traditional education control group, no random assignment, biased samples), potential benefits have documented short-term behavior change and cost effectiveness (Oosterveen, Tzelepis, Ashton, & Hutchesson, 2017). Nurses and other health care professionals have opportunities to create new roles in health promotion incorporating these information and communication technologies to promote healthy behaviors.

MEASUREMENT OF HEALTH

On the basis of the WHO definition of health, five distinct dimensions have been proposed as a minimum standard for a comprehensive measure of health: physical or functional health, mental health, social functioning, role functioning, and well-being. Multiple issues are raised when measuring these concepts, as they include both objective and subjective indicators. They are not static; they are constantly changing as life circumstances of individuals change, also challenging measurement.

One type of self-rated health assessment is the enduring self-concept or stability measurement of health. These scales measure a reflection of one's established beliefs about one's health. In this view, self-rated health is stable over time and is based on one's self-concept. Self-concept health measures may not reflect the objective indicators of health, as individuals' beliefs about their health are often incongruent with their physical status. This view is compatible with an expansive definition of health, as an individual's self-evaluation of overall health is related to an overall sense of well-being. However, if one takes the view that health depends on an individual's circumstances, then the social and physical context must also be considered when assessing health.

Measures of wellness that encompass a holistic assessment are available. Most of these measures assess the major dimensions of wellness, including physical, social, emotional, spiritual, and intellectual. Some measures also assess occupational, environmental, and financial dimensions. Many of these scales have over 100 items and the reliability and validity are not reported for others. However, the holistic approach to measuring health is a major strength. The WHO continues to convene experts to develop and test measures of health and well-being (World Health Organization, 2013a).

The focus on social determinants of health has generated the need to develop accurate, easy-to-use measures of the social and built environments. Community assessment indexes have been designed to measure policies, programs, and practices in the community that affect healthy behaviors as well as characteristics of neighborhoods. An example of one effort is the Community Healthy Living Index. This assessment identifies the extent to which the community supports active living and healthy eating across a variety of venues (Kim et al., 2010). Measures of communities that document both healthy and unhealthy food, and physical and social environments commonly include the number of grocery stores, fast-food restaurants, and convenience stores; and access to parks and/or recreational or fitness centers for physical activity; crime, and rental occupied housing (Myers, Denstel, & Broyles, 2016). Progress has also been made in measuring walkability in communities using new technologies, such as global positioning systems, smartphones, and Web-based tools. Although major challenges remain and the technology changes rapidly, the measures provide valuable health information for public policy.

The multiple components of health and its determinants point to the need for standardized, simple indicators of the health components. Decisions first need to be made about which elements of health and well-being are appropriate to measure. Often, a direct measure may not be available, so decisions have to be made about proxy measures. For example, in measuring community health, proxy measures may include the number of grocery stores, presence of health care facilities, and safe walking spaces. Measures should be relevant for the individuals who will be assessed. Important factors to consider include age, educational level, language primarily spoken, and health literacy. Multiple health measures may be needed to assess individual, family, and community levels. Measurement of health and its many determinants is complex; it becomes even more so when all perspectives are taken into account. These challenges pose multiple opportunities for developing or adapting and testing new measures.

CONSIDERATIONS FOR PRACTICE IN THE CONTEXT OF HEALTH

The definition of *health* has evolved from traditional usage in a medical, curative model to a multidimensional concept with physical, social, spiritual, environmental, and cultural dimensions. Nurses and other health care professionals need to understand and assess all dimensions in their health assessments. The assessment information can then be used to identify health needs and develop strategies to promote health. For example, a biomedical assessment may be useful in guiding genetic counseling or screening interventions. Information collected from a cultural assessment can provide valuable knowledge in developing health promotion programs in communities with diverse populations. An assessment of the social and physical environments will provide useful information about aspects of the environment that may be positively or negatively affecting the health of the individual or community. In an integrative view of health, an assessment is not complete unless it involves the individual, family, and community in which individuals live and function. Nurses work in partnership with clients to provide the knowledge and skills needed to empower them to achieve their health goals or adapt to circumstances to move toward their health goals. Health should be viewed from a positive perspective when conducting an assessment or designing health promotion strategies. This means that the focus should be on available resources, potentials, and capabilities. When health is viewed in a positive model, strategies can be developed that concentrate on strengthening resources and decreasing risks.

OPPORTUNITIES FOR RESEARCH ON HEALTH

The fundamental purpose of nursing research is to build knowledge to improve health. The contribution of nursing to health promotion depends, in part, on the way in which health knowledge is grounded in science. Nursing research has been active in knowledge development to improve the health of all. However, many questions remain unanswered. What are the gender, culture, and racial differences in the expressions of health? What interactive conditions between persons and their environment enhance or deplete health? Which social determinants are critical to assess the health of families? Which social determinants are key to improving the health of communities? How does global health security affect the health of individuals and communities? Generating knowledge will advance the scientific base to enable nurses to implement effective health-promoting interventions and begin policy discussions for change.

Multilevel models of health that incorporate ethnic, cultural, social, and environmental factors are needed to examine the determinants of health. Longitudinal studies are needed to describe the role of social determinants across the life span in diverse populations. Multidisciplinary research teams will facilitate the development and testing of multilevel interventions to address the social determinants of health. A good example is the RWJF program that is building a national culture of health.

Summary

Varying definitions of *health* have been presented to provide the foundation on which health promotion programs for individuals, families, and communities can be based. An assessment begins with learning how health is defined by the individual, family, or community and identifying realistic strategies to achieve the desired health goals. Evidence has shown that individual health cannot be separated from the health of the family, community, nation, and world. A shift to this broader perspective of health facilitates development of proactive policies to improve health. The complexity of factors known to determine the health of individuals also raises many challenges. However, the challenges are not insurmountable and are being tackled at local, national, and international levels.

Learning Activities

1. Based on the definitions provided in the chapter, write your own definition of *health* and state the rationale for the factors you considered in developing the definition.
2. Interview three persons at varying points in the life span (adolescent, young adult, elderly person) to obtain their perspective of health and the health promotion strategies they perform to stay healthy. Ask them to identify any personal, social, and environmental barriers to pursuing a healthy lifestyle.
3. Suggest health promotion strategies to help overcome the barriers stated by the interviewees in learning activity 2.
4. Develop a plan to conduct an assessment to determine the health of a family or a community using the social determinants of health.
5. Design a clinical experience for students assigned to a community-based organization that incorporates the principles of health promotion.

References

American Nurses Association. (2010). *Nursing's social policy statement: The essence of the profession* (3rd ed.). Washington, DC: Author.

Bateman, G. C., & Merryfeather, L. (2014). Newman's theory of health as expanding consciousness: A personal evolution. *Nursing Science Quarterly,* 27(1), 57–61. doi: 10.1177/0894318413509725

Bircher, J., & Kuruvilla, S. (2014). Defining health by addressing individual, social, and environmental determinants: New opportunities for healthcare and public health. *Journal of Public Health Policy,* 35(3), 363–386. doi:10.1057/jphp.2014.19

Bok, S. (2017). WHO definition of health, rethinking the. In S. R. Quah (Ed.), *International encyclopedia of public health* (2nd ed., Vol. 7, pp. 417–423). New York, NY: Elsevier.

Braveman, P., & Gottlieb, L. (2014). The social determinants of health: It's time to consider the cause of the causes. *Public Health Reports, 129*(Suppl 2), 19–31.

Caroli, E., & Weber-Baghdiguian, L. (2016). Self-reported health and gender: The role of social norms. *Social Science & Medicine, 153,* 220–229.

Chandra, A., Acosta, J. D., Carman, K. G., Dubowitz, T., Leviton, L., Martin, L. T., . . . Plough, A. L. (2016). *Building a national culture of health. Background, action framework, measures, and next steps.* Santa Monica, CA: RAND Corporation.

Chandra, A., Miller, C. E., Acosta, J. D., Weilant, S., Trujillo, M., & Plough, A. (2016). Drivers of health as a shared value: Mindset, expectations, sense of community, and civic engagement. *Health Affairs, 35*(11), 1959–1963. doi: 10.1377/hlthaff.2016.0603

de Leeuw, E., Tsouros, A. D., Dyakova, M., & Green, G. (Eds.). (2014). *Healthy cities promoting health and equity evidence for local policy and practice.* Copenhagen, Denmark: WHO Regional Office for Europe.

Diaz-Morales, J. F. (2017). Gender-based perspectives about women's and men's health. In M. Sanchez-Lopez & R. Liminana-Gras (Eds.), *The psychology of gender and health: Conceptual and applied global concerns* (pp. 55–83). St. Louis, MO: Elsevier.

Doucet, T. J., & Merlin, M. D. (2014). Conceptualization of health in nursing practice. *Nursing Science Quarterly, 27*(2), 118–125. doi: 10.1177/0894318414522665

Dubos, R. (1965). *Man adapting.* New Haven, CT: Yale University Press.

Dunn, H. L. (1959). What high-level wellness means. *Canadian Journal of Public Health, 50*(11), 447–457.

Dunn, H. L. (1980). *High-level wellness.* Thorofare, NJ: Charles B. Slack Inc.

Edington, D. W., Schultz, A. B., Pitts, J. S., & Camilleri, A. (2016). The future of health promotion in the 21st century: A focus on the working population. *American Journal of Lifestyle Medicine, 10*(4), 242–252. doi: 10.1177/1559827615605789.

Ereshefsky, M. (2009). Defining 'health' and 'disease'. *Studies in History and Philosophy of Biological and Biomedical Sciences, 40*(3), 221–227. doi:10.1016/j.shpsc.2009.06.005

Fawcett, J., & Desanto-Madeya, S. (2013). *Analysis and evaluation of nursing models and theories.* Philadelphia, PA: F.A. Davis Company.

Flannery, M. C. (2009). The mirage of health. *The American Biology Teacher, 71*(9), 558–561. doi: 10.2307/20565381

Frenk, J., Gomez-Dantes, O., & Moon, S. (2014). From sovereignty to solidarity: A renewed concept of global health for an era of complex interdependence. *The Lancet, 383,* 94–97.

Friel, S., & Marmot, M. G. (2011). Action on the social determinants of health and health inequities goes global. *American Review of Public Health, 32,* 225–236. doi: 10.1146/annurev-publhealth-031210-101220

Goddings, A., James, D. R., & Hargreaves, D. R. (2012). Distinct patterns of health engagement in adolescents and young adults: Implications for health services. *The Lancet,* published online November 23, 2012.

Golden, S. D., McLeroy, K. R., Green, L. W., Earp, J. L., & Lieberman, L. D. (2015). Upending the social ecological model to guide health promotion efforts toward policy and environmental change. *Health Education and Behavior, 42*(1S), 8S–14S. doi: 10.1177/1090198115575098

Gunther, M. (2014). King's conceptual system and theory of goal attainment in nursing practice. In M. R. Alligood (Ed.), *Nursing theory: Utilization and application* (pp. 160–180). St. Louis, MO: Elsevier.

Holaday, B. (2014). Johnson's behavioral system model in nursing practice. In M. R. Alligood (Ed.), *Nursing theory: Utilization and application* (pp. 138–159). St. Louis, MO: Elsevier.

Horton, R., & Das, P. (2015). Global health security now. *The Lancet, 385,* 1805–1806.

Huber, M., & Bok, L. (2015). Health: Definitions. In *International encyclopedia of the social and behavioral sciences* (2nd ed., Vol. 10, pp. 607–613). Amsterdam: Elsevier.

Kim, S., Adamson, K. C., Balfanz, D. R., Brownson, R. C., Wiecha, J. L., Shepard, D., & Alles, W. F. (2010). Development of the Community Healthy Living Index: A tool to foster healthy environments for the protection of obesity and chronic disease. *Preventive Medicine, 50,* S80–S85.

King, I. M. (1990). Health as the goal for nursing. *Nursing Science Quarterly, 3*(3), 123–128.

King, I. M. (2007). King's structure, process and outcome in the 21st century. In C. L. Sieloff & M. A. Frey (Eds.), *Middle range theory development using King's conceptual system* (pp. 3–11). New York: Springer.

Knowlden, A., & Sharma, M. (2016). One-year efficacy testing of enabling mothers to prevent pediatric obesity through Web-based education and reciprocal determinism (EMPOWER) randomized control trial. *Health Education & Behavior, 43*(1), 94–106. doi: 10.1177/1090198115596737

Koffi, K., & Fawcett, J. (2016). The two nursing disciplinary scientific revolutions: Florence Nightingale and Martha E. Rogers. *Nursing Science Quarterly, 29*(3), 247–250. doi: 10.1177/0894318416648782

Koplan, J. P., Bond, T. C., Merson, M. H., Reddy, K. S., Rodriguez, M. H., Sewankambo, N. K., & Wasserheit, J. N. (2009). Towards a common definition of global health. *The Lancet, 373,* 1993–1994. doi:10.1016/S0140-6736(09)60332-9

Lavizzo-Mourey, R. (2015). Why we need to build a culture of health in the United States. *Academic Medicine, 90*(7), 846–848. doi: 10.1097/ACM.0000000000000750

Mariner, W. K. (2016). Beyond lifestyle: Governing the social determinants of health. *American Journal of Law & Medicine, 42,* 284–309. doi: 10.1177/0098858816658268

Mittelmark, M. B., Kickbusch, I., Rootman, I., Scriven, A., & Tones, K. (2017). Health promotion. In S. R. Quah (Ed.), *International encyclopedia of public health* (2nd ed., Vol. 3, pp. 450–462). New York: Elsevier.

Myers, C. A., Denstel, K. D., & Broyles, S. T. (2016). The context of context: Examining the association between healthy and unhealthy measures of neighborhood food, physical activity, and social environments. *Preventive Medicine, 93,* 21–26.

Neuman, B., & Fawcett, J. (2012). Thoughts about the Neuman systems model: A dialogue. *Nursing Science Quarterly, 25*(4), 374–376. doi: 10.1177/0894318412457055

Oosterveen, E., Tzelepis, F., Ashton, L., & Hutcheson, M. J. (2017). A systematic review of eHealth behavioral interventions targeting smoking, nutrition, physical activity, and/or obesity for young adults. *Preventive Medicine, 99,* 197–206.

Orem, D. E., & Taylor, S. G. (2011). Reflections on nursing practice science: The nature, the structure, and the foundation of nursing sciences. *Nursing Science Quarterly, 24*(1), 35–41. doi: 10.1177/0894318410389061

Ortega-Navas, M. (2017). The use of new technologies as a tool for the promotion of health education. *Procedia—Social and Behavioral Sciences, 237,* 23–29. doi: 10.1016/j.sbspro.2017.02.006

Parse, R. R. (2011). The human becoming modes of inquiry: Refinements. *Nursing Science Quarterly, 24*(1), 11–18. doi: 10.1177/0894318410389066

Parsons, T. (1958). Definitions of health and illness in the light of American values and social structure. In E. G. Jaco (Ed.), *Patients, physicians and illness* (pp. 165–187). New York, NY: Free Press.

Patrick, K., Hekler, E. B., Estrin, D., Mohr, D. C., Riper, H., Crane, D., . . . Riley, W. T. (2016). The pace of technologic change: Implications for digital health behavior intervention research. *American Journal of Preventive Medicine, 51*(5), 816–824.

Plough, A. L. (2014). Building a culture of health: Challenges for the public health workforce. *American Journal of Preventive Medicine, 47*(5S3), S388–S390.

Rotegard, A. K., Moore, S. M., Fagermoen, M. S., & Ruland, C. M. (2010). Health assets: A concept analysis. *International Journal of Nursing Studies, 47,* 513–525.

Schaefer, K. M. (2014). Levine's conservation model in nursing practice. In M. R. Alligood (Ed.), *Nursing theory: Utilization and application* (5th ed., pp. 181–199). St. Louis, MO: Elsevier.

Selanders, L. C. (2010). The power of environmental adaptation. Florence Nightingale's original theory for nursing practice. *Journal of Holistic Nursing, 28*(1), 81–88. doi:10.1177/0898010109360257

Shah, M. (2015). Compare and contrast of grand theories: Orem's self-care deficit theory and Roy's adaptation model. *International Journal of Nursing Didactics, 5*(1), 39–42.

Song, M., & Kong, E. (2015). Older adults' definitions of health: A metasynthesis. *International Journal of Nursing Studies, 52,* 1097–1106.

Sorochan, W. (1970). Health concepts as a basis for orthobiosis. In E. Hart & W. Sechrist (Eds.), *The dynamics of wellness.* Belmont, CA: Wadsworth Inc.

Stanhope, M., & Lancaster, J. (Eds.). (2016). *Public health nursing: Population-centered health care in the community* (9th ed.). St. Louis, MO: Elsevier.

Tannahill, A. (2009). Health promotion: The Tannahill model revisited. *Public Health, 123,* 396–399. doi:10.1016/j.puhe.2008.05.021

Tountas, Y. (2009). The historical origins of the basic concepts of health promotion and education: The role of ancient Greek philosophy and medicine. *Health Promotion International, 24*(2), 185–192. doi:10.1093/heapro/dap006

Tremblay, M. C., Richard, L., Brousselle, A., & Beaudet, N. (2013). How can both the intervention and its evaluation fulfill health promotion principles? An example from a professional development program. *Health Promotion Practice, 14,* 563–571. doi: 10.1177/1524839912462030

Trujillo, M. D., & Plough, A. (2016). Building a culture of health: A new framework and measures for health and health care in America. *Social Science & Medicine, 165,* 206–213.

U.S. Department of Health and Human Services. (2013). *Healthy People 2020.* Washington, DC: U.S. Government Printing Office. Accessed at http://www.healthypeople.gov

U.S. Department of Health and Human Services. (2017). *Global health security.* Washington, DC: U.S. Government Printing Office.

Witt, C. M., Chiaramonte, D., Berman, S., Chesney, M. A., Kaplan, G. A., Strange, K. C., . . . Berman, B. M. (2017). Defining health in a comprehensive context: A new definition of integrative health. *American Journal of Preventive Medicine, 53*(1), 134–137. doi:10.1016/j.amepre.2016.11.029

World Health Organization. (1974). *Community health nursing: Report of a WHO expert committee*. Technical Report Series No. 558. Geneva, Switzerland: Author.

World Health Organization. (1986a). *Alma Alta 1978: Primary health care*. Geneva, Switzerland: Author.

World Health Organization. (1986b). Ottawa Charter for Health Promotion. *Health Promotion*, 1(4), ii–v.

World Health Organization. (2005). *Constitution of the World Health Organization* (55th ed.). Accessed at http://www.who.int/governance/eb/who_constitution_en.pdf

World Health Organization. (2008). *Closing the gap in a generation: Health equity through action on the social determinants of health*. Geneva, Switzerland: Author.

World Health Organization. (2013a). *Joint meeting of experts on targets and indicators for health and well-being in Health 2020*. Copenhagen, Denmark: WHO Regional Office for Europe.

World Health Organization. (2013b). *Promotion of well-being. Pursuit of happiness*. New Delhi, India: Regional Office for Southeast Asia.

World Health Organization. (2014). *Mental health: A state of well-being*. Accessed at http://www.who.int/features/factfiles/mental_health/en

World Health Organization. (2016). *Shanghai Declaration on promoting health in the 2030 agenda for sustainable development*. 9th Global Conference on Health Promotion, Shanghai, China.

CHAPTER 2

Individual Models to Promote Health Behavior

OBJECTIVES

This chapter will enable the reader to:

1. Discuss the rationale for using behavior change theory to structure interventions.
2. Describe commonalities and differences in the individual models of behavior change.
3. Apply the stages of change model to designing interventions to promote health behaviors.
4. Discuss the revised health promotion model and its usefulness for nursing practice.
5. Describe the role of behavior change theories in digital interventions.
6. Discuss theory-based strategies to promote healthy behaviors in face-to-face and mobile technology encounters.

Health promotion activities enable individuals, families, and communities to achieve their full health potential. Health promotion supports lifestyles and behaviors that enable persons to maximize their health and well-being through individual, organizational, and community change. As the number of persons who are living with a chronic illness continues to increase, health promotion in secondary prevention, which focuses on persons who are already diagnosed with a disease, is receiving more attention. While primary prevention strategies reduce the occurrence or prolong the onset of diseases, such as diabetes, secondary prevention activities promote health within the limits of an illness or disability. Health promotion and primary prevention have been shown to have substantial benefits in improving quality of life and longevity. Both health promotion and primary prevention should be based on models of health that recognize the effects of multiple systems on health outcomes.

Health protection refers to the use of regulatory measures to promote health. Historically, health protection included measures to address public health issues such as safe drinking water. However, health protection measures have extended to other aspects of the environment, such as automobile safety and consumer product safety. Health protection strategies are addressed by government regulations.

The goal of improving population health is best served by emphasizing health promotion and primary prevention throughout the life span. Progress toward this goal requires an understanding of the motivational dynamics of actions that enhance health. This chapter focuses on models and theories that have been found useful in explaining and predicting individual health behaviors. Examples of how the models and theories have been used to explain, predict, or change health behaviors are described.

Health behavior may be motivated by a desire to protect one's health by avoiding illness or a desire to increase one's level of health in the presence or absence of illness. For many health behaviors, both "approaching a positive state" and "avoiding a negative state" serve as sources of motivation. Health behaviors of middle-age and older adults can be explained by approach and avoidance. In contrast, children and young people are more likely to be motivated toward positive health behaviors. In young people, avoidance is not perceived to be relevant, as negative states (illnesses) are considered unlikely to occur for many years.

INDIVIDUAL POTENTIAL FOR CHANGE

Individuals have tremendous potential for self-directed change due to their capacity for self-knowledge, self-regulation, decision-making, and problem solving. Almost everyone has the capacity and skill to change unhealthy behaviors or modify health-related lifestyles. The nurse's role is to promote a positive climate for change, serve as a catalyst for change, assist with steps in the change process, and increase the individual's motivation to maintain change.

USE OF THEORIES AND MODELS FOR BEHAVIOR CHANGE

Theories and models of health behavior are systematic attempts to explain how or why individuals do or do not engage in health behaviors. Behavior change theories and models specify concepts (theoretical or abstract ideas) and their relationships to predict or explain health behaviors. Understanding the predictors of behavior change is necessary to develop effective health promotion programs. In addition, it is essential to understand the possible mechanisms of change by examining possible mediators and moderators (intervening variables). Mediator variables explain how the change occurs, while moderator variables help explain when or under what conditions the change occurs. Mediators and moderators help to explain the processes underlying behavior change and enable health care professionals to develop and deliver effective, theoretically driven interventions. The scientific knowledge gained from testing theories and models also informs public policy, as the research evidence is used to improve health promotion practice.

To date, no one theory or model completely predicts behavior or behavior change, so multiple theories and models are presented. The models and theories presented focus primarily on individual, intrapersonal, and interpersonal influences to promote health. These models originated in educational and social psychology and expectancy-value, social cognitive, and decision-making theories. Cognitive processing of information is important in all of the models as the perceptions and interpretations of individuals directly affect their behaviors. Knowledge of the elements and mechanisms of behavior change theories enables nurses to design programs that are more likely to produce positive outcomes. When theories have been extensively tested, and evidence exists to explain or predict health behaviors across multiple populations and conditions, they are relevant for clinical settings to plan health promotion programs.

SOCIAL COGNITION THEORIES AND MODELS

Social cognition models consider cognitive (mental) and affective (emotional) factors as the primary determinants of behavior. They are called social cognition models because of the focus on cognitive or thought processes, such as attitudes and beliefs, as the major determinants of individual health behaviors. Social cognition models attempt to account for factors that determine behavior and behavior change. The proposed determinants are amenable to change, so they are the focus of interventions. Social cognition models include the health belief model, the theory of reasoned action and planned behavior, social cognitive and self-efficacy theory, and the health promotion model. These models are similar in their determinants of health behavior, although they are described differently in the various models. The shared model concepts are described in Table 2–1. Each model describes the determinants or potential causes of health behaviors and behavior change. However, in most cases, they do not provide direction for how to change behavior. Bandura's social cognitive theory and Pender's health promotion model are the only two that incorporate the environment. However, neither model has described and operationalized these factors as major determinants of change. Lack of environmental

TABLE 2–1 Shared Psychosocial Concepts in Five Individual Theories/Models of Health Behavior

Theories/Models	Psychosocial Concepts			
	Self-Efficacy	Outcome Expectations	Evaluation of Benefits and Barriers	Health Behavior Goals
Health belief model (revised)	+	+	+	−
Theory of reasoned action	−	+	+	+
Theory of planned behavior	+	+	+	+
Health promotion model	+	+	+	+
Social cognitive model	+	+	+	+

Key: (+) Concept present; (−) concept absent in theory/model.

operational definitions is a weakness of all of the models, as they have remained static, with almost no consideration of the context in which behaviors occur.

The Health Belief Model

The health belief model (HBM) was proposed in the 1950s to describe why some people who are free of illness will take actions to prevent illness, while others fail to do so (Rosenstock, 1960). The model was developed at a time when there were public health concerns about the widespread reluctance to accept screening for tuberculosis, screening for detection of cervical cancer, immunizations, and other preventive measures that were often free or provided at a nominal charge. The model was viewed as potentially useful to predict individuals who would or would not use preventive measures and to suggest interventions that might increase the willingness of resistant individuals to engage in preventive behaviors.

The HBM originated in social psychology and Lewin's classic value-expectancy theory. Lewin, a cognitive theorist, conceptualized the life space in which an individual exists as composed of regions, some regions having negative valence, some having positive valence, and others being relatively neutral. Illnesses are considered to be regions of negative valence exerting a force that moves the person away from the regions of positive valence. Preventive behaviors are strategies for avoiding illnesses or the negative valence regions in the life space.

Research with the HBM has shown that individuals will take action if two conditions are present: (1) there is a perceived threat (illness susceptibility and severity) to personal health and (2) the individual is convinced that the benefits of taking action to protect health outweigh the barriers that will be encountered. Beliefs about personal susceptibility and the seriousness of a specific illness combine to produce the degree of threat or negative valence of that illness. Perceived susceptibility reflects feelings of personal vulnerability or risk for a specific health problem. Perceived seriousness may be judged either by the degree of emotional arousal created by the thought of having the disease or by the medical, clinical, or social difficulties (family and work life) that individuals believe the illness or disease would create for them. Perceived benefits are beliefs about the effectiveness of recommended actions (more energy, save money) in preventing the health threat. Perceived barriers are perceptions about the potential negative aspects of taking action, such as unpleasantness, inconvenience, and time requirements. Cues to action are events, either internal (symptoms experienced) or external (public media campaigns, health provider advice), that trigger action. Modifying factors, including demographic, social, psychological, and structural variables, as well as cues to action, indirectly affect an individual's tendency to take action.

Several years after it was introduced, the model was expanded to include the self-efficacy concept, described as feelings of confidence in one's ability to perform a behavior. When the HBM was first developed, it was intended for application to one-time behaviors such as screening or immunization. However, application of the model to more complex behavioral risks such as smoking and unsafe sexual practices pointed to the need to expand it to include individual self-efficacy to engage in preventive behaviors over a long period of time. Results of research with the extended model have substantiated the addition of self-efficacy. An example of how the revised HBM can be applied to a risk behavior such as smoking is presented in Figure 2–1.

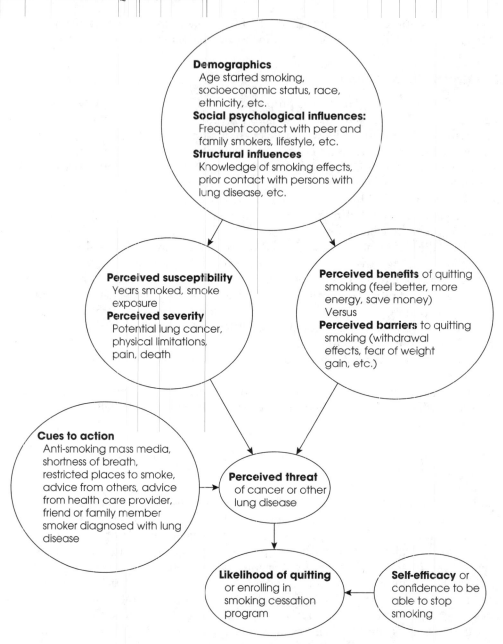

FIGURE 2–1 The Revised Health Belief Model Applied to Smoking as a Health Behavior Risk

The HBM continues to be used to explain preventive health behaviors, including breast cancer screening in different cultures (VanDyke & Shell, 2016), cyber-safety behaviors (Dodel & Mesch, 2017), human papillomavirus (HPV) vaccination among young people (Sundstrom et al., 2015), helmet use among skateboarders (Peachey, Sutton, & Cathorall, 2016), oral hygiene behaviors (Zetu, Zetu, Dogaru, Duta, &

Dumitrescu, 2014), bisphenol A (BPA) exposure during pregnancy (Che et al., 2014), and community preparedness behaviors (Ejeta, Ardalan, Paton, & Yaseri, 2016). All of these studies have been descriptive in design. The use of the HBM in cyber-safety behaviors found that self-efficacy and threat perceptions along with demographic variables predicted cyber-victimization preventive behaviors. The self-efficacy concept in the HBM was modified by Ejeta et al. (2016) to measure collective efficacy instead of individual self-efficacy. The concept was not found to be a significant predictor of community preparedness behaviors. However, perceived threat, perceived benefits and barriers, and cues to action were significant predictors. This study provides an example of how theoretical concepts can be adapted to the population of interest, as long as the rationale for the adaptation is scientifically sound (Kok & Ruiter, 2014).

The HBM has also been used to inform and test interventions. The effect of an education intervention based on HBM concepts to adopt low back pain preventive behaviors in nurses was tested by Sharafkhani, Khorsandi, Shamsi, and Ranjbaran (2016). In another study, an intervention using the HBM concepts was compared to a traditional knowledge-based intervention to increase HPV vaccinations in college men (Mehta, Sharma, & Lee, 2014). The HBM intervention was significantly more effective in changing HBM concepts and knowledge about HPV. A course based on barriers and benefits to Pap smear testing was found to be effective in increasing perceived susceptibility and severity to cervical cancer and increased participation in Pap smear testing (Daryani, Shojaeezadeh, Batebi, Charati, & Naghibi, 2016). Educational strategies based on the HBM were also implemented to increase dietary iron and folic acid intake during pregnancy (Araban, Baharzadeh, & Karimy, 2017). Dietary intake of these nutrients, increased, along with perceived susceptibility, severity, benefits, and self-efficacy. Perceived barriers to taking these nutrients decreased after the intervention.

The success of the HBM to predict behavior has been well documented since its introduction in the 1960s. However, the model concepts have varied in their predictive ability. Perceived barriers and benefits are considered to be the strongest predictors of preventive behaviors; perceived susceptibility and severity have not been consistently strong determinants. In a systematic review of studies that used the HBM to guide interventions to improve adherence, results showed moderate to strong positive effects (Jones, Smith, & Llewellyn, 2014). However, although the model informed the intervention in many studies, the HBM concepts were not integrated into the interventions. In addition, in several studies, the primary outcome was not the HBM model concepts, leading the authors of the study to conclude that evidence for the ability of the HBM to predict adherence was weak.

Theory of Reasoned Action and Theory of Planned Behavior

The theory of reasoned action (TRA) was originally developed to predict simple behaviors under an individual's control (Fishbein & Ajzen, 1975). The theory is based on the assertion that a person's intention to perform a behavior is considered the most immediate determinant and best predictor of that behavior. Attitudes and subjective norms, and intrapersonal factors are the fundamental building blocks of the theory, as they determine one's intention to perform a behavior (Fishbein & Ajzen, 1975). An individual's attitude toward a behavior is an overall positive or negative judgment of the consequences (outcomes) of performing the behavior. When the evaluation of the consequences is desirable, the result is a positive attitude, while a negative attitude results when an assessment of the consequence is undesirable. Subjective norms are beliefs about whether members of one's social network expect them to engage in the behavior—that is, whether important persons in the individual's network would approve or disapprove of performing the behavior.

The TRA is based on the assumption that both attitudes and subjective norms are amenable to change. Interventions may target attitudes by addressing an individual's beliefs about the consequences and/or subjective norms, by focusing on perceptions about normative expectations of others and their motivation to comply with what others expect. Research has shown that components of the TRA influence a range of health behaviors.

In the TRA, behavior is assumed to be under an individual's volitional control; in other words, individuals can make choices related to their behaviors. Ajzen, one of the original authors of the TRA, recognized that all behaviors are not completely under an individual's control, so a third variable, perceived behavioral control, was added as a predictor of intentions and behavior. The extended model became the *theory of planned behavior (TPB)* (Ajzen, 1991, 2011). Perceived behavioral control refers to an individual's beliefs about the perceived ease or difficulty of performing a particular behavior. Perceived behavioral control is considered similar to Bandura's self-efficacy concept. An example of the TPB applied to a weight loss behavior is described in Figure 2–2.

The TPB has been widely applied in research to explain many health behaviors, including battery recycling (Lizin, Van Dael, & Van Passel, 2017), adherence to antiretroviral therapy (Banas, Lyimo, Hospers, van der Ven, & de Bruin, 2017), and weight loss (Chung & Fong, 2015). Most studies continue to be observational and cross-sectional. In several systematic reviews and meta-analyses, the TPB has been documented to be effective in predicting behavioral intentions including dietary patterns

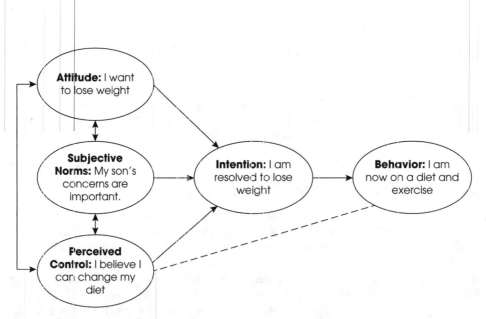

FIGURE 2–2 Example of Theory of Planned Behavior Applied to Weight Loss

(McDermott et al., 2015), nutritional behaviors in youth (Riebl et al., 2015), and physical activity (Schuz, Li, Hardinge, McEachan, & Conner, 2017).

Some authors have expanded the TPB to measure actual behavior, as behavior intention is an antecedent to performance of the behavior. The TPB was applied in research to implement a behavioral intervention to change sugar-sweetened beverage consumption (Zoellner et al., 2017). The model constructs predicted both intention and actual consumption behavior. Education was found to moderate the relationship between intention and performance of physical activity, suggesting that persons with higher education were more likely to translate intentions into behaviors (Schuz et al., 2017).

Despite the popularity of the TPB, there have been suggestions to include additional variables to further increase understanding of behavior and its actual performance. The TPB has been extended to include habit strength, which relates to behavioral factors, such as unawareness in performing the behavior (automatic), difficulty in controlling the behavior, and mental efficiency in performing the behavior. This addition acknowledges the influence of past behavior on current and future behaviors (Manstead, 2011). The relationship has been tested in several studies. Findings indicate that habit strength interacts with intentions to explain behavior (Manstead, 2011). When habit strength is strong, intentions are weakly correlated with behavior. When habit strength is weak, intention is a stronger predictor of behavior. These findings provide a beginning explanation for the limited success in breaking strong unhealthy habits.

The TPB model continues to be criticized for its parsimony, which has resulted in limited predictability of the model (Sniehotta, Presseau, & Araujo-Soares, 2014). In addition, integrating the model concepts into interventions is limited. In spite of these valid concerns, the TPB continues to be popular in nursing and the behavioral sciences. Further development and experimental testing of the model is needed to contribute to the science of behavior change.

Self-Efficacy and Social Cognitive Theory

Social cognitive theory (SCT) is based on the principle of reciprocal determinism, or the interaction of individual factors, the environment in which behaviors are performed, and actual behaviors. The core components include knowledge of health risks and benefits of reducing risks; perceived self-efficacy, or the belief that one has the ability to change one's health habits; outcome expectations or beliefs about the possible positive or negative consequences of changing behavior; personal health goals and strategies for achieving them; and perceived facilitators and structural impediments to achieving goals (Bandura, 1985, 1986, 2004). Although SCT is the only social cognition model that includes the environment, the concept is limited to the social environment, omitting the physical environment, and in general, it has been overlooked in most research with the model.

Self-efficacy plays a central role in personal change and is considered the foundation of human motivation and action. Individuals must believe they have control to change a behavior in order to take action. Health behaviors are also influenced by outcome expectancies and goals set by the individual, as they serve as incentives for change. Perceived facilitators and impediments to performing a behavior must also be taken into account when assessing self-efficacy. Bandura recognized that impediments may be outside of one's personal control. An application of the model to physical activity behavior is presented in Figure 2–3.

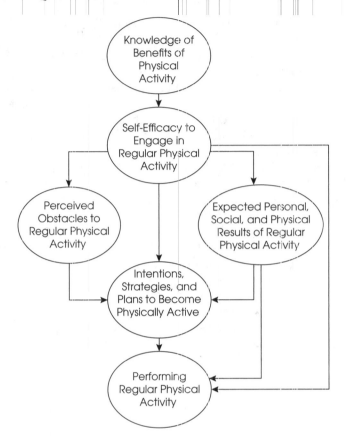

FIGURE 2–3 The Social Cognitive Theory Applied to Physical Activity Behavior

According to social cognitive theory, one's self-beliefs are formed through self-observation and self-reflective thought and greatly influence how one functions. The greater one's perceived efficacy, the more vigorously and persistently an individual will engage in a behavior, even in the face of obstacles and aversive experiences. Individuals with high levels of self-efficacy expectations are more likely to set higher goal challenges, expect that their efforts will produce favorable change, and believe that obstacles are surmountable.

Four main sources of self-efficacy beliefs have been described. *Mastery or performance* expectations are evidence of whether or not one can accomplish the tasks necessary for performing the behavior. *Vicarious experiences or modeling* refers to seeing others perform a behavior and observing the consequences of their actions. Vicarious experiences supply the strategies and techniques needed to accomplish the behavior. *Verbal persuasion*, the most widely used technique, is used to verbally convince individuals to perform a positive behavior or stop a negative behavior. *Somatic or affective states* refer to the emotional or physiological arousal or tensions created by performing an activity. For example, pain resulting from exercise is a negative somatic state that may decrease self-efficacy, while feeling energetic as a result of exercising increases one's self-efficacy.

Outcome expectations refer to perceptions of the possible consequences of performing a behavior. Outcome expectations may be physical, social, and self-evaluative.

Physical outcome expectations are the body experiences anticipated as a result of change, both positive and negative. For example, an individual who is on a weight loss program may expect cravings and hunger short term, but weight loss long term. Social outcome expectations are the anticipated responses from family and friends, such as positive comments on weight loss. Self-evaluative outcome expectations are those expected internally, such as satisfaction with one's progress or depression due to relapse. Outcome expectations are a major component of the model and are important to include with self-efficacy.

In recent years, attention has focused on self-efficacy as a motivational concept, and some authors are making the case for self-efficacy as a proxy for motivation (Williams & Rhodes, 2016). This premise is based on the literature showing that what individuals feel they are physically or mentally capable of performing is not the same as having the desire to perform the behavior. The issue has been raised due to the measurement of self-efficacy with statements that begin with "How much confidence do you have that you can. . . ." These stems lead many to believe that motivation is being measured, not one's ability to perform the behavior. Others believe these types of questions measure one's beliefs about capability to perform the behavior, independent of one's desire or one's motivation to perform the behavior. Williams and Rhodes (2016) point to the need to continue research to clarify the self-efficacy concept, as assessments need to be clear on what is being measured: the capability to perform a behavior or the motivation to perform or change the behavior.

Research continues to support the role of social cognitive theory in predicting health behaviors, and self-efficacy is one of the most commonly used concepts in theories of individual behavior. The theory has been used to predict healthy eating behaviors in adolescents (Chansukree & Rungjindarat, 2017), physical activity and nutrition behaviors (Stacey, James, Chapman, Courneya, & Lubans, 2015), condom use (Yang, Yang, Latkin, Luan, & Nelson, 2016), and many other health behaviors.

Interventions based on SCT concepts have been developed and tested to increase self-efficacy. Physical activity could be predicted by self-efficacy and intentions following a 3-month weight loss program for overweight and obese men (Young, Plotnikoff, Collins, Callister, & Morgan, 2016). An intervention for childhood obesity prevention included the environmental concept of the SCT, focusing on the home food environment (Knol et al., 2016). Both parental role modeling of healthy eating behaviors and changes in the home food environments resulted in positive changes in sedentary behaviors and food choices in preschool-age children. This study highlights the significance of including the environment concept.

Meta-analysis of physical activity interventions has shown inconsistent results. A review of physical activity and nutrition behavior change interventions for cancer survivors showed significant improvements in physical activity and at least one component of diet quality (Stacey et al., 2015). However, in a review of 18 studies, none of the SCT concepts was a significant predictor of behaviors. A review of physical activity in adolescents indicated that intentions were the most significant predictor across 23 studies (Plotnikoff, Costigan, Karunamuni, & Lubans, 2013). Using a meta-analysis of factors that predict digital piracy, the major SCT predictors were self-efficacy and outcome expectations (Lowry, Zhang, & Wu, 2017). Social learning and moral disengagement were additional factors that predicted digital piracy or copyright infringement. This study is an example of the wide applicability of the SCT.

The Health Promotion Model

The health promotion model (HPM) proposes a framework for integrating nursing and behavioral science perspectives with factors that predict health behaviors. The model provides a way to explore biopsychosocial processes that motivate individuals to engage in behaviors that enhance health and well-being.

The original HPM described the potential of seven cognitive–perceptual factors and five modifying factors to predict health behaviors. Cognitive–perceptual factors include importance of health, perceived control of health, definition of health, perceived health status, perceived self-efficacy, perceived benefits, and perceived barriers. Modifying factors include demographic and biological characteristics, interpersonal influences, situational influences, and behavioral factors.

The HPM is a competence- or approach-oriented model, as it does not include "fear" or "threat" as a source of motivation for health behavior. Although immediate threats to health have been shown to motivate action, threats in the distant future lack the same motivational strength. The HPM is applicable to any health behavior in which threat is not proposed as a major source of motivation.

THEORETICAL BASIS FOR THE HEALTH PROMOTION MODEL

The HPM describes the multidimensional nature of persons interacting with their interpersonal and physical environments as they pursue health. The HPM integrates constructs from expectancy-value theory and social cognitive theory within a holistic nursing perspective.

THE HEALTH PROMOTION MODEL (REVISED)

The revised HPM (Pender, 1996) is shown in Figure 2–4. Three new concepts were incorporated into the original model: activity-related affect, commitment to a plan of action, and immediate competing demands and preferences.

Individual Characteristics and Experiences

Individual characteristics and experiences include personal factors and prior related behavior. Personal characteristics and experiences affect subsequent actions. Their influence depends on the target behavior being considered.

PRIOR RELATED BEHAVIOR.   Research indicates that often the best predictor of behavior is the frequency of the behavior in the past. Prior behavior has both direct and indirect effects on the likelihood of engaging in health-promoting behaviors. The direct effect may be due to habit formation, which predisposes one to engage in the behavior automatically with little attention to the details of its execution. Habit strength accrues each time the behavior occurs and is strengthened by concentrated, repetitive practice.

Prior behavior is expected to indirectly influence health-promoting behavior through perceptions of self-efficacy, benefits, barriers, and activity-related affect. Bandura refers to anticipated benefits as "outcome expectations." If short-term benefits are experienced early in the course of behavior change, the behavior is more likely to be repeated. Barriers to a given behavior are experienced and stored in memory as "hurdles" to overcome to be able to engage successfully in the behavior.

Individual
Characteristics
and Experiences

Behavior-Specific
Cognitions
and Affect

Behavioral
Outcome

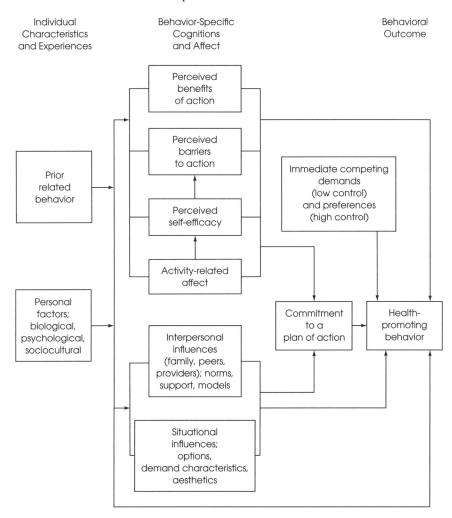

FIGURE 2–4   Health Promotion Model (Revised)

Every behavior is accompanied by emotions or affect. Positive or negative affect before, during, or following the behavior is encoded into memory. This information is retrieved when the behavior is contemplated at a later time. Prior behavior is proposed to shape all of these behavior-specific cognitions and affects. The nurse helps individuals shape positive behaviors by focusing on the benefits, teaching how to overcome hurdles to performing the behavior, and building high self-efficacy and feelings through successful performance and positive feedback.

PERSONAL FACTORS.   The relevant personal factors are shaped by the nature of the target behavior being considered. Personal factors are categorized as biological, psychological, and sociocultural. Biological factors may include age, body mass index, aerobic capacity, or strength. Psychological factors include self-esteem, self-motivation, and perceived health status. Sociocultural factors include race, ethnicity, acculturation, education, and socioeconomic status. Personal factors should be limited to those that are theoretically relevant to explain or predict a given target behavior.

Behavior-Specific Cognitions and Affect

Behavior-specific variables have major motivational significance as they can be modified through interventions. They include perceived benefits and barriers, self-efficacy, activity-related affect, interpersonal influences, and situational influences. Measuring these variables is essential to evaluating change following an intervention.

PERCEIVED BENEFITS OF ACTION.   Perceived benefits of action are beliefs about the positive or reinforcing consequences of performing a behavior. Anticipated benefits influence one's desire to engage in a particular behavior. In the HPM, perceived benefits are proposed to directly and indirectly motivate behavior through shaping the extent of commitment to a plan of action. Benefits may be intrinsic or extrinsic. Intrinsic benefits include the potential for increased energy or perceived attractiveness. Extrinsic benefits include monetary rewards or social interactions possible as a result of engaging in the behavior. Initially, extrinsic benefits may be more significant, whereas intrinsic benefits may be more powerful in motivating the sustainability of health behaviors.

PERCEIVED BARRIERS TO ACTION.   Barriers consist of beliefs about the inconvenience, expense, difficulty, or time-consuming nature of taking a particular action. Barriers are often viewed as mental blocks, hurdles, and personal costs to undertaking a given behavior. Barriers arouse motives to avoid performing a particular behavior. Anticipated barriers have been repeatedly found to affect intentions to engage in behavior. Loss of satisfaction from giving up enjoyable behaviors such as eating high-fat or high-sugar foods may also create a barrier.

When readiness to act is low and barriers are high, action is unlikely to occur. Perceived barriers in the revised HPM affect health-promoting behavior directly by preventing action as well as indirectly through decreasing commitment to a plan of action.

PERCEIVED SELF-EFFICACY.   Self-efficacy is an individual's beliefs about one's personal capability to carry out a particular behavior. Self-efficacy involves judgments of what one can do with whatever skills one possesses. Judgments of personal efficacy are distinguished from outcome expectations. Perceived self-efficacy is a judgment of one's abilities to accomplish a certain level of performance, whereas an outcome expectation is a judgment of the potential outcomes the behavior will produce. Perceptions of skill and competence motivate individuals to engage in behaviors in which they can excel.

The HPM proposes that perceived self-efficacy is influenced by activity-related affect (emotions). The more positive the affect, the greater are the perceptions of efficacy. In reality, however, this relationship is reciprocal. Greater perceptions of efficacy, in turn, increase positive affect. Self-efficacy influences perceived barriers to action, as higher efficacy results in lowered perception of barriers. Self-efficacy motivates health-promoting behavior directly by efficacy expectations and indirectly by decreasing perceived barriers and increasing level of commitment to pursuing a plan of action.

ACTIVITY-RELATED AFFECT.   Activity-related affect consists of three components: emotional arousal to the act itself (act related), self-acting (self-related), and the environment (context) in which the action takes place. The resultant feeling state is likely to determine whether an individual will repeat the behavior or maintain the behavior long term. Subjective feeling states occur prior to, during, and following an activity, based on the stimulus properties associated with the behavior. These emotional responses may be mild, moderate, or strong and are cognitively labeled, stored in memory, and associated with subsequent thoughts of performing the behavior. The affect associated with the behavior can be positive or negative—is it fun, enjoyable, disgusting, or unpleasant? Behaviors associated with positive affect are likely to be repeated, whereas those associated with negative affect are likely to be avoided. Both positive and negative feeling states are induced for some behaviors. Thus, the relative balance between positive and negative affects is important to ascertain.

For any given behavior, the full range of negative and positive feeling states in relation to the act and context for action should be measured. Negative feelings are frequently elaborated more extensively than positive feelings. This is not surprising as anxiety, fear, and depression are studied much more than positive states such as joy, elation, and calm. Emotional responses and their induced physiological states during a behavior serve as sources of efficacy information (Bandura, 1985). Thus, activity-related affect is proposed to influence health behavior directly and indirectly through self-efficacy and commitment to a plan of action.

INTERPERSONAL INFLUENCES. Interpersonal influences are cognitions (thoughts) involving the behaviors, beliefs, or attitudes of others. These thoughts or perceptions may or may not correspond with reality. Primary sources of interpersonal influence on behaviors are family, peers, and health care providers. Interpersonal influences include social norms (expectations of important others), social support, and modeling (vicarious learning through observing others). These three interpersonal influences determine individuals' predisposition to engaging in health-promoting behaviors.

Social norms set standards for performance that individuals may either adopt or reject. Modeling demonstrates the components of a health behavior and is an important strategy for behavior change. The HPM proposes that interpersonal influences affect health-promoting behavior directly as well as indirectly through social norms (pressures or encouragement to commit to a plan of action). Individuals vary in the extent to which they are sensitive to the wishes, examples, and praise of others. Susceptibility to the influence of others may vary developmentally and be particularly evident in adolescence. Some cultures place more emphasis on interpersonal influences than do others. For example, *familismo* among Hispanic populations may encourage individuals to engage in a particular behavior for the good of the family rather than for personal gain.

SITUATIONAL INFLUENCES. Personal perceptions and thoughts of any situation facilitate or impede behavior. Situational influences on health behaviors include perceptions of options available and characteristics of the environment in which a given behavior is proposed to take place. Individuals perform more competently in situations or environmental contexts in which they feel compatible, related, and safe.

In the revised HPM, situational influences have been modified to directly and indirectly influence health behavior. Situations may directly affect behaviors in an environment "loaded" with cues that trigger action. For example, a "no smoking" environment supports nonsmoking behavior. Company regulations for hearing protection mandate that employees comply with regulations. Both situations influence commitment to health actions. Situational influences are important in developing more effective strategies to facilitate the acquisition and maintenance of health-promoting behaviors.

Commitment to a Plan of Action

Commitment to a plan of action initiates a behavior, as it propels individuals into action unless there is a competing demand that cannot be avoided or a competing preference that is not resisted. In the revised HPM, *commitment to a plan of action* implies the following underlying cognitive processes: (1) commitment to carry out a specific action at a given time and place with specified persons or alone, irrespective of competing preferences, and (2) identification of strategies to initiate, perform, and reinforce the behavior. Identification of specific strategies goes beyond intention to increase the likelihood that the plan of action will be implemented. For example, the strategy of contracting consists of a mutually agreed-upon set of actions to which one party commits with the understanding that the other party will provide some tangible reward or reinforcement if the commitment is sustained. Strategies are tailored to energize and reinforce health behaviors according to individual preferences. Commitment alone without associated strategies often results in "good intentions" but failure to perform the health behavior.

Immediate Competing Demands and Preferences

Immediate competing demands or preferences refer to obstacles that intrude into consciousness immediately prior to performing a planned health-promoting behavior. Competing demands are alternative behaviors over which individuals have a relatively low level of control, such as work or family care responsibilities. Failure to respond to a competing demand may have negative effects. In contrast, competing preferences have powerful reinforcing properties over which individuals exert a relatively high level of control. The extent to which an individual resists competing preferences depends on the ability to be self-regulating. Examples of "giving in" to competing preferences are selecting a high-fat food rather than one low in fat because of taste or flavor preferences. Both competing demands and preferences can derail a plan of action. Competing preferences are differentiated from barriers such as lack of time, because competing preferences are last-minute urges based on one's preferences that disrupt a plan for positive health action.

Inhibiting competing preferences requires the exercise of self-regulation and control. Strong commitment to a plan of action may sustain dedication to complete a behavior in light of competing demands or preferences. In the HPM, immediate competing demands and preferences are proposed to directly affect the probability of performing a health behavior as well as moderate the effects of commitment.

Behavioral Outcome

HEALTH-PROMOTING BEHAVIOR. Health-promoting behavior is the positive action outcome in the HPM. Health-promoting behavior is ultimately directed toward attaining positive health outcomes. Health-promoting behaviors result in improved health, enhanced functional ability, and better quality of life at all stages of development.

Studies continue to support the HPM model concepts. Most studies have focused on testing the predictability of the model rather than integrating the theoretical concepts into interventions to test the mechanisms of change proposed in the model. Model concepts have been used to predict physical activity, nutrition, oral health, and hearing protection. An ongoing issue is that only partial testing of the HPM model is conducted in most studies. A possible reason may be the complexity of the model and large number of concepts that need to be measured to test the full model. In spite of these ongoing limitations, the HPM model continues to make significant contributions in the prediction of health behavior.

Recent research has documented the effectiveness of the model to guide health behavior interventions to improve diet quality in children (Rosario et al., 2017), change nutritional behaviors in overweight women (Khodaveisi, Omidi, Farokhi, & Soltanian, 2017), and increase dairy food intake in females (Dehdari, Yekehfallah, Rahimzadeh, Aryaeian, & Rahini, 2016). All model concepts were measured in these studies. However, the interventions were not operationalized with HPM concepts. In other words, the HPM was used to describe the basis for the research, but the theoretical HPM concepts were not integrated into the design, implementation, and evaluation of the intervention. The HPM has been used by researchers around the world, providing evidence of its usefulness across cultures. Systematic reviews and meta-analysis are needed to better understand which model concepts are consistently significant predictors of health-promoting behaviors.

STAGE MODELS OF BEHAVIOR CHANGE

The fundamental assumption underlying a stage model of change is that differences exist in people in their likelihood of action, and different explanations are necessary for different stages of change. Stage models differ from continuum models in that continuum models assume a linear relationship between predictors and behaviors, while stage models propose that individuals go through qualitatively different stages during behavior change and that predictors of behaviors change across the different stages (Sutton, 2015). Interventions can be tailored to the individual's stage of change.

The best known health behavior stage model is the transtheoretical model of change. Another stage model is the precaution adoption process model, a seven-stage model that focuses on risk and changing behavior to reduce risks (prevention). Further information on the precaution adoption process model is available in the literature.

Transtheoretical Model

The transtheoretical model, derived from psychotherapy and theories of behavior change, is an integrative framework that describes how individuals progress toward adopting and maintaining behavior change (Prochaska, Johnson, & Lee, 2009). The premise of the model is that health-related behavior change progresses through five stages, regardless of whether the client is trying to quit a health-threatening behavior or adopt a healthy behavior (Prochaska & DiClemente, 1983). These stages are as follows:

- *Precontemplation:* An individual is not thinking about quitting or adopting a particular behavior, at least not *within the next six months* (no intention to take action).
- *Contemplation:* An individual is seriously thinking about quitting or adopting a particular behavior *in the next six months* (aware of the problem and intends to change).
- *Planning or Preparation:* An individual is seriously thinking about engaging in the behavior change *within the next month* (making small or sporadic changes).
- *Action:* The individual has made the behavior change and it has persisted *for less than six months* (actively engaged in behavior change).
- *Maintenance:* The change has been in place for at least six months and is continuing (sustaining the change over time).

Individuals may not move through the stages consecutively, as they may regress back to a prior stage. Or they become stagnant in one stage for a period of time.

The model contains three concepts in addition to the five stages of change: decisional balance, situational self-efficacy, and processes of change (Di Noia & Prochaska, 2010). The concept of *decisional balance,* from Janis and Mann's decision-making model (Janis & Mann, 1977), is considered central to the model in that decision-making involves comparison of all potential pros and cons. Behavior should occur when the potential gains of engaging in a behavior outweigh the losses. Similar to previously described social cognition models, the benefits need to outweigh the barriers to change.

Situational self-efficacy also is considered a core concept in the model. Self-efficacy shifts in a predictable way across the stages of behavior change, with clients progressively becoming more self-confident. Self-efficacy is similar to the self-efficacy concept in social cognitive theory discussed earlier in the chapter.

Change processes refer to interventions used to facilitate change. Different strategies or techniques need to be used at different stages to facilitate movement through the stages and behavior change. The eight processes of change are presented in Table 2–2. They are categorized as either cognitive or behavioral processes or strategies for change.

In the early stages of change, cognitive processes are more important than behavioral processes for understanding and predicting progress. These processes are to a large extent internally focused on behavior-linked emotions, values, and cognitions. Behavioral processes are important to understand and predict the transition from preparation to action, and from action to maintenance. Behavioral processes focus directly on change. After an individual's stage has been assessed, appropriate processes are implemented to help the client progress to the next stage of change.

TABLE 2–2	Cognitive and Behavioral Processes Involved in Behavior Change
Process	**Definition**
Cognitive	
Information seeking	Exploring, reading, and learning about the desired health behavior.
Evaluating barriers and benefits	Assessing the pros and cons of the behavior change.
Acknowledging contextual influences	Recognizing the pressure of work, peer, and family attitudes on promoting healthy behaviors.
Behavioral	
Substituting behaviors	Choosing positive behaviors to replace old, unhealthy ones.
Accepting support	Obtaining help from family and friends to change the behavior.
Setting realistic goals	Creating obtainable steps to reach long-term health behavior goals.
Practicing self-discipline	Believing in one's ability to change, and actively prioritizing, committing, and performing the new behavior.
Managing environment	Rearranging one's activities and social contacts to avoid old behaviors and promote the new health behavior.

Many studies have been conducted using the transtheoretical model, including research on smoking, physical activity, stress management, bullying prevention, condom use, and obesity. Behavior change is most successful when all of the core concepts are integrated, not just the stages of change. However, the stages are more commonly used without attention to the other concepts. Evidence also supports that those who are ready to change respond more to stage-based interventions than those who are not ready. A meta-analysis of randomized trials to promote physical activity substantiated earlier research findings that interventions based on the theory improved physical activity behavior (Romain et al., 2016).

Despite the success of the model in helping predict change behavior, the model has received numerous criticisms. A major issue continues to be the lack of standardized measurement of the concepts across studies. Although there is support from cross-sectional studies, little attention has been paid to longitudinal research or randomized trials that test interventions derived from the model. Using stage-specific interventions is theoretically appealing; however, whether the stage interventions produce more effective and sustained behavior changes than non-stage interventions is not known. Last, additional concepts may be needed to increase the predictive power of the model.

THEORIES OF HEALTH BEHAVIOR IN THE DIGITAL AGE

Digital interventions have taken on a significant role in health promotion, as Internet and mobile technologies (eHealth, mHealth) have become major resources for health information, social networking, and interactive health promotion, prevention, and self-care interventions for persons of all ages. Mobile technologies and health applications (apps) are tools that enable interventions to be tailored and interact with individuals in real time in their social context (Riley et al., 2011).

Behavioral intervention technologies (BITs) refer to behavioral and psychological interventions that use a variety of technologies to target behaviors to promote health and well-being (Mohr, Schueller, Montague, Burns, & Rashidi, 2014). The advantages of BITs over face-to-face health promotion include the ability to reach and interact with large numbers of persons over and over, thereby reducing costs. They can be used anywhere the technology is available, in any language or culture. BITs can also be tailored to individuals to enhance the likelihood of successful behavior change, and they offer anonymity. In spite of the benefits, many challenges remain. Individuals must use and interact with the new technologies on an ongoing basis for the technologies to be effective. In addition, advances in technology occur rapidly, making evaluation of the effectiveness of specific BITs a major challenge.

In spite of the rapid growth of behavior change software, little attention has been paid to the theoretical base underlying the software designed to promote healthy behaviors. The integration of health behavior theory into digital technology interventions has also been limited. Theory is necessary to understand the mechanisms underlying behavior change, which strategies are more effective, and how individuals interact with the technology to change their behaviors (Schueller, Munoz, & Mohr, 2013). Some reviews indicate that theories have been reported in some cases, including social cognitive theory, theory of planned behavior, transtheoretical model, and social determination theory. Some studies used specific concepts from the theories or models, such as self-efficacy. However, there is very little information about how or if the theories were used to guide the development or evaluation of the intervention and its effects (Webb, Joseph, Yardley, & Michie, 2010). In addition, the health behavior models are considered inadequate, due to their linear, static nature, limiting their usefulness in behavioral information technologies that are interactive and changing as new data are analyzed (Riley et al., 2011). Theories are needed that can respond to individual data to tailor intervention content over the course of the intervention, adapt the timing of the intervention, and continuously interact with individuals in their context to provide ongoing feedback.

Theories of Persuasion and Digital Health Technologies

Theories of persuasion or social influence have been studied in social psychology for over 75 years. The interactional nature of behavioral information technologies has generated renewed interest in persuasion as a foundational strategy to motivate people to change behaviors. Persuasion is defined as a process that can be used to change attitudes (Barden & Petty, 2012). Changes in attitude are likely to change behaviors, as attitudes play a major role in shaping behavior. Persuasion occurs within an exchange, as one party (e.g., a software app) attempts to influence another party (e.g., the user of the app who receives the message). Theories and models of persuasion describe how people are convinced to change, as well as factors that may influence persuasion, such as motivation or ability (Gardikiotis & Crano, 2015). All of the persuasion theories emphasize the role of persuasion in changing attitudes.

   Persuasive communication is the application of persuasive theories to health communication. It is a form of influence that promotes the internalization of a specific attitude (Cassell, Jackson, & Cheuvront, 1998). For example, if a health promotion message is compatible with the individual's pre-existing attitude, the individual is more likely to accept the message, internalize the message, and perform the health behavior in the future in the absence of additional messages or reminders. Persuasion is not the same as coercion. *Coercion* uses external social influence, such as punishment or rules or laws to promote change, such as no smoking laws in public places. The behavior change may only be observed when the rules or laws are enforced. In persuasive communication, recipients of the message are voluntarily able to make their own decision about whether or not they will change their behavior.

Persuasive Technology

Any interactive computer system designed to change people's attitudes or behaviors is described as persuasive technology (Fogg, 2003). The interactive function of computer technology has expanded computers from managing data to changing behaviors. The use of persuasive technology is widespread, as multiple, commonly accessed websites are designed to influence individuals to take action, for example, to purchase goods or services, undertake new behaviors, quit harmful behaviors, or manage medical regimens. Persuasive strategies play a major role in acceptance of and intention to continue using eHealth software programs designed to change behavior.

HEALTH BEHAVIOR CHANGE SUPPORT SYSTEMS. Health behavior change support systems (hBCSS) are sociotechnical information systems designed to form, alter, or reinforce attitudes and behaviors (Langrial, Karppinen, Lehto, Harjumaa, &

Oinas-Kukkonen, 2017). They are one type of behavioral information technology and serve as frameworks to develop eHealth technologies to help people achieve their goals for health and well-being. Persuasive features that have been incorporated into hBCSS applications can be evaluated with persuasive system design (PSD) models. PSD models are tools that assist in developing and evaluating hBCSS. The models evaluate persuasive systems using four design support principles underlying hBCSS software (Kelders, Oinas-Kukkonen, Oorni, & van Gemert-Pijnen, 2016):

1. *Primary task support* reflects an individual's goals and tracks progress to achieving them.
2. *Dialogue support* promotes persuasive features that motivate, activate, and help users reach their goals.
3. *Credibility support* refers to features that ensure the system is trustworthy.
4. *Social support* specifies aspects that motivate users by leveraging social influence.

The PSD model provides a systematic approach to evaluate persuasive content in hBCSS apps. Evidence shows that persuasion plays a critical role in determining health behavior outcomes. Although theories of persuasion and social support have been integrated into the hBCSS systems, there has been a call for increased attention to behavioral theories in human–computer interactions. Evaluation of research conducted with hBCSS eHealth applications is ongoing. The PSD model is one model being used to understand which persuasive principles and behavior strategies are most effective in changing health behaviors. Other BITs and evaluation models are proliferating. Persuasive technology is widespread in health care software applications, so understanding how and what works under what condition will assist in defining concepts and building new theories of change applicable to digital technology.

STRATEGIES FOR HEALTH BEHAVIOR CHANGE

Promoting healthy behaviors and eliminating risky or health-damaging behaviors are major challenges in promoting healthy lifestyles. Health care professionals are continually searching for strategies or interventions that will enable clients to make desired changes. The strategies presented here have been found useful in traditional face-to-face health promotion programs and mobile technologies. Digital technologies (Internet and mobile telephones) have incorporated the strategies into health behavior change support systems as they are the tools for persuasion. In addition, digital technologies are integrating virtual reality, gaming, virtual coaches, and social media (Winter, Sheats, & King, 2016). The multiple technologies offer many possibilities, as they are changing the ways health professionals engage with clients to promote healthy lifestyles.

Setting Goals for Change

Individuals make a commitment to change when goals (desired behavior outcomes) are set, and action plans are developed to accomplish the goals. Setting goals for change is an effective self-regulation strategy as it demonstrates a desire to initiate a behavior change. Well-planned goals focus the client's attention on the activities necessary to change the behavior. Goals should be set by the client, with input as requested or needed and shared with the nurse and supportive others. Commitment to accomplishing goals is demonstrated with action plans. Realistic action plans are behavior specific, short term, action oriented, and can be realistically attained (Lorig, Laurent, Plant, Krishnan, & Ritter, 2014). The action plans should be quantifiable and attainable within one to two weeks so that progress can be seen. For example, a client's goal to walk five days a week may have an initial action plan to walk 10 minutes every other day for one week. If the action plan is accomplished, a new one is set. It is important for the plan to be tied to an action over which the client has control. In addition, the client must be confident that the action plan is attainable, as this increases self-efficacy. Achieving short-term, realistic action plans promotes mastery, which increases self-efficacy. If clients initially have difficulty setting action plans, the nurse should provide a menu of potential options for addressing the proposed goal. Providing options enables the client to have personal control over behaviors to accomplish the proposed goal. As goals are achieved, they should become more challenging, while remaining realistic and achievable. Goals that include specific actions or implementation intentions to implement the behavior are more likely to be achieved than those without an action implementation plan. Implementation intentions are behavioral plans that detail the where, when, and how of what one will do to achieve the goal (Sniehotta, 2009). Implementation intentions have been called "goal primes," as they specify how the goal will be carried out (van Koningbruggen, Stroebe, Papies, & Aarts, 2011). For example, one may set a short-term goal of walking 15 minutes a day for five days to reach the long-term goal of becoming more physically active. The action plan describing the implementation intention may state that the individual will use the first 15 minutes of lunch hour to walk on the path around the building at work with a co-worker each workday. Specifying implementation intentions has been shown to facilitate goal attainment of health behavior change (Kendzierski, Ritter, Stump, & Anglin, 2015).

Monitoring Progress Toward Goals to Promote Change

Self-monitoring or progress monitoring is a behavioral strategy that enables individuals to evaluate their ongoing progress relative to their goal and make changes based on the monitoring information. Monitoring goal progress, a self-regulation strategy, has consistently been shown to contribute to successful behavior change for such behaviors as weight loss or physical activity. The steps in the self-monitoring process are (1) recording behaviors, (2) self-evaluation, and (3) self-reinforcement (Laitner, Minski, & Perri, 2016). Ongoing progress is systematically and continuously evaluated in relation to target goals, and adjustments in behaviors are made based on the ongoing evaluation. The behaviors chosen to target the change or the outcomes of the behavior may be monitored, or both. For example, if one has initiated a walking program to lose weight, the time spent walking daily may be monitored, or weight may be recorded weekly to monitor the desired outcome, weight loss. It is important to distinguish between monitoring behaviors to accomplish goals (the process) and monitoring outcomes of the behaviors, as different patterns are reinforced, depending on what is monitored and reinforced (Harkin et al., 2016). Monitoring data are reviewed on a regular basis to ascertain if progress is being made toward the target goals. The information is then used to reinforce ongoing successful behaviors or make adjustments in one's behaviors. For example, if no weight loss is occurring, time spent walking may need to be increased, or walking at a greater intensity is needed. Self-monitoring of goal progress is a major strategy for behavior change and is a component of many behavioral interventions.

Some authors are calling for the addition of progress monitoring to behavioral models that specify determinants of behavior change, including the theory of planned behavior, to complete the missing link between intentions and behavior (Harkin et al., 2016).

Elements of successful self-monitoring have been identified (Harkin et al., 2016):

- Both *process* (ongoing behaviors to achieve goals) and goal *outcomes* need to be monitored. If only behaviors are monitored, the behaviors may persist; however, they may not change outcomes. Monitoring goal outcomes keeps one focused on the desired endpoint and is more likely to increase commitment to attaining goals.
- Physically *recording* behaviors is more likely to promote change than not recording one's behaviors. Visual information provides evidence or lack of evidence of ongoing behaviors, so that changes can be made if needed.
- Both *active* and *passive* monitoring are effective in meeting goals. Active or deliberate monitoring enables one to have a record of progress. Passive monitoring provides feedback from external sources, such as a change in clothing size.
- *Sharing* self-monitoring information with others (public monitoring) is more effective in meeting goals than private monitoring. Sharing information is thought to increase effort into achieving goals and may increase accountability of behaviors.
- The *frequency* of self-monitoring has an effect on meeting goals. More frequent monitoring has been shown to result in greater levels of behavior change (Reed, Struwe, Bice, & Yates, 2017).
- *Continued* self-monitoring is important. Ongoing monitoring has been shown to promote long-term behavior change (Laitner et al., 2016).

An example of a self-monitoring record of smoking behaviors is shown in Table 2–3.

Promoting Self-Efficacy

The most powerful input to self-efficacy is successful performance (mastery) of the behavior. Whenever possible, the client should receive ongoing positive feedback about successful performance of desired behaviors. Praising or rewarding clients early in the change process by focusing on small successes and progress increases self-efficacy. For

TABLE 2–3   An Example of a Self-Monitoring Record

Behavior to be recorded:	Smoking
Method of coding behavior:	E = Smoking after or during eating and drinking
	S = Smoking when stressed
	D = Smoking when driving the car
	O = Smoking at other times
Smoking record:	

Date: Tuesday, August 26

Morning	Afternoon	Evening
E E D O S S S E	O S S D S E E E	E O

Date: Wednesday, August 27

Morning	Afternoon	Evening
E E E D D S S E E	S S S S D D E E E E	S E O

example, when the client selects low-fat foods from a display of food models, providing immediate feedback on the healthy choices builds self-efficacy relevant to the particular behavior. Learning from the experiences of others as well as observing the behaviors of others is one of the most effective social cognitive strategies for enhancing self-efficacy.

Observation of others engaging in the desired behavior (vicarious experience) is important when initiating a new behavior, as this helps to refine one's performance capabilities, which will enhance self-efficacy. Modeling shows clients how to perform the behavior. This strategy is especially helpful when clients have articulated specific health goals but are uncertain about the action plans to develop to move toward the goals. The following considerations are helpful when choosing modeling as a strategy to increase self-efficacy:

- Clients should share characteristics with the model, such as gender, age, ethnicity, race, and language.
- Clients should have an opportunity to observe the desired behavior.
- Clients should have the essential knowledge and skills to engage in the behavior.
- Clients need to perceive benefits from engaging in the behavior.
- Clients need to practice the target behavior.

Enhancing Benefits of Change

Potential benefits or rewards of behavior change may be tangible, social, or self-generated. Benefits serve to reinforce desired behavior. Tangible benefits include visible objects or activities, such as a new mobile device, or time to engage in a favorite activity. Tangible benefits also include physical changes such as weight loss or lowered blood pressure as a result of a regular physical activity program. Social benefits focus on activities with families and friends. Self-generated benefits include internal rewards, such as increased self-confidence or a positive body image as a result of weight loss.

Planning for rewards is a unique way to expand the positive outcomes of behavior change. Initially rewards may be extrinsic or provided by others. After a client starts engaging in a desired behavior, intrinsic rewards, such as losing weight or feeling more energetic, have reinforcing properties. When the behavior begins to offer its own reward, extrinsic rewards to enhance the benefits of the behavior may no longer be necessary.

Managing Barriers to Change

Barriers or the perceived costs of changing behavior are central concepts in the health belief model, the social cognitive model, and the health promotion model. Behavior change is facilitated when barriers to taking action are minimized or eliminated. It is futile to encourage clients to take actions that are likely to cause frustration or are unrealistic. Early in the change process, clients need to identify potential barriers, which may include cognitive, emotional, social, behavioral, and environmental impediments to change. Potential barriers may include the following:

- Unclear short-term and long-term goals
- Lack of knowledge and/or skills needed to make change
- Lack of resources
- Lack of perceived control

TABLE 2–4   Interrelationships among Level of Readiness to Take Health Actions, Barriers, Consequences for Clients, and Nursing Interventions

Level of Readiness	Barriers to Action	Consequences for Client	Nursing Interventions
High	Low	Action	Support and encouragement; provide low-intensity cues
High	High	Conflict	Assist client in lowering barriers to action
Low	Low	Conflict	Provide high-intensity cues
Low	High	No action	Assist client in lowering barriers to action and then provide high-intensity cues

- Lack of motivation
- Lack of support

The interaction of level of readiness and barriers to action is depicted in Table 2–4. Consequences and appropriate interventions are also presented. When clients have a high level of readiness to engage in health-promoting behaviors and barriers are low, a low-intensity cue, such as a telephone or e-mail reminder, is sufficient to activate behavior. When readiness is high and barriers to action are also high, barriers must be reduced or eliminated. When both readiness and barriers are low, promoting readiness for change should be the initial focus by clarifying misconceptions or concerns, and providing information and access to resources. When readiness is low and barriers are high, both factors should be addressed.

Family members or friends may be barriers to changing behaviors. As noted in the TPB and the HPM, social norms play a pivotal role in behavior change. When family members or other persons disagree or are neutral or apathetic toward health behaviors, the constraints created depend on the following factors:

- Importance of disagreeing persons to the client: Is this person influential in the client's life?
- Extent of disagreement of important persons: Is this person voicing a large disagreement or is it a minor concern?
- Number of persons important to the client who disagree with the behavior: How many important persons are against the action?
- Extent to which the client is self-directed rather than other dependent: Is it a significant concern to the client if important others are not on board with the change?

Membership in support groups may be beneficial if support is not available from family or friends to suggest strategies to overcome the identified constraints.

TAILORING COMMUNICATION FOR BEHAVIOR CHANGE

Tailoring information is a process for creating individualized communication to meet the unique needs and interests of an individual. The aim of tailoring is to increase the relevance of the information to increase the likelihood of behavior change (Kim, Shin, &

Yoon, 2017). Tailored health information is personalized, based on characteristics of the individual and the behavior outcome of interest. Information that will be used to tailor communication is obtained from an individual assessment. Tailored materials are considered more effective than generic or targeted communication, as tailoring engages individuals, builds self-efficacy, and improves health behaviors; and tailored communication is more likely to be read, remembered, and viewed more positively, as it is personally relevant.

"One-size-fits-all" health education information has become outdated as information technology expands the range of possibilities for using interactive behavior change strategies relevant to clients. The one-size-fits-all approach does not address the range of details that vary from person to person to effectively guide individuals as they attempt new health behaviors.

A tailored health message is health information that is based on an assessment of a client's health profile and behavior change models. The message is matched to the individual's needs, interests, and preferences. Behavior change models guide the development of health messages to maximize readiness for change or to motivate maintenance of the new behavior. For example, if the transtheoretical stages of change model is the basis for the intervention, health messages tailored to the individual's current stage is more likely to promote change. With the HBM, tailored information is developed to reduce perceived threats and barriers and increase perceived benefits. A tailored message using the TPB targets an individual's attitudes, subjective norms, and perceived behavioral control. In social cognitive theory, tailored health messages might focus on changing efficacy expectations to meet the desired outcomes (outcome expectations). The selected theory provides the conceptual structure for designing the communication messages to match client characteristics. Tailored health messages may be delivered through many channels: print, face-to-face, and digital. Tailored health communication is popular in interactive digital media.

Tailoring strategies that increase the likelihood of meetings one's goals have been described (Hawkins, Kreuter, Resnicow, Fishbein, & Dijkstra, 2008). First, *personalization* uses the individual's preferences to make them feel like the information is specifically designed for them. An example is identifying the client by name to increase attention to the health information. *Overt tailoring*, such as "This is especially for you, Jane," also focuses attention on the communication message. When the information is framed in a context meaningful for the client, such as one's culture, ethnic or educational background, or gender, it is more likely to influence behavior.

Another tailoring strategy is to provide feedback about the information obtained during the client's assessment to target the psychological determinants of behavior (Hawkins et al., 2008). *Descriptive feedback* uses information from the initial assessment to motivate an individual to focus on a particular behavior. For example, calling attention to an elevated blood cholesterol level may stimulate the client to think about dietary changes. *Comparative feedback,* in which a client is compared with others, is also effective. For example, the client's cholesterol level may be compared to the normal value for his age or peer group. *Evaluative feedback* adds a judgment of the assessment findings, such as noting that the client's reported diet intake is high in fats and sugars, being consistent with the elevated blood cholesterol. The evaluative judgment can then open the door to suggesting actions to change dietary behaviors. *Content matching* in tailoring refers to ensuring that the information is based on the individual's knowledge, beliefs, and outcome expectancies. In other words, the message targets the major determinants of the individual's behavior.

Tailored communication has been widely used in health behavior change and is a major component in interactive technologies today. As the use in technology increases, research is needed to understand how tailored health messages change behaviors, and which tailoring strategies are most effective for change.

Behavior Change Strategies in Persuasive Technology

Persuasive strategies are considered foundational to the behavioral change technologies available for mobile health app users. Persuasion technology has resulted in multiple "persuasive tools" that target attitudes and behaviors (Fogg, 2003). These tools have been refined and expanded and described as persuasion principles. Persuasive tools or principles refer to interactive persuasive strategies that have been built into the software to change behaviors (Langrial et al., 2017). Fogg (2003) originally identified seven tools or strategies, including reduction, tunneling, tailoring, suggestion, self-monitoring, surveillance, and conditioning. They were expanded to support the persuasive system design model mentioned earlier in the chapter. The strategies are expected to increase a user's interaction with the system, leading to continuous engagement with the intervention, which is thought to result in greater task adherence and task completion (Langrial et al., 2017). The commonly used principles or strategies and their definitions are listed in Table 2–5 (Fogg, 2003; Langrial et al., 2017; Wildeboer, Kelders, & van Gemert-Pijnen, 2016). Research has documented the significance of self-monitoring reminders, tunneling, social support, and unobtrusiveness in persuasive technology interventions (Karppinen et al., 2016).

TABLE 2–5   Persuasive Strategies or Principles in Persuasive System Design

Persuasive Strategy	Definition
Reduction	Lowering client's effort in performing target behavior by decreasing complex tasks to simple tasks
Tunneling	Guiding users through a process or experience to make the process easier and consistent; guided persuasion
Tailoring	Providing information relevant to user based on user's needs, interests, personality, and usage context
Self-monitoring	Providing a system for user to track performance toward goals
Suggestion	Offering user compelling, optional behaviors at opportune moments to try out
Reminders	Providing users prompts about their target behavior such as text messages
Social comparisons	Enabling user to compare own performance with the performance of others
Normative influence	Providing ways to bring together peers with similar goals to share information

ETHICS AND HEALTH BEHAVIOR CHANGE

Although the Ottawa Charter is considered the ethical cornerstone for world health promotion, the charter does not address the ethical issues facing individual health promotion. Ethical issues in health promotion are found in all aspects of behavior change, beginning with defining the health problems, setting goals, developing interventions to change behavior, and assessing outcomes. Common ethical issues include personal responsibility versus government obligation, persuasion tactics, cultural sensitivity, and labeling and stigmatization.

Personal responsibility, an underlying assumption in the social cognition and stage theories, is based on the premise that individuals are free to make choices about their health behavior practices, and therefore should take responsibility for changing behaviors. Although targeting individuals can be empowering and promote autonomy, it may also result in blaming the victim. Victim blaming, or locating the source of the problem within individuals or shaming individuals for not adopting change, de-emphasizes the role of social and environmental factors in behavior change (Carter, 2017).

Potential ethical issues may also be present in behavior change strategies, such as communication tactics (persuasion), cultural insensitivity, and stigmatization. Often, clients may not have the desire to change, so they need to be persuaded to do so. Persuasion becomes an ethical issue when information is emotionally manipulating, exaggerated, omitted, or misrepresented. Cultural beliefs and customs must be taken into consideration when designing change strategies for individuals. However, culture becomes an ethical concern when change strategies ignore or contradict cultural values or are viewed as offensive by the cultural group. Last, stigmatization, which links individuals to negative stereotypes and results in prejudice and discrimination, labels individuals in ways that promote shame. Obesity stigma is an ongoing example. Negative attitudes toward obese people are common in the United States. Obesity stigma is similar to other examples throughout history when individuals and groups have been blamed for their disease and considered immoral, unclean, or lazy. However, it is well known that obesity must be framed within the social and environmental conditions that have played a major role in creating the problem.

Health promotion digital technologies offer many possibilities for health care professionals. The technologies present potential ethical issues as well. In spite of the increased availability of mobile telephones and texting in low-income populations and low-income countries, these technologies have not addressed health inequities. Disadvantaged social groups have limited health literacy and limited digital literacy, which hinder their ability to access and interact with mHealth apps (Lupton, 2014). In addition, the focus of health change software is on the individual, with no attention to the social context of health and health behavior. The interactive nature of the technologies raises potential privacy, confidentiality, and security issues about personal digital data shared by individuals.

Nurses must recognize the potential ethical issues that may arise in face-to-face and digital health promotion. Steps must be developed and implemented to ensure that ethical principles are applied in all types of health promotion interventions and evaluations, as ethically sensitive interventions gain the respect and trust of individuals. Most authors recognize the need to address the social, environmental, and political context as well as individual factors. Expansion of the models will facilitate attention to many of the ethical issues.

CONSIDERATIONS FOR PRACTICE IN HEALTH BEHAVIOR CHANGE

Knowledge of individual theories and models of health behavior enables the nurse to select one that is appropriate to guide health promotion programs. One's choice of theory takes into account the needs of the individual. For example, barriers such as travel or cost may be significant for a rural woman who needs to obtain mammography. The health belief model is appropriate to identify perceived barriers and benefits, as well as the perceived threat of breast cancer to be able to design effective strategies to enable her to participate in health screenings. In contrast, self-efficacy may need attention for individuals who desire to develop new patterns of food shopping and preparation to change eating patterns. Interactive mobile technology is available to extend the efforts of the nurse, especially for youth and adolescents.

Intervention strategies vary for different stages of change. Raising consciousness has been shown to be effective in making clients aware of the benefits of behavior change. This strategy is more effective in the early stages when individuals are beginning to either think about change or have not considered making a change. Restructuring the environment to provide cues to trigger new behaviors is effective when individuals are ready to implement change. The availability of healthy foods, such as fruits and vegetables, in the house serves as a trigger for healthy family eating. Smoke-free environments are triggers for tobacco avoidance. Community walking paths and bike lanes are visible cues for individuals and families to motivate regular physical activity habits.

Existing theories, models, and strategies enable the nurse to engage in evidence-based counseling and implement tailored interventions for health promotion. Tailoring enhances the effectiveness of health promotion when knowledge level, perceived needs, and health literacy are taken into account. Additional information on evidence-based counseling strategies can be found at the Agency for Healthcare Research and Quality (AHRQ) website.

Self-monitoring is a very useful strategy when counseling clients to change behaviors, so teaching clients how to monitor their behaviors, both short term and long term, will more likely result in successful behavior change.

OPPORTUNITIES FOR RESEARCH WITH HEALTH BEHAVIOR THEORIES AND MODELS

All of the behavior change models described in this chapter need further testing and expansion to provide a better understanding of the mechanisms that promote behavior change. The following are suggested avenues of research:

1. Continue to perform meta-analysis and systematic research reviews to identify models and concepts that consistently predict or explain health behaviors across social and cultural contexts.
2. Identify the major sociocultural–environmental concepts that can be integrated into social cognition models and develop hypotheses to test these models in diverse groups and geographic settings.

3. Design studies to identify the most effective strategies for tailoring eHealth communication to change behavior.
4. Develop reliable and valid measures of concepts identified to expand the social cognition models.
5. Identify the most effective persuasive strategies that are used in digital technologies to promote change.

Research requires collaboration of scientists from multiple disciplines to design and test the effectiveness of expanded models that integrate the context, including social and environmental determinants.

Summary

This chapter presents an overview of models and theories relevant to individual health behaviors. Theories that incorporate a wider range of powerful explanatory and predictive variables for effective health promotion interventions, including contextual variables, continue to be a priority. Although two of the models include the social context, these concepts are defined narrowly in these models. Application of the models into digital technology interventions has not been fully explored.

Theory-based behavior change strategies described in this chapter are useful in implementing both face-to-face and Internet and mobile interventions. The potential ethical issues need to be addressed in the expanding role of technology in health promotion, including the ethics of persuasion technology in tailoring interventions to individuals as well as the security issues that arise with data sharing.

Learning Activities

1. Choose one social cognition theory described in the chapter and use it as a guide to develop an intervention to address a selected behavior change for you. Identify the stage of change you are in currently as it relates to the selected behavior.
2. Describe potential barriers that you will face in maintaining your behavior change and identify strategies to overcome them.
3. Write one long-term goal to obtain the behavior selected in the learning activity above and two short-term realistic, measurable implementation strategies to begin to achieve the goal.
4. Use the behavioral-specific cognitions described in Pender's health promotion model to perform an individual assessment and develop an intervention to change one's behavior based on the assessment.

References

Ajzen, I. (1991). The theory of planned behavior. *Organizational Behavior and Human Decision Processes, 50*(2), 179–211. doi:10.1016/0749-5978(91)90020-T

Ajzen, I. (2011). The theory of planned behavior: Reactions and reflections. *Psychology and Health, 29*(9), 1113–1127. doi:10.1080/08870446.2011.613995

Araban, M., Baharzadeh, K., & Karimy, M. (2017). Nutrition modification aimed at enhancing dietary iron and folic acid intake: An application of health belief model in practice. *European Journal of Public Health, 27*(2), 287–292. doi:10.1093/eurpub/ckw238

Banas, K., Lyimo, R. A., Hospers, H. J., van der Ven, A., & de Bruin, M. (2017). Predicting adherence to combination antiretroviral therapy for HIV in Tanzania: A test of the extended theory of planned behavior. *Psychology & Health*, doi:10.1080/08870446.2017.1283037

Bandura, A. (1985). Model of causality in social learning theory. In M. J. Mahoney & A. Freeman (Eds.), *Cognition and psychotherapy* (pp. 81–99). New York, NY: Plenum Publishing Corporation.

Bandura, A. (1986). *Social foundations of thought and action: A social cognitive theory*. Englewood Cliffs, NJ: Prentice Hall.

Bandura, A. (2004). Health promotion by social cognitive means. *Health Education & Behavior*, 31(2), 143–164. doi:10.1177/1090198104263660

Barden, J., & Petty, R. E. (2012). Persuasion. In V. Ramachandran (Ed.), *Encyclopedia of human behavior* (2nd ed., Vol. 2, pp. 96–102). Oxford, UK: Elsevier Science & Technology.

Carter, S. M. (2017). Ethics and health promotion. In S. R. Quah (Ed.), *International encyclopedia of public health* (2nd ed., Vol. 3, pp. 1–6). New York, NY: Elsevier.

Cassell, M. M., Jackson, C., & Cheuvront, B. (1998). Health communication on the Internet: An effective channel for health behavior change? *Journal of Health Communication*, 3(1), 71–79. doi:10.1080/108107398127517

Chansukree, P., & Rungjindarat, N. (2017). Social cognitive determinants of healthy eating behaviors in late adolescents: A gender perspective. *Journal of Nutrition Education and Behavior*, 49(3), 204–210. doi:10.1016/j.jneb.2016.10.019

Che, S., Barrett, E. S., Velez, M., Conn, K., Heinert, S., & Qiu, X. (2014). Using the health belief model to illustrate factors that influence risk assessment during pregnancy and implications for prenatal education about endocrine disruptors. *Policy Futures in Education*, 12(7), 961–974. doi:10.2304/pfie.2014.12.7.961

Chung, L., & Fong, S. (2015). Predicting actual weight loss: A review of the determinants according to the theory of planned behavior. *Health Psychology Open*, January–June, 1–9. doi:10.1177/2055102914567972

Daryani, S., Shojaeezadeh, D., Batebi, A., Charati, J. Y., & Naghibi, A. (2016). The effect of education based on a health belief model in women's practice with regard to the Pap smear test. *Journal of Cancer Policy*, 8, 51–56. doi:10.1016/j.jcpo.2015.11.001

Dehdari, T., Yekehfallah, F., Rahimzadeh, M., Aryaeian, N., & Rahini, T. (2016). Dairy food intake among female Iranian students: A nutrition education intervention using a health promotion model. *Global Journal of Health Sciences*, 8(10), 192–199. doi:10.5539/gjhs.v8n10p192

Di Noia, J., & Prochaska, J. O. (2010). Mediating variables in a transtheoretical model dietary intervention program. *Health Education & Behavior*, 37(5), 753–762. doi:10.1177/1090198109334897

Dodel, M., & Mesch, G. (2017). Cyber-victimization preventive behavior: A health belief model approach. *Computers in Human Health*, 68, 359–367. doi:10.1016/j.chb.2016.11.044

Ejeta, L. T., Ardalan, A., Paton, D., & Yaseri, M. (2016). Predictors of community preparedness for flood in Dire-Dawa town, Eastern Ethiopia: Applying adapted version of health belief model. *International Journal of Disaster Risk Reduction*, 19, 341–354. doi:10.1016/j.ijdrr.2016.09.005

Fishbein, M., & Ajzen, I. (1975). *Belief, attitude, intention and behavior: An introduction to theory and research*. Boston, MA: Addison-Wesley Publishing Company, Inc.

Fogg, B. J. (2003). *Persuasive technology: Using computers to change what we think and do*. Amsterdam, The Netherlands: Morgan Kaufmann Publishers.

Gardikiotis, A., & Crano, W. D. (2015). Persuasion theories. In J. Wright (Ed.), *International encyclopedia of the social and behavioral sciences* (2nd ed., Vol. 17, pp. 941–947). New York, NY: Elsevier.

Harkin, B., Webb, T. L., Chang, B. P., Prestwich, A., Conner, M., Kellar, I., . . . Sheeran, P. (2016). Does monitoring goal progress promote goal attainment? A meta-analysis of the experimental evidence. *Psychological Bulletin*, 142(2), 198–229. doi:10.1037/bul0000025

Hawkins, R. P., Kreuter, M., Resnicow, K., Fishbein, M., & Dijkstra, A. (2008). Understanding tailoring in communicating about health. *Health Education Research*, 23(3), 454–466. doi:10.1093/her/cyn004

Janis, I. L., & Mann, L. (1977). *Decision making: A psychological analysis of conflict, choice and commitment*. New York, NY: Free Press.

Jones, C. J., Smith, H., & Llewellyn, C. (2014). Evaluating the effectiveness of health belief model interventions in improving adherence: A systematic review. *Health Psychology Review*, 8(3), 253–269. doi:10.1080/17437199.2013.802623

Karppinen, P., Oinas-Kukkonen, H., Alahaivala, T., Jokelainen, T., Keranen, A., Salonurmi, T., & Savolainen, M. (2016). Persuasive user experiences of a health behavior change support system: A 12-month study for prevention of metabolic syndrome. *International Journal of Medical Informatics*, 96, 51–61. doi:10.1016/j.ijmedinf.2016.02.005

Kelders, S. M., Oinas-Kukkonen, H., Oorni, A., & van Gemert-Pijnen, J. (2016). Health behavior change support systems as a research discipline: A viewpoint. *International Journal of Medical Informatics, 96*, 3–10. doi:10.1016/j.ijmedinf.2016.06.022

Kendzierski, D., Ritter, R. L., Stump, T. M., & Anglin, C. L. (2015). The effectiveness of an implementation intentions intervention for fruit and vegetable consumption as moderated by self-schema status. *Appetite, 95*, 228–238. doi:10.1016/j.appet.2015.07.007

Khodaveisi, M., Omidi, A., Farokhi, S., & Soltanian, A. (2017). The effect of Pender's health promotion model in improving the nutritional behavior of overweight and obese women. *International Journal of Community Based Nursing and Midwifery, 5*(2), 165–174.

Kim, K. J., Shin, D., & Yoon, H. (2017). Information tailoring and framing in wearable health communication. *Information Processing and Management, 53*(2), 351–358. doi:10.1016/j.ipm.2016.11.005

Knol, L. L., Meyers, H. H., Black, S., Robinson, D., Awololo, Y., Clark, D., . . . Higginbotham, J. C. (2016). Development and feasibility of a childhood obesity prevention program for rural families: Application of the social cognitive theory. *American Journal of Health Education, 47*(4), 204–214. doi:10.1080/19325037.2016.1179607

Kok, G., & Ruiter, R. A. (2014). Who has the authority to change a theory? Everyone! A commentary on Head and Noar. *Health Psychology Review, 8*(1), 61–64. doi:10.1080/17437199.2013.840955

Laitner, M. H., Minski, S. A., & Perri, M. G. (2016). The role of self-monitoring in the maintenance of weight loss success. *Eating Behaviors, 21*, 193–197. doi:10.1016/j.eatbeh.2016.03.005

Langrial, S., Karppinen, P., Lehto, T., Harjumaa, M., & Oinas-Kukkonen, H. (2017). Evaluating mobile-based behavior change support systems for health and well-being. In L. Little, E. Sillence, & A. Joinson (Eds.), *Behavior change research and theory: Psychological and technological perspectives* (pp. 69–86). New York, NY: Elsevier.

Lizin, S., Van Dael, M., & Van Passel, S. (2017). Battery pack recycling: Behavior change interventions derived from an integrative theory of planned behavior study. *Resources, Conservation and Recycling, 122*, 66–82. doi:10.1016/j.resconrec.2017.02.003

Lorig, K., Laurent, D. D., Plant, K., Krishnan, E., & Ritter, P. L. (2014). The components of action planning and their associations with behavior and health outcomes. *Chronic Illness, 10*(1), 50–59. doi:10.1177/1742395313495572

Lowry, P. B., Zhang, J., & Wu, T. (2017). Nature or nurture? A meta-analysis of the factors that maximize the prediction of digital piracy by using social cognitive theory as a framework. *Computers in Human Behavior, 68*, 104–120. doi:10.1016/j.chb.2016.11.015

Lupton, D. (2014). Health promotion in the digital era: A critical commentary. *Health Promotion International, 30*(1), 174–183. doi:10.1093/heapro/dau091

Manstead, A. S. R. (2011). The benefits of a critical stance: A reflection on past papers on the theories of reasoned action and planned behavior. *British Journal of Social Psychology, 50*(3), 366–373. doi:10.1111/j.2044-8309.2011.02043.x

McDermott, M. S., Oliver, M., Simnadis, T., Beck, E. J., Coltman, T., Iverson, D., & Sharma, R. (2015). The theory of planning behavior and dietary patterns: A systematic review and meta-analysis. *Preventive Medicine, 81*, 150–156. doi:10.1016/j.ypmed.2015.08.020

Mehta, P., Sharma, M., & Lee, R. C. (2014). Designing and evaluating a health belief model-based intervention to increase intent of HPV vaccination among college males. *Quarterly of Community Health Education, 34*(1), 101–117. doi:10.2190/IQ.34.1.h

Mohr, D. C., Schueller, S. M., Montague, E., Burns, M. N., & Rashidi, P. (2014). The behavioral intervention model: An integrated conceptual and technical framework for eHealth and mHealth interventions. *Journal of Medical Internet Research, 16*(6), 1–22. doi:10.2196/jmir.3077

Peachey, A. A., Sutton, D. L., & Cathorall, M. L. (2016). Helmet ownership and use among skateboarders: Utilization of the health belief model. *Health Education Journal, 75*(5), 565–576. doi:10.1177/0017896915607912

Pender, N. J. (1996). *Health promotion in nursing practice* (3rd ed.). Stamford, CT: Appleton & Lange.

Plotnikoff, R. C., Costigan, S. A., Karunamuni, N., & Lubans, D. R. (2013). Social cognitive theories used to explain physical activity behavior in adolescents: A systematic review and meta-analysis. *Preventive Medicine, 56*(5), 245–253. doi:10.1016/j.ypmed.2013.01.013

Prochaska, J. O., & DiClemente, C. C. (1983). Stages and processes of self-change of smoking: Toward an integrative model of change. *Journal of Consulting and Clinical Psychology, 51*(3), 390–395. doi:10.1037/0022-006X.51.3.390

Prochaska, J. O., Johnson, S., & Lee, P. (2009). The transtheoretical model of change. In S. Shumaker, J. Ockene, & K. Riekert (Eds.), *The handbook of behavior change* (3rd ed., pp. 59–84). New York, NY: Springer Publishing Company.

Reed, J. R., Struwe, L., Bice, M. R., & Yates, B. C. (2017). The impact of self-monitoring food intake on motivation, physical activity and weight loss in rural adults. *Applied Nursing Research, 35*, 36–41. doi:10.1016/j.apnr.2017.02.008

Riebl, S. K., Estabrooks, P. A., Dunsmore, J. C., Savla, J., Frisard, M. H., Dietrich, A. M., . . . Davy, B. M. (2015). A systematic literature review and meta-analysis: The theory of planned behavior's application to understand and predict nutrition-related behaviors in youth. *Eating Behaviors, 18*, 160–178. doi:10.1016/j.eatbeh.2015.05.016

Riley, W. T., Rivera, D. E., Atienza, A. A., Nilsen, W., Allison, S. M., & Mermelstein, R. (2011). Health behavior models in the age of mobile interventions: Are our theories up to the task? *Translational Behavioral Medicine, 1*(1), 53–71. doi:10.1007/s13142-011-0021-7

Romain, A. J., Bortolon, C., Gourlan, M., Carayol, M., Decker, E., Lareyre, O., . . . Bernard, P. (2016). Matched or nonmatched interventions based on the transtheoretical model to promote physical activity. A meta-analysis of randomized controlled trials. *Journal of Sport and Health Science*, 1–8. doi:10.1016/j.jshs.2016.10.007

Rosario, R., Araujo, A., Padrao, P., Lopes, O., Moreira, A., Pereira, B., & Moreira, P. (2017). Health promotion intervention to improve diet quality in children: A randomized trial. *Health Promotion Practice, 18*(2), 253–262. doi:10.1177/1524839916634096

Rosenstock, I. M. (1960). What research in motivation suggests for public health. *American Journal of Public Health, 50*(3 Pt 1), 295–303.

Schueller, S. M., Munoz, R. F., & Mohr, D. C. (2013). Realizing the potential of behavioral intervention technologies. *Current Directions in Psychological Science, 22*(6), 478–483. doi:10.1177/0963721413495872

Schuz, B., Li, A. S., Hardinge, A., McEachan, R., & Conner, M. (2017). Socioeconomic status as a moderator between social cognitions and physical activity: Systematic review and meta-analysis based on the theory of planned behavior. *Psychology of Sport and Exercise, 30*, 186–195. doi:10.1016/j.psychsport.2017.03.004

Sharafkhani, N., Khorsandi, M., Shamsi, M., & Ranjbaran, M. (2016). The effect of an educational intervention program on the adoption of low back pain preventive behaviors in nurses: An application of the health belief model. *Global Spine Journal, 6*(1), 29–34. doi:10.1055/s-0035-1555658

Sniehotta, F. F. (2009). Towards a theory of intentional behavioral change: Plans, planning and self-regulation. *British Journal of Health Psychology, 14*(2), 261–273. doi:10.1348/135910708X389042

Sniehotta, F. F., Presseau, J., & Araujo-Soares, V. (2014). Time to retire the theory of planned behavior. *Health Psychology Review, 8*(1), 1–7. doi:10.1080/17437199.2013.869710

Stacey, F. G., James, E. L., Chapman, K., Courneya, K. S., & Lubans, D. R. (2015). A systematic review and meta-analysis of social cognitive theory-based physical activity and/or nutrition behavior change interventions for cancer survivors. *Journal of Cancer Survivorship, 9*(2), 305–338. doi:10.1007/s11764-014-0413-z

Sundstrom, B., Carr, L. A., DeMaria, A. L., Korte, J. E., Modesitt, S. C., & Pierce, J. Y. (2015). Protecting the next generation: Elaborating the health belief model to increase HPV vaccination among college-age women. *Social Marketing Quarterly, 21*(3), 173–188. doi:10.1177/1524500415598984

Sutton, S. (2015). Health behavior: Psychosocial theories. In J. D. Wright (Ed.), *International encyclopedia of the social and behavioral sciences* (2nd ed., Vol. 10, pp. 577–581). New York, NY: Elsevier.

VanDyke, S. D., & Shell, M. D. (2016). Health beliefs and breast cancer screening in rural Appalachia: An evaluation of the health belief model. *Journal of Rural Health*, 1–11. doi:10.1111/jrh.12204

van Koningbruggen, G. M., Stroebe, W., Papies, E. K., & Aarts, H. (2011). Implementation intentions as goal primes: Boosting self-control in tempting environments. *European Journal of Social Psychology, 41*(5), 551–557. doi:10.1002/ejsp.799

Webb, T. L., Joseph, J., Yardley, L., & Michie, S. (2010). Using the Internet to promote health behavior change: A systematic review and meta-analysis of the impact of theoretical basis, use of behavior change techniques, and mode of delivery on efficacy. *Journal of Medical Internet Research, 12*(1), e4. doi:10.2196/jmir.1376

Wildeboer, G., Kelders, S. M., & van Gemert-Pijnen, J. (2016). The relationship between persuasive technology principles, adherence and effect of Web-based interventions for mental health: A meta-analysis. *International Journal of Medical Informatics, 96*, 71–85. doi:10.1016/j.ijmedinf.2016.04.005

Williams, D., & Rhodes, R. E. (2016). The confounded self-efficacy construct: Conceptual analysis and recommendations for future research. *Health Psychology Review, 10*(2), 113–128. doi:10.1080/17437199.2014.941998

Winter, S. J., Sheats, J. L., & King, A. C. (2016). The use of behavior change techniques and theory in technologies for cardiovascular disease prevention and treatment in adults: A comprehensive review. *Progress in Cardiovascular Disease, 58*(6), 605–612. doi:10.1016/j.pcad.2016.02.005

Yang, Y., Yang, C., Latkin, C. A., Luan, R., & Nelson, K. E. (2016). Condom use during commercial sex among male clients of female sex workers in Sichuan, China: A social cognitive theory analysis. *AIDS and Behavior, 20*, 2309–2317. doi:10.1007/s10461-015-1239-z

Young, M. D., Plotnikoff, R. C., Collins, C. E., Callister, R., & Morgan, P. J. (2016). A test of social cognitive theory to explain men's physical activity during a gender-tailored weight loss program. *American Journal of Men's Health, 10*(6), N176–N187. doi:10.1177/1557988315600063

Zetu, L., Zetu, I., Dogaru, C. B., Duta, C., & Dumitrescu, A. L. (2014). Gender variations in the psychological factors as defined by the extended health belief model of oral hygiene behaviors. *Procedia—Social and Behavioral Sciences, 127*, 358–362. doi:10.1016/j.sbspro.2014.03.271

Zoellner, J. M., Porter, K. J., Chen, Y., Hedrick, V. E., You, W., Hickman, M., & Estabrooks, P. A. (2017). Predicting sugar-sweetened behaviors with theory of planned behavior constructs: Outcome and process results from the SIP*smart*ER behavioral intervention. *Psychology and Health, 32*(5), 509–529. doi:10.1080/08870446.2017.1283038

CHAPTER 3

Community Models to Promote Health

OBJECTIVES

This chapter will enable the reader to:

1. Describe commonalities and differences in the various definitions of communities.

2. Discuss the key concepts in social-ecological models of health promotion.

3. Describe the characteristics of social capital and the role of social support in this approach.

4. Define the steps in the PRECEDE–PROCEED model in planning health promotion programs.

5. Discuss characteristics that determine the diffusion of innovations.

6. Contrast upstream and downstream social marketing models.

Health professionals' attention to community-based approaches to promote health and prevent disease has dramatically increased in recent years. The increased emphasis is due to many factors, including a greater understanding of the complex etiologies of health problems, an appreciation of the relationship of individuals with their environment, and recognition of the limitations of focusing only on individual behaviors to promote health. A greater understanding of the role of the sociocultural, physical, and political environments in achieving health has resulted in multiple approaches to promoting wellness. Individual approaches to health promotion identify a finite number of lifestyle areas that can be targeted for intervention. Community-based models move beyond individual lifestyles to distal factors that influence health, such as working and living conditions. In a community-based view, the social, political, institutional, legislative, and physical environments in which behavior occurs can be targeted to promote health. Community approaches emphasize populations and communities as clients and acknowledge that the greater environment influences individual health behaviors.

Although health care professionals recognize that attention to the social, physical, and political environments is necessary for health promotion, community-based models are not intended to neglect the individual. Individuals make up communities, so although the community may be targeted, individuals play a critical role in providing leadership. Community-based strategies for health promotion are community-led strategies, as control is placed with individuals who reside in the community. This chapter introduces the concepts in community models and provides an overview of the commonly cited community models and theories.

THE CONCEPT OF COMMUNITY

Community has been defined in multiple ways. The World Health Organization (WHO) was a pioneer in defining the community as a collective body of individuals identified by geography, common interests, concerns, characteristics, or values (World Health Organization, 1974). A community can be considered a self-generated gathering of common people or citizens who have the creativity and capacity to solve problems. The definition of community has evolved from a structural focus on geographic boundaries to a functional focus on people interacting in social units and sharing common interests. Whatever the definition of *community*, residents have a sense of identity, shared values, social norms, communication modes, and helping patterns, and identify themselves as being of the same community.

The community in which individuals live, work, and play is critical to health promotion and prevention. The community context refers to the interdependence that exists between selected aspects of a given environment or setting. The context includes personal, physical, cultural, and social aspects of environments and the relationship between them that may influence an individual's mental and physical health, opportunities, achievement, and developmental outcomes. The relationship between individuals and the social system in which they interact is reciprocal, as individuals may work to change their neighborhood context, just as the context influences individuals. For example, lack of street lighting may prevent persons from walking later in the evening. However, individuals can work together to get appropriate lighting installed in their community to facilitate safe walking environments.

The community context includes social institutions and resources within a community, its surroundings, and social relationships. Social institutions include cultural and religious organizations, economic systems, and political structures. Surroundings include neighborhoods, workplaces, towns, and cities; and social relationships include one's position in the social hierarchy, social group, and social networks. Health care professionals need to take all of these aspects into consideration to understand how the community context influences one's health.

A risk environment is an example of a context in which factors present may increase the chances of unhealthy behaviors and harm. Physical environments that may increase risks include lack of safe running water, inadequate public transportation, and unsafe housing. Social environments, such as high crime, high poverty, and residentially segregated neighborhoods, have been associated with higher rates of obesity in children and adults (Suglia et al., 2016). Knowledge of the environmental context is necessary to create an enabling environmental context in which risks are reduced to maximize healthy behavior.

The client becomes the community when the focus is on the collective or the common good of the population. In the community models discussed in this chapter, the nurse works with individuals and groups. However, the outcomes of health promotion programs are expected to affect the entire community. For example, the nurse may work with parents to get safe walking tracks for adults and recreational parks for children. These changes improve the health of the community. In community health promotion, change occurs at multiple levels, beginning with individuals and moving to the community as a whole. Healthy individuals result in healthier communities. Policy changes may be necessary at the societal level for community-wide change to occur. When the community is the client, the nurse and the community work together to achieve mutual goals, as community members are at the heart of the process.

COMMUNITY INTERVENTIONS AND HEALTH PROMOTION

Community interventions differ from interventions within a community. Community interventions target either the majority of the population in a community or the community as a whole, as the goal is to change the entire setting. Community interventions have multiple advantages. First, they have the potential to make large-scale changes. Interventions based on community models focus on both high-risk persons and the larger community to promote health. The interventions are relevant for the population in the community. Other benefits include a high level of exposure to the intervention and increased generalizability of the intervention to other communities. The interventions are also likely to be valuable in the development of public health policies. Community changes are integrated into existing structures within the community, thereby changing the system that influences health behaviors.

Community models are based on four underlying assumptions (Minkler & Wallerstein, 2012):

1. Communities shape individual behaviors through community values and norms.
2. Communities can be mobilized to change individual behaviors by legitimizing the desirable behaviors and changing environments to facilitate the new behaviors.
3. Participation of community leaders is crucial for community ownership.
4. Members of the community must have a sense of responsibility and control over the planned change.

In other words, community members must own the planned change for it to be successful. People are more likely to commit to and sustain change if they participate in identifying the problem, as well as in developing and implementing the program to address the problem. Community interventions must engage participants to guide the change. Members are engaged early in the planning process to identify needs, develop priorities, and plan programs to promote health. Community-based models take into consideration individuals in interaction with their families, cultures, and social structures, as well as the actual physical environment.

Community empowerment and community participation were identified decades ago as the twin pillars of community-based programs, and they are still considered the cornerstone for effective community change. *Community empowerment* is a social action process by which people and communities are enabled to participate and act to transform their lives and their environments (Minkler, 2000). The concept of empowerment refers to a process by which people and communities work together to gain mastery over factors that shape their lives and health. Empowerment principles are essential components in health promotion. Empowered communities are visible when people within the community participate in equal partnership with health professionals and organizations to define their health problems and develop solutions. In addition, community members receive the benefits of the interventions and are partners in evaluating the effectiveness of the intervention. Community empowerment is not new in public health; public health nurses have long recognized the need for members to take control of the health of their community.

Community participation is the process of taking part in activities, programs, or discussions to promote change to improve the community. Community participation is a basic principle in health education. Community participation empowers individuals and communities through group decision-making and knowledge of resources, as well as creating new networks and opportunities. Participation of community members results in greater buy-in, higher participation, and greater sustainability. Empowerment and community participation go hand in hand, as empowered members participate in the health agenda for the community.

Community participation varies from little or no participation and control to high participation or engagement with leadership and control over the proposed action (Dooris & Heritage, 2013). The amount of community participation can be viewed on a continuum, which describes participation ranging from manipulation (no control) to empowerment (complete control over the project) (Dooris & Heritage, 2013). As Figure 3–1 depicts, empowering people enables the community to fully participate and have control of the project or program, including identifying the problem and making all key decisions for the program. Community empowerment involves shifts in power relations among individuals, groups, and institutions within a community. These shifts occur as people and institutions come together for social action. The nurse's role is to create opportunities to enable community members to become empowered to gain control over the factors that determine their health.

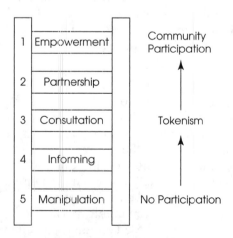

FIGURE 3–1 Continuum of Community Involvement in Decisions

COMMUNITY SOCIAL-ECOLOGICAL MODELS AND THEORIES

Ecological models recognize the role of the environment in the health of individuals and emphasize the social, physical, and cultural contexts of individuals in interaction with their environment. The term *ecology* refers to the interrelations between organisms and their environments. The concept has evolved to provide an understanding of the interactions of people with their physical and sociocultural environments. As mentioned in Chapter 2, a major limitation of individual models of health promotion is the lack of attention to factors beyond an individual's control that may influence health behaviors. In ecological theories, individuals cannot be separated from their environment.

Papers describing ecological perspectives have been present in the literature for over 75 years. In the social sciences, Bronfenbrenner (1977) developed a systems perspective based on the theories of Kurt Lewin. Lewin described his approach as the ecology of human development, in which individuals are constantly interacting with the environment in a reciprocal relationship. Individuals are influenced by their environments, and they also influence their environments. Lewin considered the ecological environment to have successive levels of influence, ranging from microsystems to macrosystems. In other words, individuals are influenced by multiple elements in their environments, including family, friends, workplace, neighborhood, community, institutions, and the wider cultural context. These levels of influence, or factors that determine health behaviors, were later described by McLeroy, Bibeau, Steckler, and Glanz (1988) as:

1. Intrapersonal (individual)
2. Interpersonal (relationships)
3. Institutional
4. Community
5. Public policy (societal)

These factors are present in almost all social-ecological theories.

Social-Ecological Model

The concept of an ecology model was expanded to a social-ecological approach to health promotion by Stokols (1992, 2000) and Stokols, Lejano, & Hipp (2013) who viewed environments as complex systems. Stokols believed that efforts to promote well-being must take into account the interdependence among all components and levels of the environment.

In a social-ecological perspective, health promotion interventions target multiple levels: intrapersonal, interpersonal, organizational, community, and public policy. Intrapersonal factors include knowledge, beliefs, and other personal attributes described in the individual models covered in Chapter 2. Interpersonal factors target social relationships, and organizational factors focus on institutional environments. At the community level, partnerships are developed with churches, schools, and neighborhoods for community participation. Community participation is necessary to build community capacity and empower citizens. Community participation also facilitates the development, implementation, and maintenance of health promotion programs. At the public policy level, implementation of policies to promote or improve health is targeted.

The social-ecological perspective suggests that the effectiveness of health promotion interventions can be increased through multilevel interventions, which combine multiple behavioral and environmental strategies. In a social-ecological approach to

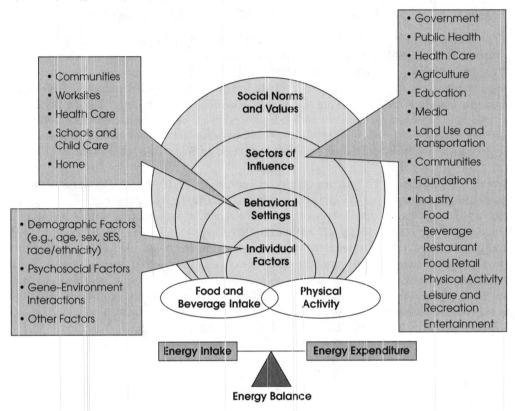

FIGURE 3–2 A Social-Ecological Model Describing a Comprehensive Approach for Preventing and Addressing Childhood Obesity

Source: Institute of Medicine (IOM) (2005).

health promotion, the interplay between environmental resources and the health habits of individuals is assessed to identify features of the environment that promote or hinder well-being. Identifying the interdependent links helps define both environmental components and individual characteristics that must be targeted to promote healthy lifestyles. Figure 3–2 is an example of a social-ecological model developed to describe a comprehensive approach for preventing childhood obesity (Koplan, Liverman, Kraak, & Wisham, 2007). Ecological factors that influence individual eating and activity behaviors include interpersonal processes (social norms, values), behavioral settings, and community and institutional factors and settings.

Social-ecological models go beyond a focus solely on environmental factors to include individuals and groups together with the environment. This is a key feature and major strength, as strategies for specific behavior change are integrated with specific environmental change strategies. However, it is also a challenge to identify the critical environmental determinants that can be realistically targeted for change.

Social-ecological approaches are guided by principles that facilitate program development (Sallis & Owens, 2008). Some of the principles relevant for health promotion programs are listed in Table 3–1. Ecological models have been applied to research

TABLE 3–1   Principles of Ecological Models for Health and Well-Being

- The physical, psychological, and social dimensions of health and well-being interact with and are influenced by the social and physical environments.
- Both individual (intrapersonal, interpersonal) and environmental (institutional, community, public policy) factors influence health and well-being.
- Health and well-being are dependent on the congruence between individual needs and environmental resources.
- Multidisciplinary, multilevel approaches contribute to the understanding of health and well-being.

with physical activity, nutrition, tobacco use, sexual behaviour and health screening. Despite the widespread acceptance of the social-ecological approach and support for multilevel interventions, individual characteristics continue to be the major focus of research. In a 20-year review of health behavior research, two-thirds of the articles targeted only one or two levels. Interventions in schools and workplaces were more likely to target institutional-level factors (Golden & Earp, 2012). Other reviews of research have reported similar findings. Most studies were more likely to target the individual, interpersonal, and organizational levels, with few studies aimed at the community and political levels.

Barriers to social-ecological intervention include multiple factors, such as the complexity of targeting multiple levels, the cost and feasibility of implementing complex interventions, and often the lack of theoretical understanding of the number and levels of environmental factors to target (Scholmerich & Kawachi, 2016). Targeting one level (intrapersonal) may influence another level (family) either positively or negatively, so more attention to the links between the environmental factors is important. In a review of the social-ecological model applied to diet and physical activity in children, results indicated that characteristics of children moderate the influence of their childcare environments on physical activity and diet (Gubbels, Van Kann, de Vries, Thijs, & Kremers, 2014). Although the number of studies reviewed was small, findings support the need to understand and examine the relationships between the levels of environmental influences as well as the interactions of individual characteristics with environmental influences. When planning interventions nurses need to understand which environmental levels need to be targeted, and which individual factors interact with the environmental levels being targeted to ensure the success of the intervention.

The expertise of nurses and other health care professionals is needed at all levels of influence in social-ecological models. At the intrapersonal and interpersonal levels, attention to an individual's characteristics and support systems are assessed prior to planning interventions. At the institutional level, nurses can focus on changes in the workplace or school environments that influence health, such as working to improve nutrition and physical activity resources. At the community level, health care professionals can engage churches, volunteer organizations, and neighborhood groups to plan and implement interventions. Skills in community organizing strategies to engage and empower community participants are essential. Last, at the public policy or societal level, nurses should have the expertise to communicate policy changes and evaluate their implementation within the community. In addition, nurses need to understand how to build coalitions to advocate for healthier communities and health equity for all community members (Golden, McLeroy, Green, Earp, & Lieberman, 2015).

Social Capital Theory

Social capital refers to factors in the social environment that influence health. The theory of social capital focuses on how individuals, groups, and communities interact and how these interactions result in benefits for individuals as well as their communities (Brunie, 2009). The theory focuses on actions taken to either maintain or gain resources or valued goods in a society.

Although definitions of social capital vary, in most definitions, trust and reciprocity are central components. Currently, two major approaches to the measurement of social capital are accepted: the *social cohesion* approach and the *network-based* approach (Alvarez, Kawachi, & Romani, 2017). The *social cohesion* approach is defined as the extent of closeness within groups and is measured as a sense of belonging, trust, and norms of reciprocity. The *network-based* approach focuses on the resources accessed by individuals in their social structures, including their social networks, social relationships, and social support. In addition, there are two levels of social capital: *individual* and *collective*. *Collective* social capital focuses on characteristics of the community, including families, neighborhoods, and workplace in terms of social participation, trust, and reciprocity norms (Kawachi & Berkman, 2014). *Individual* social capital refers to the level of trust, social networks, and support an individual has within a given family, neighborhood, or community, whereas *collective* social capital is the amount of trust, networks, or cooperation within a neighborhood or community (Yoon & Brown, 2011).

Social capital has also been described by five types of assets needed to promote the health of communities (Manzi, Lucas, Lloyd-Jones, & Allen, 2010). These five capital assets include the following:

- Human capital (skills and education)
- Social capital (social networks)
- Built capital (access to amenities)
- Natural capital (access to green space)
- Economic capital (income and resources).

Three types of social capital that are important for health include *bonding* (within groups) social capital, *bridging* (across groups) social capital, and *linking* social capital (Beaudoin, 2009; Putnam, 2000; Szreter & Woolcock, 2004). *Bonding* social capital refers to the trusting and cooperative relations between persons who have similar identities. *Bonding* social capital builds strong ties within communities, but it can also build higher barriers that may exclude those who are different. *Bonding* social capital is considered a critical factor in creating and nurturing the group solidarity seen in close neighborhoods and among some ethnic groups. *Bridging* social capital refers to respect and mutuality between persons or groups who are not alike, for example, different ethnic groups or groups of different socioeconomic status. *Bridging* social capital facilitates linkages among different groups or organizations in a community around a common purpose. *Linking* social capital refers to how communities are vertically networked with institutions and political structures. For example, political participation and political activation, two types of linking social capital, are associated with the health of a community. Linking social capital has also been described as respect and trust across authority gradients in a community, for example, ties between citizens and government officials or professional resources (lawyers, journalists, etc.) in a community (Dahl & Malmberg-Heimonen, 2010).

Bonding and *bridging* social capital, measured as social cohesion, civic participation, heterogeneous socioeconomic relationships, political efficacy, and trust have been found to be associated with community health and self-rated health (Poortinga, 2012). In an intervention to increase social networking in young adult cancer survivors, those who were identified with weak bonding social capital were taught to use their network to fulfill needs that were not being met (McLaughlin et al., 2012). This study is an example of interventions that can be implemented when social capital is found to be low. Table 3–2 provides examples of components that have been used to assess bonding, bridging, and linking social capital.

TABLE 3–2   Social Capital: Characteristics and Examples

Characteristics	Example
Bonding	
Neighborhood cohesion	Extent to which individuals in a neighborhood pull together to improve the neighborhood
Neighborhood trust and belonging	Extent to which individuals trust others in the neighborhood; the extent of feeling a sense of belonging to the neighborhood
Civic participation	Extent to which individuals in a neighborhood are involved with groups, clubs, or organizations on an ongoing basis
Bridging	
Social cohesion	Extent to which people from multiple backgrounds in a community interact
Mutual respect	Extent to which racial/ethnic differences in a community are recognized and valued
Heterogeneity	Extent to which an individual's friends are of different racial/ethnic groups and have dissimilar income and educational backgrounds
Linking	
Political participation and activism	Amount of contact community members have with people in their local political organization; the extent to which individuals attend public meetings or have signed a petition
Political influence	Extent to which citizens believe they can influence decisions affecting their community
Political trust	Amount of trust members of a community have in their local government, law enforcement, and the federal government

A key ingredient of *network* social capital is social support, as this is the initial informal relationship among individuals. The social support component of social capital draws attention to the significant role of family and social connections as a builder and source of social capital through nurturance, caregiving, socialization, values, attitudes, and expectations. Participation in social networks has been linked to health, positive social relationships, and increased social capital. Family relationships and behavior also help establish the principle of reciprocity, the idea of receiving and giving in return, which is another component of social capital.

Why is social capital important in health promotion? Evidence has consistently shown that higher social capital has been associated with higher rated health and positive health outcomes. For example, social capital has been shown to play a role in the relationship between neighborhood income equality and body mass index (BMI) in adults (Mackenbach et al., 2017). Greater income inequality (low neighborhood social capital) has also been associated with higher BMI. High neighborhood social capital has also been associated with higher self-rated health, lower obesity risks, and greater fruit consumption (Mackenbach et al., 2016). Higher community social capital has been associated with a reduction in obesity risks, with a larger effect on persons with higher education (Yoon & Brown, 2011). Potential explanations for the positive association of social capital and health have been suggested. Shared behavior patterns, social norms (bonding social capital), and social support may reinforce positive health behaviors and, through collective efficacy, promote access to health care or health-promoting places in the community. Measurement of social capital provides valuable information to plan interventions for individuals and communities. Multiple strategies may be needed to design programs to address areas identified in the measurement of social capital.

Inconsistency in defining and measuring social capital is an ongoing issue. While it is acceptable to measure either individual or collective social capital, measures need to be consistent across studies and programs and generalizable across populations. Social capital is a complex concept and warrants continued refinement to better understand how it influences the health of individuals and communities and to provide information for program development.

COMMUNITY PLANNING MODELS FOR HEALTH PROMOTION

The PRECEDE–PROCEED Model

The PRECEDE–PROCEED model was initially designed in 1974 to guide the planning, development, and evaluation of health education programs (Green, 1974; Green & Kreuter, 2005). The policy and environmental components (PROCEED) were later added. The model (Figure 3–3) provides a structure to identify and implement the most appropriate health promotion program. It is a planning model, a road map that provides practice-based evidence for the choice among possible evidence-based practices. In contrast, theories suggest specific routes to follow. Program planners choose theories of their choice during the planning process to best guide the program under development. Two fundamental propositions of the model are the following: (1) health and health risks have multiple determinants, and (2) efforts to change the behavioral, physical, and social environments must be multidimensional and participatory.

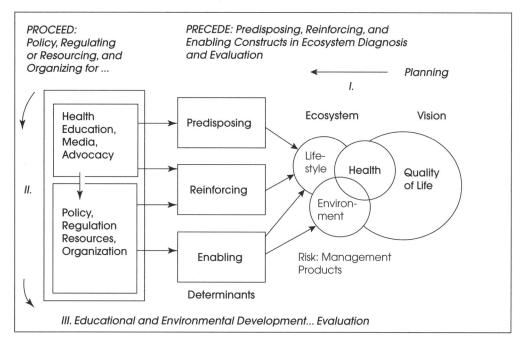

FIGURE 3–3   The PRECEDE–PROCEED Model for Health Promotion Planning and Evaluation

Source: Green, L. W. & Kreuter, M. W. (2005). The PRECEDE-PROCEED model of health program planning and evaluation. Retrieved from http://www.lgreen.net/precede.htm. Used with permission.

The model consists of two separate components, *PRECEDE* and *PROCEED*. *PRECEDE* stands for Predisposing, Reinforcing, and Enabling Constructs in Educational/Ecological Diagnosis and Evaluation. *PROCEED* stands for Policy, Regulatory, and Organizational Constructs in Educational and Environmental Development. The *PROCEED* framework can be considered an ecological planning model as it takes into consideration individuals as well as their physical and social environments. *PRECEDE* has four assessment and planning stages, and *PROCEED* has four phases that describe implementation and evaluation.

The planning and assessment process consists of three phases in sequential order. Planning begins with a social assessment to learn people's perceptions of their needs and life quality. This step involves a community assessment that includes problem-solving capacity, strengths, and readiness for change. In step 2, an epidemiologic assessment is performed to identify the most important health problems. Secondary sources of data (e.g., state and national surveys) can be used to identify major health problems in the community. Step 3 consists of an educational and ecological assessment to identify the predisposing, reinforcing, and enabling factors that must be in place to initiate and sustain the proposed program. Predisposing and reinforcing factors target individual-level factors, whereas enabling factors focus on community-level factors such as programs, services, and resources needed. In step 4, administration and policy assessment and intervention alignment, development of intervention strategies, and planning for implementation occur. Resources needed, barriers to implementation, and organization policies that may affect implementation are assessed. In step 5, implementation of the planned program takes place, and both impact and outcome evaluations are performed in steps 6–8. Objectives, which are written at each step, are the basis for evaluating accomplishments.

The PRECEDE–PROCEED model has been widely used to plan health promotion programs. Despite its success, several limitations have been identified. Application of the model requires significant human and financial resources, as the model is data driven. The planning process is time intensive, which may dampen enthusiasm of community members who want to implement change strategies quickly. Cole and Horacek (2009) developed a consolidated version to shorten the time frame needed to implement the assessment. Demographic, behavioral, organizational, and administrative data are obtained with a single survey instead of in distinct steps. Focus groups, made up of planning and steering committee members, are conducted to obtain environmental, organizational, and policy assessment data. The consolidated PRECEDE–PROCEED model overcomes the time needed to conduct the assessment while remaining a participatory planning model.

A major strength of the PRECEDE–PROCEED model is its comprehensive ecological approach, as the model incorporates individual and community perspectives in a participatory process, accounts for the social and physical environment, and can be used in many types of settings (Porter, 2016). Evidence for the usefulness of the model in health promotion includes its application to workplace health promotion (Post, Daniel, Misan, & Haren, 2015), health promotion professional education (Tapley & Patel, 2016), prediabetes preventive behaviors (Moshki, Dehnoalian, & Alami, 2017), and smoking cessation programs (Aldiabat & Le Navenec, 2013). For a searchable bibliography of the 1,100+ published applications of the model, see www.lgreen.net.

COMMUNITY DISSEMINATION MODELS TO PROMOTE HEALTH

Diffusion of Innovations Model

The diffusion of innovations model was developed to help disseminate health behavior interventions that have been successfully tested into the mainstream for practical use (Rogers, 2003). The framework describes the process of innovation diffusion and the various stages involved in adopting a new idea, thereby narrowing the gap between what has been tested in research and what is put to use.

In the diffusion of innovations model, *diffusion* is considered a process through which an innovation (new idea) is communicated through certain channels, over time, among a group or community (Rogers, 2003). It is a special kind of communication to spread messages about new ideas that might represent a certain degree of uncertainty to individuals or organizations. Diffusion is a type of social change, as social changes often occur when new ideas are adopted. The terms *dissemination* and *diffusion* are used interchangeably in the diffusion of innovations model.

Four elements characterize the diffusion of new ideas:

- Innovation
- Communication channels
- Time
- Social system

These elements are found in every diffusion program. An *innovation* is an idea that is thought to be new. An innovation is broad and can be almost any new idea or a novel approach to an old way of doing things. An example of an innovation is electronic books instead of traditional hard copies of books. It does not matter if the idea is not new, as it is perceived newness that decides how individuals will react. Individuals progress through five stages, known as the innovation decision process, as they are evaluating an innovation for adoption. These stages are *knowledge, persuasion, decision, implementation*, and *confirmation*. In the persuasion stage, potential adopters form either a positive or a negative attitude toward the innovation. According to Rogers (2003), the perceived characteristics of the innovation influence the adopter's attitudes.

Characteristics that also help explain the relative speed of adoption of an innovation include relative advantage, compatibility, complexity, trialability, and observability. *Relative advantage* is the degree to which the innovation is perceived to be better than the current, older idea. It does not matter if the innovation has no true advantage. What matters is whether an individual thinks the innovation will be better. Relative advantage may be perceived in economic terms or as social prestige, convenience, or satisfaction. *Compatibility* is the degree to which an innovation is perceived to fit with existing values and past experiences. Innovations that are consistent with the existing values and norms of the individual or group are more likely to be adopted. For example, an incompatible innovation might be the use of contraceptives in a traditionally conservative, religious community, as it is unlikely that the majority would adopt it. *Complexity* is the degree to which the innovation is thought to be difficult to understand or use. In general, new ideas that are simple to understand are more easily adopted than complex ones. *Trialability* is the extent to which the innovation may be experimented with and considered tentative for a limited time period. Ideas that can be tried in installments are usually adopted more quickly than those that cannot be divided. Last, *observability* is the degree to which the results of the innovation are visible to others. The easier it is to see results, the more likely the idea will be adopted. *Relative advantage, compatibility*, and *complexity* have been found to be most important in the rate of adoption of an innovation (Reinhardt, Hietschold, & Spyridonidis, 2015). Additional considerations in adoption of the innovation include the influence of the innovation on social relationships, the ability to reverse the innovation, the ability to easily communicate the innovation, the time and commitment needed to adopt the innovation, and the ability to modify the innovation over time.

Communication must take place for an innovation to spread. Mass media channels (television, newspapers, and technology channels) are used to reach large audiences to provide initial information about the innovation. Because diffusion is a process of people talking to people, interpersonal or face-to-face communication channels are effective in persuading individuals to change their attitudes toward a new idea. Social media, the "participative Internet," is a cost-effective communication strategy for reaching large numbers of people (Korda & Itani, 2013). Social media include Internet-based social network services (Facebook, MySpace), Twitter, blogs, and mobile messaging platforms. As with other types of communication, social media requires careful application to achieve the desired outcomes.

Innovativeness refers to the degree to which individuals, organizations, or communities adopt new ideas or practices. Five adopter categories have been described: innovators, early adopters, early majority, late majority, and laggards (see Figure 3–4). These

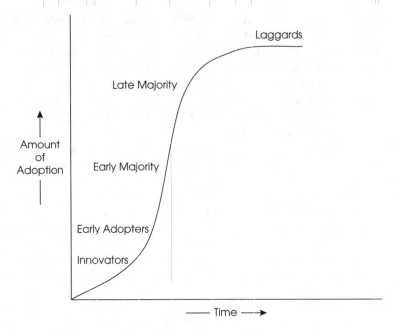

FIGURE 3–4   The Diffusion Process for Adoption of an Innovation

patterns of adoption have been shown to be predictable in many populations and settings. *Innovators* are active information seekers and can cope with high levels of uncertainty about a new idea. They are open to taking risks and the first to adopt a new idea. Innovators are role models for others in the social system. *Early adopters* have the greatest degree of opinion leadership in most social systems and are considered to be the persons to check with before adopting the innovation. The *early majority* may deliberate before adopting, so they seldom lead in adoption of an idea. The *late majority* view innovations with skepticism and may adopt only because of increasing pressure from peers, or because they feel it is safe to adopt. The *laggards* tend to be suspicious of innovations and change. They want to be sure that the innovation will not fail before they adopt and often slow down the innovation diffusion process.

Identification of adopter categories facilitates implementing new health behavior programs, as it is important to know that not everyone will accept the change in the same time frame. *Laggards*, for example, will need more time and evidence that the program is effective and safe. Early adopters, the opinion leaders in a social system who can influence others, should be identified early in the process, as they will help facilitate change. When a *critical mass* is reached, the number of adopters of the innovation has reached a point at which further rate of adoption becomes self-sustaining. To reach this point, efforts need to be focused on early adopters, persons who are the opinion leaders and role models for individuals who are hesitant to adopt the innovation. Thus, adoption is a process that leads to sustainability, not a specific point in time.

Preventive innovations are defined as new ideas that require action at one point in time in order to avoid unwanted consequences at a future point in time (Rogers, 2002). The rewards of adopting a preventive innovation are delayed and intangible, and unwanted consequences may never occur, resulting in a low relative advantage of the innovation. Because relative advantage is one of the important predictors of the rate of adoption of an innovation, it is understandable why preventive innovations may be slow or fail to be adopted. To increase the rate of adoption of a preventive innovation, perceived relative advantages should be identified and made as visible as possible. For example, the relative advantage of dietary changes for those at risk for hypertension is low, as hypertension does not have immediate or obvious symptoms. Other relative advantages, such as weight loss, should be identified and communicated. Strategies to speed up the adoption of preventive innovations include:

1. Increasing the relative advantage
2. Using role models to devote personal influence to promote the innovation
3. Changing the system norms through peer support
4. Placing educational ideas in entertainment messages
5. Activating peer and social media communication networks.

The innovation diffusion model has been used for many years with varying success. One possible reason for unsuccessful outcomes is that the nature of the innovation receives priority without attending to resource constraints. Another possible reason is that authority may be confused with influence. Persons with formal authority may not be the influential leaders. The solution is to find the informal authority leaders and seek their advice on diffusing the intervention. It is crucial to distinguish between change agents, authority figures, opinion leaders, and innovation champions. An evaluation or assessment process will enable these role functions to be evident so that the right people are on board to increase innovation adoption success.

Diffusion of an innovation is a complex, multilevel change process, as change must occur at multiple levels across different settings, using multiple strategies to promote widespread behavior change. Understanding the diffusion process enables nurses to implement behavior changes at multiple levels. The theory is based on many years of research in diffusion of innovations to change behaviors, programs, and policies to promote health. The theory incorporates strategies to promote widespread, long-term change and takes into account social structures and communication systems, as well as characteristics of the innovation.

Current Internet communication trends can facilitate the adoption of innovations, as mentioned earlier. The diffusion of innovations model presents communication channels as either mass media or interpersonal. Communication channels that capture current communication trends, such as YouTube, will lead to new forms of diffusion of health innovations. The diffusion of innovations model has been used successfully to understand the diffusion of new technologies, including adoption of electronic records, consumer e-appointment services, and online health information. In a study of the adoption of electronic health appointments, factors that explained why consumers did not use electronic appointments included incompatibility of the innovation with consumer preferences, insufficient communication of the innovation, and little relative advantage of the new innovation (Zhang, Yu, Yan, & Spil, 2015). These findings provide an example of how the evaluation of an innovation diffusion process can be used to increase the success of diffusion of the desired innovation, in this case, the use of electronic appointments by consumers.

Social Marketing Model

Social marketing, an expansion of commercial marketing, involves the application of marketing tools to solve problems that will bring about social change rather than monetary gains (Dibb, 2014). In social marketing, commercial marketing techniques are adapted to program planning, implementation, and evaluation to change or maintain behaviors for the benefit of individuals and society. Social marketing may be conducted by individuals, as well as commercial, not-for-profit, institutional, and government organizations (Kennedy, 2016). Until recently, social marketing interventions focused on individual behavior change; however, community, national, and global changes may also be targeted. The consensus definition of social marketing is the development and integration of marketing concepts with other approaches to change behaviors that will benefit individuals and communities for the greater social good (see the International Social Marketing Association website, http://www.i-socialmarketing.org).

Compared to traditional models of behavior change, social marketing promotes voluntary behavior change by offering potential benefits, reducing barriers, and using persuasion to change behaviors. Marketing practices that have traditionally been used in business advertising are applied to social purposes to adopt an idea, product, or new behavior. Guidelines or benchmarks are adhered to in social marketing (Andreasen, 2002; French & Russell-Bennett, 2015). The guidelines help ensure that social marketing is employed in a change intervention and to differentiate social marketing from other behavior change approaches (Kubacki, Rundle-Thiele, Pang, & Buyucek, 2015). The benchmarks are listed in Table 3–3 with their definitions.

The consumer orientation in social marketing distinguishes it from other approaches in health promotion. In a consumer orientation, one must understand

TABLE 3–3   Benchmark Criteria for Social Marketing

Benchmark	Definition
Behavior change	Defining goals to change behavior for individuals (downstream) or decision makers (upstream)
Citizen orientation	Conducting marketing and consumer research to understand the audience, using data from multiple sources
Segmentation	Strategically defining the target audience to tailor intervention to ensure maximum effectiveness and efficiency of resources
Exchange	Considering the costs and benefits of adopting the new behavior and offering incentives and rewards
Market mix	Implementing multiple intervention strategies to change behavior
Competition	Paying attention to pressures that compete for target audience's time and attention and developing strategies to minimize competition
Theory	Integrating behavioral (downstream) or social-ecological (upstream) theories to assist with designing and evaluating the intervention
Insight	Gaining an understanding of what motivates the target group and the relevant issues/barriers influencing current behavior

Source: Based on criteria described by Andreasen (2002) and French and Russell-Bennett (2015).

individuals' perception of factors that may influence their behavior. Social marketing uses audience segmentation to select target groups, a process of dividing the population into distinct segments based on characteristics that might influence their response to the behavior change. Segments identify smaller groups that may require different marketing strategies. Group profiles help decide which groups to target and the best way to reach them. A marketing approach goes beyond education to change behavior, as social marketers attempt to increase the attractiveness of the desired behavior so that it becomes preferable to the old behavior. Efforts are made to provide immediate effects, as immediate reinforcement has a greater potential to shape behavior.

The social marketing model is a set of principles rather than a theory. The framework considers the "Four Ps": product, price, place, and promotion. The *product* is the desired health behavior change, such as eating five fruits and vegetables daily. *Price* refers to the social, emotional, and monetary costs associated with adoption of the program or behavior, in this case, the costs of eating increased fruits and vegetables. Higher-priced changes are more difficult to implement than less expensive ones. *Place* is the location of the intervention program. The more convenient the place, the more likely adoption of the change will occur. *Promotion* refers to promoting the new behavior and using strategies to persuade adoption of the desired behavior. Both mass media and interpersonal communication channels are used to promote change. An additional concept is the product's *competition*, or the existing behavior that must be changed. In the case of increasing consumption of fruits and vegetables, the competition is the old way of eating or a long-term habit or a preference for other foods that will need to change.

The interrelated components and basic principles serve as guides to design implementation strategies for individuals or communities. The product must provide a solution to problems that individuals believe are important to them. Individuals are confronted with choosing between the new behavior and the current risk behavior, so the benefits of the new behavior must outweigh those of the current risk behavior. Price, from the consumer's perspective, is the cost, such as the cost of joining a health club to exercise. Costs may also be time, effort, and emotional discomfort in changing behaviors such as smoking cessation. Place is also an important component, and social marketers must assess when and where the target group will be most receptive to messages, or where and when they are ready to change. Promotion to motivate change includes designing attention-getting, effective messages, and using credible, trustworthy spokespersons. Strategies may include mass communication, public information, education, direct mail, public relations, and printed materials. Two additional approaches are "edutainment," or the use of traditional entertainment media for educational purposes, and media advocacy, defined as the strategic use of mass media to increase public support to address the change.

In social marketing, programs should be monitored continuously to evaluate their effectiveness in promoting change. Continuous monitoring also enables identification of activities that need to be revised as well as activities that are most effective. The target audience is constantly checked for their responsiveness to the intervention. The evaluation of social marketing is multidimensional and consists of multiple measures. Criteria include impact, reach, sustainability, cost effectiveness, acceptability, and equity (Langford & Panter-Brick, 2013). Qualitative and quantitative strategies are used for both formative and outcome evaluations.

Although social marketing has been defined as an approach to produce social change, the predominant focus has been changing individuals (Wood, 2016). In recent years, there has been a call to move from individual or downstream interventions to consider the social determinants that influence individual behaviors to reduce health inequities. *Downstream social marketing* interventions help bring about social change by focusing on individuals. *Upstream social marketing* interventions focus on changing the behaviors of decision makers and opinion leaders who have the ability to change policies or economic conditions to create healthy environments (Gordon, 2013). Examples of the target audiences for change in upstream social marketing include politicians, policy makers, educators, and the mass media. Upstream social marketing interventions have been implemented successfully to prevent obesity (Venturini, 2016), reduce sexually transmitted diseases (Friedman, Kachur, Noar, & McFarlane, 2016), and decrease alcohol use (Kubacki et al., 2015).

Social-ecological models are ideal for integrating into upstream social marketing interventions, as multilevel interventions are necessary to bring about successful social change (Wood, 2016). As with social-ecological approaches, upstream social marketing models need to include individuals (downstream), communities (midstream), and social structures (upstream) in interventions to successfully change behaviors. Upstream social marketing, while complex, facilitates sustained change when social marketers align with decision makers to reduce health inequities.

CONSIDERATIONS FOR PRACTICE USING COMMUNITY MODELS OF HEALTH

The concepts and principles of community models of health promotion are relevant for assessing, planning, designing, and evaluating interventions and programs. Communities must be assessed prior to implementing health promotion programs. Assessment of an individual's physical and social environments, including social capital, will provide helpful information about facilitators and barriers to healthy lifestyle practices in the community. Knowledge of the physical environment sheds light on the resources (or lack of) in a neighborhood—such as safe walking areas and access to grocery stores or transportation—that influence one's ability to practice healthy behaviors. Focus groups that incorporate concepts and principles of social capital are appropriate to gain an understanding of factors to consider in planning programs. The diffusion of innovations model, as well as the social marketing approach, is useful in implementing change within communities. Learning to identify individual characteristics of adopters will enable the nurse to choose specific strategies, based on the type of adopter, for example, whether one is an innovator or laggard. Social marketing strategies that target specific populations as well as their environments offer opportunities for large-scale health promotion changes. As the nurse gains a broader understanding of the role of the community and greater social system in promoting health, small-scale interventions can be piloted to develop evidence to gain support for larger-scale, more complex programs.

OPPORTUNITIES FOR RESEARCH WITH COMMUNITY-BASED MODELS

The limited success of individual-level theories and models in achieving long-term changes in health behavior has led to a growing trend to use community theories and models in health promotion. Community-level theories and models are complex, as multiple dimensions of both the individual and the environment are addressed. The costs and complexity of designing and testing multilevel programs have resulted in their limited use. Research is needed to develop consistent measures of social capital concepts as well as social and environmental concepts. Community level research requires a team partnership among health disciplines. Additional research in the following areas is recommended:

1. Perform state-of-the-science reviews and meta-analyses to identify the consistently significant concepts in the social-ecological model that promote behavior change.
2. Develop and test reliable and valid measures of social capital.
3. Identify culturally sensitive and measurable community outcomes of health promotion.
4. Design and test multilevel community models of behavior change.
5. Test the effectiveness of upstream social marketing intervention to produce community-level changes in high-risk behaviors.

Summary

The increased attention on community-based models to promote healthy behaviors has occurred because of a greater need to understand the complex etiologies of health problems, an appreciation of the relationship of individuals and their social and physical environments, and recognition of the limited effectiveness of individual models in promoting health. Community-based models focus on contextual factors that influence health, such as social conditions, and the political, institutional, legislative, and physical environments in which behaviors occur. Tests of community-level interventions show promising results. Additional research is needed to identify the most effective models to guide health promotion interventions. Diffusion of innovations and social marketing models have the potential to promote widespread change.

Learning Activities

1. Design three strategies that can be applied to empower individuals to increase health resources to facilitate healthy behaviors in their communities.
2. What elements in a community would you assess using a social-ecological model for health behavior?
3. Apply the eight steps in the PRECEDE–PROCEED model to design a program to improve a specific health behavior such as physical activity for adolescents. Which individual and community theories would you choose to implement the program?
4. Using principles or benchmarks described in the social marketing framework, how would you develop an upstream social marketing intervention to prevent underage alcohol use? Who is your target audience to promote change? What theory or theories would be appropriate to integrate to inform the intervention?

References

Aldiabat, K. M., & Le Navenec, C. (2013). Developing smoking cessation program for older Canadian people: An application of Precede–Proceed model. *American Journal of Nursing Science, 2*(3), 33–39. doi:10.11648/j.ajns.20130203.13

Alvarez, E. C., Kawachi, I., & Romani, J. R. (2017). Family social capital and health – A systematic review and redirection. *Sociology of Health & Illness, 39*(1), 5–29. doi:10.1111/1467-9566.12506

Andreasen, A. R. (2002). Marketing social marketing in the social change marketplace. *Journal of Public Policy & Marketing, 21*(1), 3–13. doi:10.1509/jppm.21.1.3.17602

Beaudoin, C. E. (2009). Bonding and bridging neighborliness: An individual-level study in the context of health. *Social Science & Medicine, 68*(12), 2129–2136. doi:10.1016/j.socscimed.2009.04.015

Bronfenbrenner, U. (1977). Toward an experimental ecology of human development. *American Psychologist, 32*(7), 513–531. doi:10.1037/0003-066X.32.7.513

Brunie, A. (2009). Meaningful distinctions within a concept: Relational, collective, and generalized social capital. *Social Science Research, 38*(2), 251–265. doi:10.1016/j.ssresearch.2009.01.005

Cole, R. E., & Horacek, T. (2009). Applying PRECEDE–PROCEED to an intuitive eating nondieting approach to weight management pilot program. *Journal of Nutrition Education and Behavior, 41*(2), 120–126. doi:10.1016/j.jneb.2008.03.006

Dahl, E., & Malmberg-Heimonen, I. (2010). Social inequality and health: The role of social capital. *Sociology of Health & Illness, 32*(7), 1102–1119. doi:10.1111/j.1467-9566.2010.01270.x

Dibb, S. (2014). Up, up, and away: Social marketing breaks free. *Journal of Marketing Management, 30*(11–12), 1159–1185. doi:10.1080/0267257X.2014.943264

Dooris, M., & Heritage, Z. (2013). Healthy cities: Facilitating the active participation and empowerment of local people. *Journal of Urban Health, 90*(Suppl 1), 74–91. doi:10.1007/s11524-011-9623-0

French, J., & Russell-Bennett, R. (2015). A hierarchical model of social marketing. *Journal of Social Marketing, 5*(2), 139–159. doi:10.1108/JSOCM-06-2014-0042

Friedman, A. L., Kachur, R. E., Noar, S. M., & McFarlane, M. (2016). Health communication and social marketing campaigns for sexually transmitted disease prevention and control: What is the evidence of their effectiveness? *Sexually Transmitted Diseases, 43*(Suppl 1) S83–S101. doi:10.1097/OLQ.0000000000000286

Golden, S. D., & Earp, J. A. (2012). Social ecological approaches to individuals and their contexts: Twenty years of health education & behavior health promotion interventions. *Health Education & Behavior, 39*(3), 364–372. doi:10.1177/1090198111418634

Golden, S. D., McLeroy, K. R., Green, L. W., Earp, J. L., & Lieberman L. D. (2015). Upending the social ecological model to guide health promotion efforts toward policy and environmental change. *Health Education & Behavior, 42*(1S), 8S–14S. doi:10.1177/1090198115575098

Gordon, R. (2013). Unlocking the potential of upstream social marketing. *European Journal of Marketing, 47*(9), 1525–1547. doi:10.1108/EJM-09-2011-0523

Green, L. W. (1974). Toward cost-benefit evaluations of health education: Some concepts, methods and examples. *Health Educ. Monographs. 2*(Suppl 2), 34–64.

Green, L. W., & Kreuter, M. W. (2005). *Health promotion program planning: An educational and ecological approach* (4th ed.). Boston, MA: McGraw-Hill.

Gubbels, J. S., Van Kann, D. H., de Vries, N. K., Thijs, C., & Kremers, S. P. (2014). The next step in health behavior research: The need for ecological moderation analysis – An application to diet and physical activity at childcare. *International Journal of Behavioral Nutrition and Physical Activity, 11*, 52. doi:10.1186/1479-5868-11-52

Institute of Medicine (IOM). (2005). *Preventing childhood obesity: Health in the balance.* Washington, DC: The National Academies Press.

Kawachi, I., & Berkman, L. (2014). Social cohesion, social capital and health. In L. Berkman, I. Kawachi, & M. Glymour (Eds.), *Social epidemiology* (2nd ed.). New York, NY: Oxford University Press.

Kennedy, A. (2016). Macro-social marketing. *Journal of Macromarketing, 36*(3), 354–365. doi:10.1177/0276146715617509

Koplan, J. P., Liverman, C. T., Kraak, V. I., & Wisham, S. L. (Eds.). (2007). *Progress in preventing childhood obesity: How do we measure up?* Washington, DC: The National Academies Press.

Korda, H., & Itani, Z. (2013). Harnessing social media for health promotion and behavior change. *Health Promotion Practice, 14*(1), 15–23. doi:10.1177/1524839911405850

Kubacki, K., Rundle-Thiele, S., Pang, B., & Buyucek, N. (2015). Minimizing alcohol harm: A systematic social marketing review (2000–2014). *Journal of Business Research, 68*(10), 2214–2222. doi:10.1016/j.jbusres.2015.03.023

Langford, R., & Panter-Brick, C. (2013). A health equity critique of social marketing: Where interventions have impact but insufficient reach. *Social*

Science & Medicine, *83*, 133–141. doi:10.1016/j.socscimed.2013.01.036

Mackenbach, J. D., Lakerveld, J., van Lenthe, F. J., Kawachi, I., McKee, M., Rutter, H., . . . Brug, J. (2016). Neighborhood social capital: Measurement issues and associations with health outcomes. *Obesity Reviews*, *17*(Suppl 1), 96–107. doi:10.1111/obr.12373

Mackenbach, J. D., Lakerveld, J., van Oostveen, Y., Compernolle, S., De Bourdeaudhuij, I., Bardos, H., . . . Nijpels, G. (2017). The mediating role of social capital in the association between neighborhood income inequality and body mass index. *European Journal of Public Health*, *27*(2), 218–223. doi:10.1093/eurpub/ckw157

Manzi, T., Lucas, K., Lloyd-Jones, T., & Allen, J. (Eds.). (2010). *Social sustainability in urban areas: Communities, connectivity, and the urban fabric*. London: Earthscan.

McLaughlin, M., Nam, Y., Gould, J., Pade, C., Meeske, K. A., Ruccione, K. S., & Fulk, J. (2012). A videosharing social networking intervention for young adult cancer survivors. *Computers in Human Health*, *28*(2), 631–641. doi:10.1016/j.chb.2011.11.009

McLeroy, K. R., Bibeau, D., Steckler, A., & Glanz, K. (1988). An ecological perspective on health promotion programs. *Health Education Quarterly*, *15*(4), 351–377.

Minkler, M. (2000). Health promotion at the dawn of the 21st century: Challenges and dilemmas. In M. S. Jamner & D. Stokols (Eds.), *Promoting human wellness* (pp. 349–377). Berkeley, CA: University of California Press.

Minkler, M., & Wallerstein, N. (2012). Improving health through community organization and community building: Perspectives from health education and social work. In M. Minkler (Ed.), *Community organizing and community building for health and welfare* (3rd ed., pp. 37–58). New Brunswick, NJ: Rutgers University Press.

Moshki, M., Dehnoalian, A., & Alami, A. (2017). Effect of Precede–Proceed model on preventive behaviors for type 2 diabetes mellitus in high-risk individuals. *Clinical Nursing Research*, *26*(2), 241–253. doi:10.1177/1054773815621026

Poortinga, W. (2012). Community resilience and health: The role of bonding, bridging, and linking aspects of social capital. *Health & Place*, *18*, 286–295. doi:10.1016/j.healthplace.2011.09.017

Porter, C. (2016). Revisiting Precede–Proceed: A leading model for ecological and ethical health promotion. *Health Education Journal*, *75*(6), 753–764. doi:10.1177/0017896915619645

Post, D. K., Daniel, M., Misan, G., & Haren, M. T. (2015). A workplace health promotion application of the Precede–Proceed model in a regional and remote mining company in Whyalla, South Australia. *International Journal of Workplace Health Management*, *8*(3), 154–174. doi:10.1108/IJWHM-08-2014-0028

Putnam, R. (2000). *Bowling alone: The collapse and revival of American community*. New York, NY: Simon & Schuster.

Reinhardt, R., Hietschold, N., & Spyridonidis, D. (2015). Adoption and diffusion of innovations in health care. In S. Gurtner & K. Soyez (Eds.), *Challenges and opportunities in health care* (pp. 211–221). New York, NY: Springer.

Rogers, E. M. (2002). Diffusion of preventive innovations. *Addictive Behaviors*, *27*(6), 989–993.

Rogers, E. M. (2003). *Diffusions of innovations* (5th ed., pp. 5–34). New York, NY: Free Press.

Sallis, J. F., & Owens, N. (2008). Ecological models of health behavior. In K. Glanz, B. K. Rimer, & K. Viswanath (Eds.), *Health behavior and health education theory, research and practice* (4th ed., pp. 464–484). San Francisco, CA: Jossey-Bass.

Scholmerich, V. L., & Kawachi, I. (2016). Translating the socio-ecological perspective into multilevel interventions: Gaps between theory and practice. *Health Education & Behavior*, *43*(1), 17–20. doi:10.1177/1090198115605309

Stokols, D. (1992). Establishing and maintaining healthy environments: Toward a social ecology of health promotion. *American Psychologist*, *47*(1), 6–22. doi:10.1037/0003-066X.47.1.6

Stokols, D. (2000). The socio ecological paradigm of wellness promotion. In M. S. Jamner & D. Stokols (Eds.), *Promoting human wellness: New frontiers for research, practice and policy* (pp. 21–37). Berkeley, CA: University of California Press.

Stokols, D., Lejano, R. P., & Hipp, J. (2013). Enhancing the resilience of human–environment systems: A social ecological perspective. *Ecology and Society*, *18*(1), 7. doi:10.5751/ES-05301-180107

Suglia, S. F., Shelton, R. C., Hsiao, A., Wang, Y. C., Rundle, A., & Link, B. G. (2016). Why the neighborhood environment is critical in obesity prevention. *Journal of Urban Health: Bulletin of the New York Academy of Medicine*, *93*(1), 206–212. doi:10.1007/s11524-015-0017-6

Szreter, S., & Woolcock, M. (2004). Health by association? Social capital, social theory, and the political economy of public health. *International Journal of Epidemiology*, *33*(4), 650–667. doi:10.1093/ije/dyh013

Tapley, H., & Patel, R. (2016). Using the PRECEDE–PROCEED model and service-learning to teach health promotion and wellness: An innovative approach for physical therapist professional education. *Journal of Physical Therapy Education*, *30*(1), 47–59.

Venturini, R. (2016). Social marketing and big social change: Personal social marketing insights from a complex system obesity prevention intervention. *Journal of Marketing Management, 32*(11–12), 1190–1199. doi:10.1080/0267257X.2016.1191240

Wood, M. (2016). Social marketing for social change. *Social Marketing Quarterly, 22*(2), 107–118. doi:10.1177/1524500416633429

World Health Organization. (1974). *Community health nursing: Report of a WHO expert committee*. Report No. 558. Geneva: Author.

Yoon, J., & Brown, T. T. (2011). Does the promotion of community social capital reduce obesity risks? *The Journal of Socio-Economics, 40*(3), 296–305. doi:10.1016/j.socec.2011.01.002

Zhang, X., Yu, P., Yan, J., & Spil, I. (2015). Using diffusion of innovation theory to understand the factors impacting patient acceptance and use of consumer e-health innovations: A case study in a primary care clinic. *BMC Health Services Research, 15*, 1–15. doi:10.1186/s12913-015-0726-2

PART 2

Planning for Health Promotion and Prevention

CHAPTER 4

Assessing Health and Health Behaviors

OBJECTIVES

This chapter will enable the reader to:

1. Describe emerging technologies that influence a nursing health assessment.
2. Discuss expected outcomes of a nursing health assessment.
3. Identify components of a nursing health assessment conducted for an individual client.
4. Examine life span, language, literacy, and culturally appropriate nursing health assessment tools for children, adults, and older adults.
5. Compare various approaches to assessing family, mindful of cultural and literacy influences.
6. Evaluate criteria for conducting a community screening.
7. Describe different approaches to community assessment.

A thorough assessment of health and health behaviors is the foundation for tailoring a health promotion–prevention plan. Assessment provides the basis for making clinical judgments about clients' health strengths, health problems, nursing diagnoses, and desired health and/or behavioral outcomes, as well as interventions likely to be effective. This information also determines components of the client–nurse partnership, such as the frequency and mode of contact, that is, electronic devices or face-to-face, and coordination and/or collaboration with other health professionals.

Client characteristics, including developmental stage, cultural orientation, language, and literacy, determine the choice of assessment measures. The enhanced National Standards for Culturally and Linguistically Appropriate Services (CLAS), based on an expanded definition of culture to include age, geography, spirituality, language, race, ethnicity, and biology, provide a practical guide to culturally and linguistically sensitive care (Office of Minority Health, 2013). Disability has also been suggested to be included in the definition by some authors.

Ethnically and racially diverse groups whose primary language is not English are growing rapidly (Office of Minority Health, 2017). Tailoring care to an individual's culture and language preference is the cornerstone of nursing assessment. The nurse's awareness of clients' health beliefs, practices, and health status, with particular attention to literacy level, is critical to meet the challenges of advancing health equity at every point of contact (Ali & Johnson, 2017; Silva, Rodrigues, de la Torre Diez, & Lopez-Coronado, 2015).

Recognizing that diversity in educational level, socioeconomic status, religion, rural/urban residence, and individual and family characteristics exists in all cultures ensures the best client outcomes regardless of cultural or linguistic preference. An online cultural educational program, designed specifically for nurses and other direct service providers, features videotaped case studies and interactive tools to support the delivery of client-centered care. This program is available on the Office of Minority Health, U.S. Department of Health and Human Services website.

EMERGING TECHNOLOGIES AND NURSING ASSESSMENT

eHealth (electronic health) increases the options for clients' involvement in their health care. mHealth, a subset of eHealth, is the use of mobile communication devices to provide or enhance health services/outcomes. The electronic health record (EHR), for example, promotes involvement of the client in developing a dynamic, tailored database. The EHR offers great promise to improve health and increase clients' satisfaction with care. Data aggregation, cross-continuum coordination, and clinical care plan management are critical components of the EHR. It allows storage and almost instantaneous access to data while improving quality and efficiency, and improving communication among providers, insurers, and consumers (Figure 4–1).

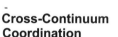

Data Aggregation

- Data acquisition and exchange platforms for ADT feeds, claims, and clinical data
- Ability to import provider directory files
- Algorithms and analytics for inclusion/exclusion criteria by population
- Processes, algorithms for patient–provider attribution

Cross-Continuum Coordination

- Shared care plans
- Activity tracking and real-time notification of encounters (ED, admission, discharge)
- Disease registries
- Health information exchanges
- Enhanced communication aids for care team connectivity
- Patient outreach and messaging

Clinical Care Plan Management

- EMR, case, and utilization management systems
- Workflow automation and rules engines
- Assessment tools, clinical care protocols, and work lists
- Analytics for high-risk patient identification
- Telehealth and home monitoring capabilities

FIGURE 4–1 IT Support for Care Management Progresses Beyond EHR Functionality

Sources: Comstock, J. (2013). Asthmapolis, now Propeller, moves beyond asthma. *Mobilhealthnews,* September 10; Propeller Health, available at http://propellerhealth.com/, accessed September 25, 2013. www.HealthIT.gov.

Promising developments in EHRs are facilitating widespread implementation. Cooperation among health care providers, health care organizations, and technology companies to create standards for seamless communication, regardless of vendor, is essential. The Centers for Medicare & Medicaid Services' (CMS) cost subsidization and incentives encourage EHR implementation. This major stimulus occurred as a result of the Health Information Technology for Economic and Clinical Health (HITECH) Act of 2009 (Centers for Medicare & Medicaid Services, 2009).

One objective of the HITECH Act is to provide electronic copies of health information to clients who request it within three business days. In many systems, health care visit data including laboratory results, medications, and health history are available immediately online through a password-protected patient portal. Clients' access or request for electronic health information is critical, as they can address missing data or correct errors. Eighty-three percent of participating physicians use some of the basic functions of the EHR, while only 49% use all available functions of the EHR (Office of the National Coordinator for Health IT, 2017). The long-term goal of the EHR is to enable clients to access their entire health record across systems digitally, using password-protected portals. The status of implementation of the EHR nationwide suggests that meeting this goal is only likely in the distant future due to the lack of EHR standardization, complexity of implementation, and evaluation issues (Cook, Ellis, & Hildebrand, 2016; Report to Congress, 2016).

While the EHR has many benefits, concerns have been raised about best practices for the successful implementation of client-accessible EHRs. These concerns include cost, security, privacy, consumer and provider technology education, and user-friendly systems. Older individuals (born 1954 or earlier) are more suspicious of online security and have less confidence in the system to protect their personal information (File & Ryan, 2014). Unless health care providers are in the same health care system or use the same health record software, clients are likely to have more than one EHR and portal. Multiple EHRs and access portals increase security concerns and may hinder a client's participation. Tamper-resistant, portable health folders and evidence-based designs are examples of security strategies to encourage participation in EHRs (Chen, Lu, & Jan, 2012; Kreps & Neuhauser, 2010).

As the science of biometric identifiers (e.g., fingerprints, iris scans, DNA, facial features, and voice) advances, clients are more likely to believe that their health information is more secure (Huston, 2013). While biometric markers are unique to each individual, markers such as fingerprints left on public surfaces, images captured on public security cameras, embedded cameras, social media sites, and voice recordings left on phones are in the public domain. In addition, electronic files including health applications often contain critical security vulnerabilities and are susceptible to data breaches of personal information (Leventhal, 2016).

Health care providers who are willing to open their records via secure, password-protected patient portals create greater transparency between provider and client. This ensures more open communication and shared responsibility for the client's health. Many clients are willing to accept some compromise to privacy in order to have online access to health records, to have records more transparent, and to have increased access to their health care provider through patient portal messaging (Bagwell, 2014; Robert Wood Johnson Foundation, 2009).

During clinic visits, EHRs enable health care professionals to input relevant clinical data into a tablet or laptop as the client responds to questions and discusses health

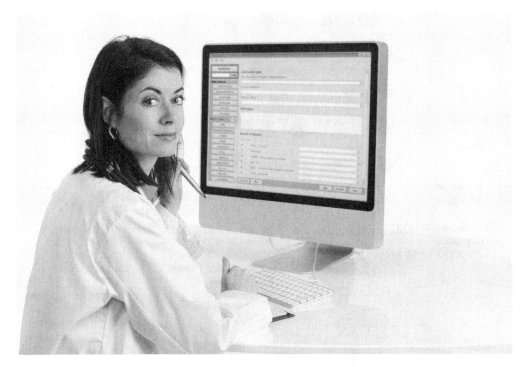

FIGURE 4–2 Nurse Maintains Eye Contact with Client While Entering Health Data into Electronic Health Record

issues. A computer in the examination room is a potential barrier to a meaningful provider–client relationship. Health care providers should face the client while they are entering data, being careful to maintain eye contact and engage the client. To do otherwise is to focus on the technology and not the client (see Figure 4–2).

The personal health record (PHR) is another application to help consumers take charge of their health. The PHR has the potential to improve care, lower costs, and help clients obtain and manage the care they need. The PHR belongs to the user and is distinct from physician records. With an increase in direct secure messaging standards (consumer-mediated exchange), clients are more likely to be involved in their own health decisions even when their physician or care provider does not participate in HITECH (Bagwell, 2014) (Figure 4–3).

The CMS PHR program for Medicare fee-for-service beneficiaries allows the addition of supplemental information to clients' health records, authorizes access to third parties such as family members, and tracks claims. Evaluation showed that consumers preferred downloadable data, direct online communication between clients and providers, simplified access, and strong, ongoing technical support (Office of the Assistant Secretary for Planning and Evaluation, 2009).

There is tremendous growth in the number of wireless and mobile technology applications. Applications (apps) such as those that help clients monitor high-risk issues, such as potential skin cancers, or provide health care providers with mobile data, may reduce health care costs (Kelli, Witbrodt, & Shah, 2017). Although 40% of physicians agree that apps might improve client outcomes, they would not prescribe health care apps for specific health problems due to major obstacles, including finding

Data Sources for PHR

Patient
- Chronic condition management data, from patient or connected devices
- Appointment requests
- Allergies
- Medications
- Family history
- Proxy access, consent data

Insurance Company
- Claims data
- Disease management profile
- Medications
- Risk score

Personal Health Record

Provider
- Physician visits
- Hospitalizations
- Lab, test results
- Medications
- Pre-visit intake forms
- Reminders, messages
- Billing information
- Referral information

FIGURE 4–3   PHRs: Allowing Patients to Actively Manage Their Data

Source: Future of Care Management. *PHRs allowing patients to actively manage their data.* HEALTH CARE ADVISORY BOARD. Copyright © 2013. The Advisory Board Company. All rights reserved.

the right app, lack of regulatory oversight, and absence of testing for efficacy. While physicians are cautious about prescribing apps, a 2015 survey found that 91% of teens used mobile apps and 25% reported downloading health care apps (Cook, Ellis, & Hildebrand, 2016). Most of the more than 165,000 mobile health and medical apps on the market in 2015 focused on diet, exercise/fitness, lifestyle, and stress reduction (Misra, 2015). A more recent category of apps is the client–provider app. Used by clients and monitored by health care providers, this app increases regular communication between clients and providers with the goal that clients assume more responsibility for management of their chronic conditions (Hughes, 2017).

E-mail, text, and social media sites such as Facebook and Twitter optimize communication possibilities with clients. Health care providers are in positions to suggest trusted health care apps and websites, and encourage clients to discuss website findings with their health care professionals. Tailored health information delivered through technology can enhance self-efficacy, improve decision-making, increase healthy behaviors, and foster self-responsibility (Cook, Ellis, & Hildebrand, 2016).

The potential for consumers to be involved in ownership and maintenance of their health record with "cradle-to-grave" information is especially relevant for computer users and technology-savvy consumers who interface technologically with providers and health systems. Age, race, education, health literacy, and income are significant predictors of households who own computers and use the Internet. The presence of a computer in the home supports technology skill development more so than occasional use or access alone (Hicks, 2017). Less than two-thirds of householders 65 years and older use the Internet compared to over 80% in all other younger age groups. Asian households have the highest percentage of Internet use, while Whites are more likely to use a home computer to connect to the Internet than Hispanics or Blacks. The higher the income level, the more likely the household has Internet connectivity. Differences exist also in the types of connections households use to access the Internet, with cable modem service the most common (File & Ryan, 2014) (see Figure 4–4).

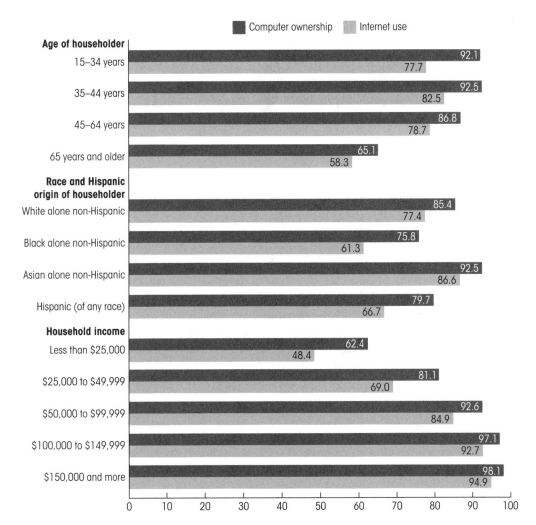

FIGURE 4–4 Percentage of Households with Computers and Internet Use, 2013

(Data based on sample. For information on confidentiality protection, sampling error, nonsampling error, and definitions, see www.census.gov/acs/www/)

Note: About 4.2% of all households reported household Internet use without a subscription. These households are not included in this figure.

Source: U.S. Census Bureau (2013).

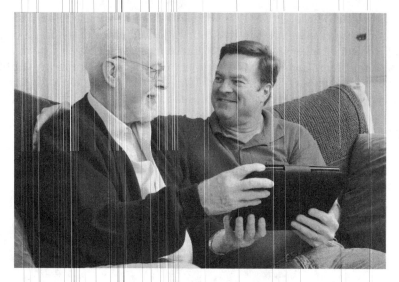

FIGURE 4–5   Older Client Gets Assistance with Online Health Assessment

Non-computer/Internet users, including the elderly and culturally and ethnically diverse populations, are at greater risk for exacerbation of health inequities unless a safeguard system enables these groups to have greater access. Although health care providers may offer detailed instructions/information, clients' reading, writing, language, and technology skills may be inadequate to make appropriate health decisions (see Figure 4–5). Strategies to increase computer use for non-computer/Internet users include the following:

1. Develop the concept of health care partners.
2. Assess the degree to which these groups have the health literacy and technology skills to obtain, process, and understand basic health information.
3. Offer educational and training opportunities for clients to learn to access health information through the Internet.
4. Provide staff to help clients with low health or technology literacy become more comfortable using online tools.
5. Offer community-wide access to wireless mobile broadband Internet service (Bagwell, 2014; Cornett, 2009).

Telehealth is another advancing technology in health promotion. Telehealth is the use of various telecommunication technologies to deliver health care, health information, and/or health education at a distance. Before engaging in telehealth services, it is important for providers to review and understand legal and regulatory requirements of their practice acts (Brous, 2016).

Health services via telehealth are available in a variety of settings, including clinics, offices, community centers, schools, and homes. In one study, cancer patients reported that they liked the flexibility and convenience of telehealth. The negative aspects of this modality were lack of computer competency and the inability of some to use phone-based services due to hearing problems (Cox et al., 2017).

As technology continues to improve the delivery of telehealth, it is likely to have an even greater impact on health promotion outcomes. Telehealth increases access to

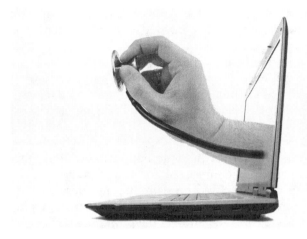

FIGURE 4–6   Telehealth Improves Access to Care

Source: http://www.telehealth.va.gov

providers but may not necessarily decrease overall cost. According to one study, direct-to-consumer telehealth decreased office and emergency room visits, but increased the number of virtual visits. The desire for increased visits demonstrated unmet demand and resulted in increased utilization costs (Ashwood, Mehrotra, Cowling, & Uscher-Pines, 2017) (see Figure 4–6). Three factors that spur adoption of telehealth include:

- Governmental support (primarily Veterans Administration) and integration into health care organizations
- Technological innovation
- Consumer demand for increased access to providers

NURSING FRAMEWORKS FOR HEALTH ASSESSMENT

Health assessment is a collaborative partnership between the client and nurse to promote mutual input into decision-making and planning to improve the client's health and well-being. The initial assessment provides a valuable baseline to compare subsequent assessments.

Health assessments describe the following:

1. Health assets
2. Health problems
3. Health-related lifestyle strengths
4. Key health-related beliefs
5. Risky health behaviors
6. Proposed changes that enhance quality of life

A nursing assessment is the systematic collection of data about a client's health status, beliefs, and behaviors relevant to developing a health promotion–prevention plan. An evidence-based framework should guide the assessment to determine nursing diagnoses. Nursing diagnostic classification systems (taxonomies) primarily focus on the individual and aspects of illness and less on positive health states (or strengths) of the individual, family, or community. As health promotion and prevention knowledge expands, taxonomies continue to include new definitions supportive of a health promotion/wellness perspective.

The NANDA International (formerly the North American Nursing Diagnosis Association) nursing diagnosis taxonomy defines the patient as individual, family, and community and includes nine human response patterns: exchanging, communicating, relating, valuing, choosing, moving, perceiving, knowing, and feeling. The defining characteristics of each diagnosis, as well as related positive and risk factors, provide direction for critical assessment areas. The NANDA-I classification provides a way to diagnose and intervene in selected health promotion and wellness processes and problems across the life span. For example, risk for powerlessness occurs when the client presents with feelings of tension and pressure that interfere with effective decision-making, resulting in physical or psychological distress. Active listening and supportive decision-making reduce tension and address the powerlessness diagnosis (Minthorn & Lunney, 2012).

Other examples of wellness nursing diagnoses/processes include:

1. Nutrition adequate to meet or maintain body requirements
2. Exercise level appropriate to maintain wellness state
3. Strength derived from one's spirituality

Gordon (2014) groups the NANDA-I diagnoses into 11 functional health patterns to assist in classifying nursing diagnoses: health perception–health management; nutritional–metabolic; elimination; activity–exercise; sleep–rest; cognitive–perceptual; self-perception–self-concept; role–relationship; sexuality–reproductive; coping–stress tolerance; and value–belief. She provides guidelines to conduct a nursing history and examination to assess clients' functional health patterns. As the assessment proceeds, diagnostic hypotheses generate more detailed data collection. Refer to Gordon's *Manual of Nursing Diagnosis* (2014) for recommended formats to assess functional health patterns in infants and young children, adults, families, and communities.

The Omaha Visiting Nurse Association System is a useful guide for community health nursing practice, as it provides a method of documentation and a framework for community management. The Omaha System incorporates the needs of individuals and families in four categories: environment, psychosocial, physiological, and health behavior needs. Nurse researchers have shown the usefulness of the Omaha System in quantifying nursing practice in community health, rural nursing practice, primary care, and wellness centers (Olsen, Thorson, Baisch, & Monsen, 2017). One difficulty in developing nursing classification systems for communities is that nursing diagnoses/problem classifications focus on nursing practice, whereas community diagnoses focus on interdisciplinary practice.

The Nursing Interventions Classification (NIC), a system that generates standardized nursing actions and interventions for providing care, is relevant for community health nursing. NIC categorizes and links nursing services to direct reimbursement (Bulechek, Butcher, Dochterman, & Wagner, 2013), which is a major issue in community health. However, NIC does not have categories for the health of communities. The Nursing Outcomes Classification (NOC) system measures the responses of an individual, family, and community behavior/perception to a nursing intervention and is useful in all settings (Moorhead, Johnson, Maas, & Swanson, 2013).

The next phase of knowledge generation in nursing is the integration of terminologies into electronic information systems to support standards of health promotion across settings. Integration of nursing terminologies makes it easier to describe and share interventions that work or do not work to improve health and reduce cost. Research using information system data embedded with nursing standards and terminologies builds nursing knowledge and documents the contribution of nursing to health promotion.

GUIDELINES FOR PREVENTIVE SERVICES AND SCREENINGS

Guidelines for preventive services across the life span for individuals, families, and communities focus on clinical care to prevent specific diseases such as cardiovascular disease and behavioral morbidity such as substance abuse.

The *Guide to Clinical Preventive Services* (U.S. Preventive Services Task Force, 2014) is an authoritative source for recommending decisions about preventive services. For example, in 2016, the Task Force recommendations, based on scientific evidence, reinforced its controversial 2009 screening mammography guidelines, recommending biennial screening for women ages 50–74 years, with voluntary choice for those ages 40–49 years.

Although breast cancer rates are lower in women ages 40–49 years and false positives persist in this age group, several organization have continued to recommend annual screening for women younger than age 50, including the American Cancer Society, the American Radiology Association, and the U.S. Congress (Lin & Gostin, 2016). The recommendations have had political ramification and brought into question the role of politics in science. Experts reported that over 30 years screenings detected 1.3 million tumors that would not lead to clinical symptoms (Bleyer & Welsh, 2012). In the survey results of women who underwent screening mammography before and after the 2009 guidelines, 1.2% of women ages 40–49 years did not have a mammogram after the guidelines, with reductions greater in younger women (Qin, Tangka, Guy, & Howard, 2017).

Screenings assess the presence of a disease before symptoms are present. Early detection usually results in early treatment and better outcomes. Screening may not be appropriate for everyone or every health problem, but detection of unrecognized health problems in individuals in at-risk groups reduces false alarms and produces more cost-effective outcomes. Data are not sufficient to address all the uncertainties of general screenings. However, screenings do uncover health problems in an efficient and economically feasible manner when the following factors are present:

1. The specific population has a high prevalence of the disease or health problem.
2. Identified conditions or diseases have available treatment.
3. Screening instruments are valid and reliable.

The cost of conducting screenings bears on the decision to offer large-scale screenings. For example, conducting a screening to detect osteoporosis requires special equipment, and the cost may be too high due to the number of machines needed to screen a large number of individuals in a timely, efficient manner. In addition to cost, large-scale screenings should consider race/ethnicity, age, health literacy, and socioeconomic level. These factors influence the willingness of individuals to participate in screenings, along with risks and benefits (Kressin et al., 2010).

The Agency for Healthcare Research and Quality's (AHRQ's) electronic Preventive Services Selector (ePSS) is a quick, hands-on tool available to primary care providers to identify screening services that are appropriate for clients based on the recommendations of the U.S. Preventive Services Task Force. The recommendations, based on client characteristics, such as age, sex, and behavioral risk factors, are available as Web and wireless apps for smartphones and other mobile devices. These apps provide nurses and other clinicians with preventive information and recommendations, clinical considerations, and selected practice tools at the point of care. *Guide to Clinical Preventive Services* (U.S. Preventive Services Task Force, 2014) and *Bright Futures: Guidelines for Health Supervision of Infants, Children, and Adolescents* (Hagan, Shaw, & Duncan, 2017) are also important guidelines for nurses to ensure that clients across the life span benefit from state-of-the-art preventive screenings.

ASSESSMENT OF THE INDIVIDUAL CLIENT

Assessment of the individual client in the context of health promotion includes a comprehensive examination of health parameters and health behaviors. The client's characteristics, such as setting, culture, and age, determine the components of health assessment. Rapidly changing technology, that is, telehealth, health care apps, and online surveys, influences the selection of the most reliable forms of assessment. Due to lack of standardized development and evaluation of technology-delivered measures, traditional formats, for example, questionnaires, interviews, and surveys, continue to be the most valid and reliable instruments for assessment. This is rapidly changing as attention is now focused on development of standards for technology-delivered measures. The overarching components of an individual assessment are as follows:

- Functional health patterns
- Physical fitness
- Nutrition
- Life stress
- Spiritual health
- Social support systems
- Health beliefs and lifestyle

Functional Health Patterns

Functional assessment of health patterns comprises health history, including hereditary and family characteristics, and physical assessment.

Physical Fitness

Physical fitness is an essential component of health assessment to optimize the fit of an exercise prescription to the physical capabilities of the client. A sedentary lifestyle often begins early in childhood and continues into adulthood. A physical fitness assessment is applicable to clients of all ages, with restrictions for physically compromised individuals. Skill-related physical fitness and health-related physical fitness focus on different qualities.

Skill-related fitness focuses on qualities that contribute to successful athletic performance: agility, speed, power, and reaction time. *Health-related fitness* focuses on qualities that contribute to general health and include cardiorespiratory endurance (aerobic capacity); muscular endurance, strength and flexibility; and body composition. This section focuses on assessment of health-related fitness.

CARDIORESPIRATORY (CR) ENDURANCE (AEROBIC CAPACITY). *Aerobic capacity* is related to the amount of physiological work an individual can perform, measured by oxygen consumption. It is the most important measure of fitness. Fitness reflects the ability of the CR system to efficiently adjust to and recover from exercise. Individuals with an acceptable aerobic capacity have a reduced risk of chronic diseases, including obesity, diabetes, and hypertension.

MUSCULAR ENDURANCE, STRENGTH, AND FLEXIBILITY. The goal of *muscular endurance, strength, and flexibility* tests is to determine the functional health status of the musculo-skeletal system. Strong muscles maintain body structure and endurance. The strength and endurance of the upper body muscles are good indicators of overall fitness. Flexibility, the ability to move muscles and joints through their maximum range of motion, is important for physical fitness. Flexibility decreases with age and chronic illness. Lack of ability to flex or extend muscles or joints often indicates poor health habits, such as sedentary lifestyle, poor posture, or faulty body mechanics. Loss of flexibility greatly decreases one's ability to move about with ease and comfort, and overall quality of life.

BODY COMPOSITION. Estimates of body fat include underwater weighing, dual X-ray absorptiometry (DXA), now the gold standard in adults, bioelectrical impedance analysis (BIA), and anthropometry measures such as skin-fold measurement, waist size, waist–hip ratio, and body mass index (BMI). The DXA is safe, easy to use, and very accurate, when used correctly. However, it is costly and cannot be used for very obese clients. The other methods also have limitations leading to measurement errors of 2% to 3% for estimates of body fat; the BMI error rate may be as great as 6% because body weight includes bone and muscle mass and not just fat composition (American College of Sports Medicine, 2013). In addition, the BMI has different cut offs for different ethnic groups, due to differences in body fat for a given BMI.

BIA is useful in healthy, normally hydrated adolescents and adults and for monitoring these groups for changes over time, due to its low cost. However, it has been found to produce lower measures than DXA. Although commercially available BIA scales are becoming popular for home use, the accuracy of these measures may not be known. In addition, the method should not be used with persons who have cardiac pacemakers or pregnant women.

Anthropometric (measures of body fat) methods are simple, convenient, and inexpensive. Skin-fold estimates, conducted while maintaining standards and using high-quality skin-fold calipers, and waist size provide accurate measures of body fat and compare favorably with BIA. The combination of body weight, anthropometric methods and BIA is an excellent predictor of total body fat composition.

The waist-to-hip ratio assesses the amount of fat distributed in the abdomen versus fat distributed below the waist. The ratio is the waist circumference over the hip circumference. The higher the value of the waist-to-hip ratio, the greater potential that health problems are present or will occur. The ratio has been associated with increased risk of mortality. Waist size has replaced the waist-to-hip ratio in many settings due to inconsistency in measuring techniques of the waist and hip. Some practitioners are also decreasing their dependence on BMI as an indicator of health risk in favor of waist circumference and body fat percentage (Chen et al., 2017; Seidell, 2010). A large waist circumference is more dangerous than being overweight. Among women 70–79 years

TABLE 4-1   Classification of Overweight and Obesity by BMI, Waist Circumference, and Associated Disease Risks

	BMI (kg/m^2)	Obesity Class	Disease Risk* Relative to Normal Weight and Waist Circumference	
			Men 102 cm (40 in.) or less Women 88 cm (35 in.) or less	Men > 102 cm (40 in.) Women > 88 cm (35 in.)
Underweight	<18.5		—	—
Normal	18.5–24.9		—	—
Overweight	25.0–29.9		Increased	High
Obesity	30.0–34.9	I	High	Very high
	35.0–39.9	II	Very high	Very high
Extreme obesity	40.0[†]	III	Extremely high	Extremely high

*Disease risk for type 2 diabetes, hypertension, and CVD.

[†]Increased waist circumference also can be a marker for increased risk, even in persons of normal weight.

Source: Classification of overweight and obesity by BMI, waist circumference, and associated disease. National Heart, Lung, and Blood Institute. Retrieved from https://www.nhlbi.nih.gov/health/educational/lose_wt/BMI/bmi_dis.htm

old, carrying extra weight around the waist or being underweight is associated with a shorten life span (Chen et al., 2017). Body weight categories and disease risks in adults relative to normal weight and waist circumference are available in Table 4–1.

Nutrition

Good nutrition is a primary determinant of good health. Effective planning for health promotion requires an assessment of the nutritional status of the client to establish a baseline. Body fat measurement, laboratory values, and dietary history are useful tools to assess nutritional status, and many are readily available online (see Chapter 7). BMI does not assess body fat composition or fat distribution, but it is the best method to assess healthy weight (American College of Sports Medicine, 2013) and a useful screening tool for overweight or obesity (see Table 4–2).

Biochemical analyses of blood and urine assess nutritional status. In addition to laboratory tests for cholesterol, triglycerides, glucose, and high-density lipoproteins, tests for protein (creatinine index, serum protein, serum albumin, total lymphocyte count, blood urea nitrogen, uric acid), serum or plasma vitamin levels (water-soluble, fat-soluble), and minerals (calcium, sodium, potassium, iron, phosphorus, magnesium) assess nutritional status. Assessment of HbA1c levels is also useful to determine average blood glucose levels as a measure of prediabetes in overweight and obese clients. Three particularly important values in assessing nutritional status are serum albumin less than 3.5 g/dL, total lymphocyte count less than 1800/mm^3, and an involuntary loss of body weight greater than 15%. These three indicators correlate significantly with nutritional status and require follow-up (Gupta & Lis, 2010; Nishida & Sakakibara, 2010).

A large body of evidence shows that healthy eating patterns contribute to good health and reduce risk of chronic diseases. A dietary diary, paper or Web-based, is

TABLE 4–2 Healthy and Unhealthy Weight Guidelines

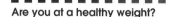

Are you at a healthy weight?

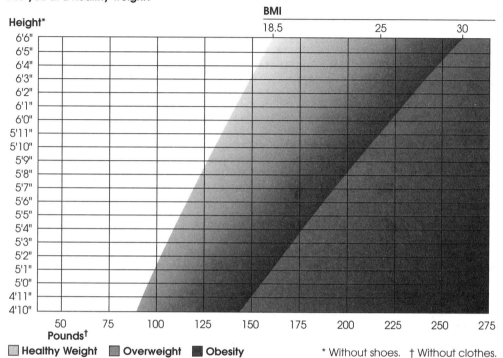

☐ **Healthy Weight**   ▨ **Overweight**   ▇ **Obesity**   * Without shoes.   † Without clothes.

The BMI (weight-for-height) ranges shown are for adults. They are not exact ranges of healthy and unhealthy weights. However, they show that health risk increases at higher levels of overweight and obesity. Even within the healthy BMI range, weight gains can carry health risks for adults.

Directions: Find your weight on the bottom of the graph. Go straight up from that point until you come to the line that matches your height. Then look to find your weight group.

BMI of 24.9 defines the upper boundary of healthy weight.
BMI of 25 to 29.9 defines overweight.
BMI of 30 or higher defines obesity.

Source: Report of the Dietary Guidelines Advisory Committee on the Dietary Guidelines for Americans. (2000).
http://www.cnpp.usda.gov/Publications/DietaryGuidelines/2000/2000DGCommitteeReport.pdf, p. 11.

helpful in assessing nutritional status. The paper dietary diary requires clients to keep a record of everything eaten for three days during the week prior to the assessment. Daily food choices, compared with published daily food guides or a computerized dietary analysis package, identify unusual or poor dietary patterns (see Chapter 7). It is important to recognize that underreporting of food eaten is a major source of error with self-report measures of dietary intake. SuperTracker, a Web-based assessment measure, helps plan, analyze, and track diet and physical activity. Easy to access and use, it incorporates both the 2015–2020 Dietary Guidelines for Americans and the 2008 Physical Activity Guidelines. After the requested dietary information is entered, the results are used to tailor a nutrition plan that empowers the client to choose healthier eating patterns. ChooseMyPlate.gov is a resource that provides information about healthy eating. It uses an illustration of a dinner plate to identify the five food groups that are the building blocks of a healthy diet. ChooseMyPlate offers information in multiple languages (U.S. Department of Agriculture, 2017).

The United States is a highly diverse country with many cultures, traditions, and personal food preferences, all influencing eating patterns, weight, and malnutrition. Assessment of nutritional status and dietary habits is a critical part of a comprehensive health assessment for individuals. An analysis of assessment data determines which interventions are most appropriate to improve a client's nutritional status.

Life Stress

Stress is a potential threat to mental health and physical well-being and is associated with risk for cardiovascular disease, cancer, gastrointestinal disorders, depression, poor sleep patterns, and inability to carry out daily activities at an effective level. Assessment begins with helping the client identify sources of stress. One strategy is to have clients explore the issues, concerns, and challenges that trigger stress responses in their lives. Stressors are both internal and external events. Internal stressors are self-induced thoughts and feelings. External stressors are events and situations that happen to people.

Examples of external stressors include the following:

1. Happy events such as marriage, birth of a child, and a new home; and negative events, such as death of a loved one, loss of a job, and an unplanned pregnancy. Stress results from both positive and negative events.
2. Unplanned, unpredictable events such as unexpected guests, increase in rent, or a sick child.
3. Family interactions, such as conflicts and arguments between children and spouses, issues resulting from health problems of family members, and multigenerational households.
4. Workplace issues such as long working hours, difficult supervisors and coworkers, and urgent deadlines.
5. Social demands such as pressure from peers, and commitments to family, friends, and organizations competing with personal time.

Internal stressors lead to unrest, anxiety, and depression. Examples of internal stressors include the following:

1. Public speaking, fear of flying and heights
2. Attitudes and expectations regarding job loss and family issues
3. Relationship issues
4. Balancing daily activities

Despite the high prevalence of stress-related health problems, including substance abuse, anxiety, and depression, health care providers do not regularly screen clients for life stress. Regular screenings enable early identification and treatment of stress-related problems. Nurses have an important role to ensure that life stress screenings are conducted. Screening tools include the following.

STRESS SCALES. Assessing a person's vulnerability to stress and strength to cope provides an essential measure of mental and physical well-being. The Derogatis Stress Profile (Derogatis & Fleming, 1997) assesses environmental events, personality mediators, and emotional responses in adolescents and adults. The Perceived Stress Scale (Cohen, Kessler, & Gordon, 1997) measures moods and feelings about everyday life stressors and is a measure of an individual's stress level.

HASSLES AND UPLIFTS MEASURES. Hassles are the irritating, frustrating, distressing demands such as traffic jams, losing items, or arguments that characterize everyday life. Uplifts, the counterpart of hassles, are the positive experiences or joys of life, such as getting a good night's rest, receiving a text from a friend, or playing with a pet. The assessment of daily hassles and uplifts is considered a better predictor of health or illness than the assessment of life events. Examples of hassles and uplifts scales are the Adolescent Hassle Scale (AHS; Wright, Creed, & Zimmer-Gembeck, 2010) and the Daily Hassles and Uplifts (Kanner, Coyne, Schaefer, & Lazarus, 1981).

ANXIETY INVENTORY. The State–Trait Anxiety Inventory consists of 20 items that assess the extent of anxiety one feels at that moment (state anxiety) and 20 items that assess how one generally feels (trait anxiety; Spielberger, Gorsuch, Lushene, & Vagg, 1983). A State–Trait Anxiety Inventory is available for children ("How I Feel Questionnaire"; Spielberger et al., 1983). Both instruments and administration manuals are available from Mind Garden, Palo Alto, California.

STRESS WARNING SIGNALS INVENTORY. Clients should understand and be aware of the symptoms of an elevated stress level. When clients are aware of their own stress signals, they can use stress management techniques (see Chapter 8) more effectively. Symptoms of stress may be physical, behavioral, emotional, or cognitive as shown in Figure 4–7.

COPING MEASURES. Coping is an individual's ongoing effort to manage specific internal and external demands that exceed personal resources. A commonly used tool to measure coping is the Ways of Coping Questionnaire developed by Folkman and Lazarus (1988). The scale measures both emotion- and problem-focused coping strategies an individual uses when responding to a stress situation. The Schoolagers' Coping Strategies Inventory measures the type, frequency, and effectiveness of children's stress-coping strategies.

The Patient Health Questionnaire (PHQ-2) is a two-item screening scale that consists of the first two questions of the Patient Health Questionnaire (PHQ-9), a tool to assist providers in diagnosing depressive symptoms. A PHQ-2 score ranges from 0 to 6. Clients with scores of 3 or more on the PHQ-2 require further evaluation using the remaining items on the PHQ-9 (Li, Friedman, Conwell, & Fiscella, 2007). The PHQ-2 is an effective screening instrument to detect undiagnosed depressive symptoms.

Spiritual Health

Spiritual health is the ability to develop one's inner self to its fullest potential. Spiritual health includes the ability to discover and articulate one's basic purpose in life; to learn how to experience love, joy, peace, and fulfillment; and to help oneself and others achieve their fullest potential.

Stress Warning Signals

PHYSICAL SYMPTOMS

☐ Headaches	☐ Back pain
☐ Indigestion	☐ Tight neck, shoulders
☐ Stomachaches	☐ Racing heart
☐ Sweaty palms	☐ Restlessness
☐ Sleep difficulties	☐ Tiredness
☐ Dizziness	☐ Ringing in ears

BEHAVIORAL SYMPTOMS

☐ Excess smoking	☐ Grinding teeth at night
☐ Bossiness	☐ Overuse of alcohol
☐ Compulsive gum chewing	☐ Compulsive eating
☐ Attitude critical of others	☐ Inability to get things done

EMOTIONAL SYMPTOMS

☐ Crying	☐ Overwhelming sense of pressure
☐ Nervousness, anxiety	☐ Anger
☐ Boredom—no meaning to things	☐ Loneliness
☐ Edginess—ready to explode	☐ Unhappiness for no reason
☐ Feeling powerless to change things	☐ Easily upset

COGNITIVE SYMPTOMS

☐ Trouble thinking clearly	☐ Inability to make decisions
☐ Forgetfulness	☐ Thoughts of running away
☐ Lack of creativity	☐ Constant worry
☐ Memory loss	☐ Loss of sense of humor

FIGURE 4–7   Stress Warning Signals

Source: Modified from Stress Warning Signals Checklist. Retrieved from http://www.instituteoflifestyle medicine.org/wp-content/uploads/2015/04/StressWarningSignalsChecklist.pdf

Assessment of spiritual health is critical in a holistic approach to health, as spiritual beliefs influence a client's interpretations of life events, health, and death. Acquiring a better understanding of clients' spiritual needs enables health care providers to develop tailored and effective individualized, spiritual interventions (Monod, Rochat, Bula, & Spencer, 2010; Taylor, Mamier, Ricci-Allegra, & Foith, 2017). Examples of spirituality measures include the following:

- The Spiritual Needs Assessment for Patients (SNAP) is a 23-item multidimensional survey that describes and measures spiritual needs (Sharma, Astrow, Texeira, & Sulmasy, 2012). Results provide information for addressing the client's spiritual beliefs about health issues.
- The Spiritual Involvement and Beliefs Scale (SIBS) measures actions as well as beliefs across religious traditions (Litwinczuk & Groh, 2007). The SIBS results provide supportive data for understanding the client's spiritual beliefs and their impact on health needs and care.
- The Spiritual Perspective Scale (SPS) is a 10-item instrument that measures clients' perceptions of the extent to which their spiritual beliefs and their daily interactions are consistent (Chung, Wong, & Chan, 2007).

Social Support Systems

A review of sources of social support enables the client to recognize current sources of support and identify barriers in social relationships that may block desirable health actions. When assessing the adequacy of support systems, it is important to be cognizant of factors such as the client's culture, age, social context (school, home, work), and role context (parent, student, occupation) (see Chapter 9).

One straightforward, useful approach to assess support systems is to ask the client to list individuals who provide emotional, instrumental, informational, and appraisal support. The client is also asked to indicate the relationship with the persons listed and to identify persons who have been sources of support for five years or more. This list enables the client to become aware of the stability of personal support systems. Last, they identify the frequency and types of contacts. These may be face-to-face or interactive e-mail/text communication.

After reviewing the client's social support systems, answers to the following questions provide the nurse important information:

- In what areas do you need more support: informational, emotional, instrumental, appraisal?
- Who within your present support system might provide the needed support?
- Who else do you think needs to become a part of your support system?
- What can you do to add the people you believe you need to your support system?

Examining the social network helps the client and nurse assess the adequacy of support available to the client. If it is inadequate, focusing on strategies to enhance the existing social network are priorities. Social media has become a significant resource to maintain and expand social contacts and can be useful in identifying possible additions to a client's social support network. While social media sites have gained significant popularity, if used to the exclusion of face-to-face contact, they may lead to social isolation.

Diagrams are also effective in assessing the strength and sources of support. Figure 4–8 presents a sample emotional support diagram that indicates strong, moderate, and weak sources of support, as well as conflicts with supportive individuals. The length of each line indicates geographical proximity to the client. This approach is particularly appropriate for clients who need a visual presentation of their emotional support system to take action to sustain or enhance emotionally satisfying relationships.

The nurse must always be alert to situations in which the client's social support is minimal or nonexistent. Extensive review of support systems may cause anxiety and/or depression, and in this case, a more informal, nonthreatening approach is useful.

SOCIAL SUPPORT QUESTIONNAIRE. The Social Support Questionnaire is a six-item measure of perceived social support and satisfaction with social support. Each item presents a specific scenario for which respondents list the people who would be available for support in that situation. Respondents are also asked to rate their satisfaction with the support available (Pierce, Sarason, & Sarason, 1991; Sarason, Sarason, Shearin, & Pierce, 1987).

Lifestyle

In the context of health, *lifestyle* defines activities that are a regular part of one's daily pattern of living and significantly influences health status. Methods for assessing

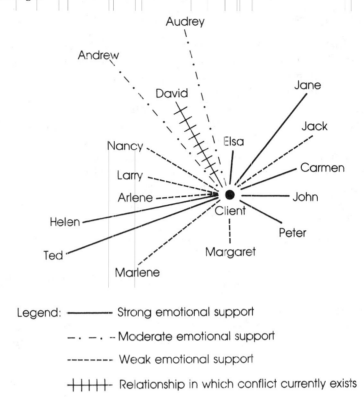

Legend: ———— Strong emotional support

—.—.— Moderate emotional support

------- Weak emotional support

+++++ Relationship in which conflict currently exists

FIGURE 4–8 Emotional Support Diagram for Client

lifestyle health behaviors include questionnaires, interviews, diary log techniques, observation, and technology-driven and physiological measures. Assessment of lifestyle health behaviors requires a combination of different methods and modes of data gathering (Renner, Klusmann, & Sproesser, 2015).

HEALTH-PROMOTING LIFESTYLE PROFILE II (HPLP-II). One example of a lifestyle assessment tool is the 52-item Health-Promoting Lifestyle Profile II. A revision of the original instrument, it consists of six subscales to measure major components of a health-promoting lifestyle: health responsibility, physical activity, nutrition, interpersonal relations, spiritual growth, and stress management. Scores are obtained for each subscale, or a total scale score can be calculated to measure overall health-promoting lifestyle (Sechrist, Walker, & Pender, 1987). An HPLP-II profile provides information to develop an individualized health promotion plan that identifies lifestyle strengths and resources as well as areas for further growth. A Spanish-language version of the HPLP-II is available. The Adolescent Lifestyle Profile (ALP) measures seven domains of health-promoting lifestyle (Hendricks, Murdaugh, & Pender, 2006) and is useful for measuring health-promoting behaviors in adolescents.

TABLE 4–3 True–False Statements for Assessing Stages of Behavior Change

1. I currently do not (specify exact behavior, e.g., exercise 30 minutes three times a week, eat 2 to 4 servings of fruit daily) and do not intend to start in the next 6 months. (Precontemplation)
2. I currently do not (specify behavior), but I am thinking about starting to do so in the next 6 months. (Contemplation)
3. I have tried several times to (specify behavior) but am seriously thinking of trying again in the next month. (Planning)
4. I have (specify behavior) regularly for less than 6 months. (Action)
5. I have (specify behavior) regularly for more than 6 months. (Maintenance)

STAGE OF CHANGE ASSESSMENT. The characteristic hallmark of lifestyle behaviors is that they are amenable to change. Given that behavior change is a function of the individual, it is essential that the individual be involved and engaged in their health care. Clients may be at one of several stages in relation to any given behavior change. Recognizing the different stages of change in relation to various health behaviors allows for more tailored interventions. Table 4–3 shows the stages of change to empower and achieve positive health behaviors.

LIFE'S SIMPLE 7 (LS7). The American Heart Association has formulated seven items to assess healthy living behaviors (Arena, McNeil, Sagner, & Lavie, 2017). The LS7 is considered an indicator of positive health, as a higher score has been associated with a more positive health outcome. It assesses four health behaviors: physical activity, diet, tobacco use, and body weight; and three health risk factors: cholesterol, blood pressure, and blood sugar. An assessment of these seven factors provides valuable information for planning lifestyle change interventions for clients.

ASSESSMENT OF THE FAMILY

The contemporary family and the reciprocal influence of family health on individual family members reconfirm the family as the primary social structure for health promotion. The family is a system of interrelated individuals whose actions and changes influence other family members. Health-promoting as well as health-damaging behaviors and lifestyle learned and reinforced within the context of the family are powerful mediating factors in determining how individual members cope with health concerns and challenges (see Figure 4–9). The family has the primary responsibility for the following:

1. Developing self-responsibility and health care competencies of its members
2. Fostering resilience of family members through shared values and goals
3. Providing social and economic resources to meet basic family needs
4. Recognizing individual differences and maintaining family cohesion
5. Mainstreaming health and healthy behaviors (Kaakinen & Webb, 2016).

The milieu for health promotion is likely to differ significantly across families, depending on their composition, structure, socioeconomic status, living environment,

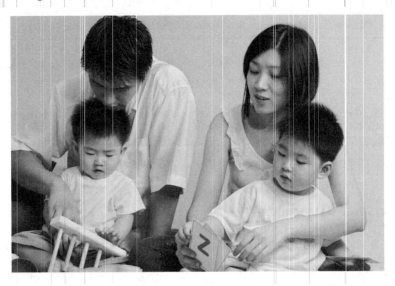

FIGURE 4–9   Young Family Spends Time Together, Teaching and Playing Together

cultural context, and family history. Variations in family units influence assessment as well. One-parent families, blended families, unmarried parents with children, and gay and lesbian families are examples of variation in family units.

Family history offers an invaluable insight into the risk of inheriting specific diseases, shared environmental factors, and individual health concerns. *My Family Health Portrait* (HHS.gov) is an excellent example of a Web-based family health tool that can be completed online or downloaded. The nurse may print a copy for the family if they do not have access to a computer or skills to download the form. The program assembles information and builds a family tree. Families may share information with other family members and/or enter the information into individual family members' PHRs.

There are limitations of the family history representation when applied to nontraditional families. *GenoPro Free* (GenoPro.com) is an example of a commercial application that may be more useful to assess nontraditional family units. Healthy family traits and family strengths have many different modes of expression.

The Calgary Family Assessment Model has been adapted for nurses to assess families. The model includes family structural assessment, family developmental assessment, and family functional assessment. Structural assessment includes internal structure (family composition, rank order, subsystem, and boundary) and external structure (culture, religion, socioeconomic level, mobility, and extended family). Family development focuses primarily on the traditional family developmental cycle, but also includes assessment of alterations brought about by separation, divorce, death, single parenthood, and remarriage (Wright & Leahey, 2012).

A significant gap in conducting family assessments is the lack of measures to assess family dimensions of a healthy lifestyle. Family assessment and individual assessment are interrelated processes and complement each other. Suggested assessment areas include nutrition, physical activity, stress control and management, health responsibility, family resilience and resources, and family support. To provide further guidance, Chapter 5 presents a format for developing such a family health plan.

ASSESSMENT OF THE COMMUNITY

A third essential component of assessing the health of individuals is an assessment of the communities in which they live, work, and play. Community assessment is complicated and time consuming, hence the need to have defined boundaries. However, community assessment is critical to identify community strengths and resources as well as to diagnose community problems and deficits.

Several trends make community assessment a priority. These include economic concerns; mandated assessment requirements of accrediting agencies and granting agencies; and the Institute of Medicine (IOM) Future of Nursing progress report recommendation for nurses' involvement in addressing population health. (Evans-Agnew, Reyes, Primomo, Meyer, & Matlock-Hightower, 2016; National Academies of Science, Engineering, and Medicine, 2016; U.S. Centers for Disease Control and Prevention, 2013).

A community analysis performed *with* community leadership and involvement, and *not on* or *for* the community, increases the likelihood of success. Gathering data and input on what the community needs gives voice to citizens' concerns and issues and allows the "voice" to influence the program design (Stanhope & Lancaster, 2016). A team or coalition of local citizens and organizations involved in the assessment process encourages community "ownership" of the assessment, planning, and implementation. Collaboration is required among community leaders, individual citizens, and community organizations, as well as health professionals.

There are four objectives for conducting a community assessment:

1. Identify community strengths and areas for improvement.
2. Identify the priorities of the community.
3. Define plans to guide the community toward implementing changes for healthy living.
4. Assist with prioritizing appropriate allocation of available resources (Rosenbaum, 2013; U.S. Centers for Disease Control and Prevention, 2013).

Successful implementation and sustainability of community health promotion–prevention programs depend in large part on a well-developed community plan. For example, an effort to improve family food choices is sustainable only if healthy, affordable, and accessible food locations are available in the community.

Community-based action may improve the overall health of the community, but certain groups may feel disenfranchised based on income level, occupation, race, or culture, exacerbating health disparities. Achieving health equity may be at odds with improving the overall health of the community, and priorities must be determined (Institute of Medicine, 2012). The need for transparency is paramount between the decision makers and the community to ensure that the implementation plan reflects the priorities, values, and preferences of all groups within a community.

CONSIDERATIONS FOR PRACTICE IN ASSESSING HEALTH AND HEALTH BEHAVIOR

Assessments document areas to enhance the health status of individuals, families, and communities and are an important responsibility of the nurse. Assessment data about health status and behaviors provide the basis for planning appropriate interventions. Nurses' knowledge and influence can ensure that a portfolio of user-friendly assessment instruments is available. The nurse must be capable of conducting assessment measures and demonstrating the value of the information obtained to the client. The use of detailed individual assessments may require significant time to administer and follow up. One strategy to manage the time issue is to seek innovative ways to incorporate wireless devices, social media sites, and simple, printed materials that explain assessment procedures. Computerized assessment measures are available in the health care setting, so clients are able to complete self-assessments at home and transmit the information electronically prior to a health care visit.

Practicing nurses must be computer literate and continually updating their skills and knowledge of assessment measures and strategies. Nurses influence the quality of health promotion plans of individuals, families, and communities through a commitment to systematic assessments of health and health behaviors and openness to new methods and technologies.

OPPORTUNITIES FOR RESEARCH IN HEALTH ASSESSMENT AND HEALTH BEHAVIOR

Technological changes have significant implications for research in nursing and health care. New research methods are emerging to replace the era of self-reported data. Digital intervention apps and instruments for assessing health and health behaviors of individuals, families, and communities require evidence-based support. Many researchers hesitate to put aside old theories of health promotion in order to speed development and evaluation of new methods and theories. Computationally intensive health behavior interventions are likely to be the method of the future to address the global health consequences (chronic diseases) of lifestyle behaviors (Patrick et al., 2016). Nurse researchers must move from the periphery of technological change to the forefront of exploring and using different designs and methods of assessments to improve nursing outcomes.

Summary

Assessment is time intensive and costly but a necessary priority to diagnose client needs and plan health promotion programs and interventions. Continuous assessment and evaluation lead to implementation strategies that improve the health of individuals, families, and communities. The rapid pace of the digital age is changing the infrastructure of health promotion, such that new assessment strategies are integral to the health promotion planning process.

Learning Activities

1. Visit the My Family Health Portrait website and record a traditional family health portrait.
2. Develop a list of strategies to ensure that non-computer users are included in the health care technology environment.
3. Develop an assessment plan based on age-specific instruments for a child, a young adult, and an older adult.
4. Using Table 4–1, determine your BMI and set a personal goal based on the results.
5. Design one approach to assessing a nontraditional family unit and discuss its strengths and weaknesses for use in clinical settings.

References

Ali, P. A., & Johnson, S. (2017). Speaking my patient's language: Bilingual nurses' perspective about provision of language concordant care to patients with limited English proficiency. *Journal of Advanced Nursing*, 73(2), 421–432. doi:10.1111/jan.13143

American College of Sports Medicine (ACSM). (2013). *ACSM's resource manual for guidelines for exercise testing and prescription* (7th ed.). Baltimore, MD: Lippincott Williams and Wilkins.

Arena, R., McNeil, A., Sagner, M., & Lavie, C. J. (2017). Healthy living: The universal and timeless medicine for healthspan. *Progress in Cardiovascular Diseases*, 59(5), 419–421. doi:10.1016/j.pcad.2017.01.007

Ashwood, J., Mehrotra, A., Cowling, D., & Uscher-Pines, L. (2017). Direct-to-consumer telehealth may increase access to care but does not decrease spending. *Health Affairs*, 36(3), 485–491. doi:10.1377/hlthaff.2016.1130

Bagwell, J. (2014). *Summary report on the PHR Ignite Project: Advancing consumer-mediated exchange*. Research Triangle Park, NC: RTI International. Retrieved from https://www.healthit.gov/sites/default/files/onc_shpc_phrignite_summaryreport.pdf

Bleyer, A., & Welsh, H. (2012). Effect of three decades of screening mammography on breast cancer incidence. *New England Journal of Medicine*, 367(21), 1998–2005. doi:10.1056/NEJMoa1206809

Brous, E. (2016). Legal considerations in telehealth and telemedicine. *American Journal of Nursing*, 116(9), 64–67. doi:10.1097/01.NAJ0000494700.786.16.d3

Bulechek, G., Butcher, H., Dochterman, J., & Wagner, C. (2013). *Nursing Interventions Classification (NIC)* (6th ed.). St. Louis, MO: Mosby.

Centers for Medicare & Medicaid Services. (2009). *Medicare and Medicaid health information technology: Title IV of the American recovery and reinvestment act*. Retrieved on August 10, 2017, from https://www.cms.gov/Newsroom/MediaReleaseDatabase/Fact-sheets/2009-Fact-sheets-items/2009-06-16.html

Chen, Y., Lu, J. C., & Jan, J. K. (2012). A secure EHR system based on hybrid clouds. *Journal of Medical Systems*, 3(5), 3375–3384. doi:10.1007/s10916-012-9830-6

Chen, Z., Klimentidis, Y., Bea, J., Ernst, K., Hu, C., Jackson, R., & Thomson, C. (2017). Body mass index, waist circumference, and mortality in a large multiethnic postmenopausal cohort: Results from the Women's Health Initiative. *Journal of the American Geriatrics Society*, 65(9), 1907–1915. doi:10.1111/jgs.14790

Chung, L., Wong, F., & Chan, M. (2007). Relationship of nurses' spirituality to their understanding and practice of spiritual care. *Journal of Advanced Nursing*, 58(2), 158–170. doi:10.1111/j.1365-2648.2007.04225.xb

Cohen, S., Kessler, R., & Gordon, L. (Eds.). (1997). *Measuring stress: A guide for health and social scientists*. New York, NY: Oxford University Press.

Cook, V., Ellis, A., & Hildebrand, K. (2016). Mobile health applications in clinical practice: Pearls, pitfalls, and key considerations. *Annals of Allergy, Asthma, & Immunology*, 117(2), 143–149. doi:10.1016/j.anai.2016.01.012

Cornett, S. (2009). Assessing and addressing health literacy. *The Online Journal of Issues in Nursing*, 14(3), Manuscript 2. doi:10.3912/OJIN.Vol14No03Man02.

Cox, A., Lucas, G., Marcu, A., Piano, M., Grosvenor, W., Mold, F., . . . Ream, E. (2017). Cancer survivors' experience with telehealth: A systematic review and thematic synthesis. *Journal of Medical Internet Research*, 19(1), e11. doi: 10.2196/jmir.6575

Derogatis, L., & Fleming, M. (1997). The Derogatis Stress Profile: A theory driven approach to stress measurement. In C. P. Zalaquett & R. J. Wood (Eds.), *Evaluating stress: A book of resources* (pp. 113–140). Lanham, MD: Scarecrow Press.

Evans-Agnew, R., Reyes, D., Primomo, J., Meyer, K., & Matlock-Hightower, C. (2016). Community health needs assessments: Expanding the boundaries of nursing education in population health. *Public Health Nursing, 34*(1), 69–77. doi:10.1111/phn.12298

File, T., & Ryan, C. (2014). *Computer and Internet use in the United States: 2013*. U.S. Department of Commerce, U.S. Census Bureau.

Folkman, S., & Lazarus, R. (1988). Coping as a mediator of emotion. *Journal of Personality and Social Psychology, 54*(3), 466–475. doi:10.1037/0022-3514.54.3.466

Gordon, M. (2014). *Manual of nursing diagnosis* (13th ed.). Sudbury, MA: Jones and Bartlett Learning.

Gupta, D., & Lis, C. (2010). Pretreatment serum albumin as a predictor of cancer survival: A systematic review of the epidemiological literature. *Nutrition Journal, 9*, 69. doi:10.1186/1475-2891-9-69

Hagan, J. F., Jr., Shaw, J. S., & Duncan, P. M. (Eds.). (2017). *Bright futures: Guidelines for health supervision of infants, children, and adolescents* (4th ed.). Elk Grove Village, IL: American Academy of Pediatrics.

Hendricks, C., Murdaugh, C., & Pender, N. (2006). The Adolescent Lifestyle Profile: Development and psychometric characteristics. *Journal of National Black Nurses Association, 17*(2), 1–5.

Hicks, E. (2017). Digital citizenship and health promotion programs: The power of knowing. *Health Promotion Practice, 18*(1), 8–10. doi:10.1177/1524839916676263

Hughes, J. (2017). Reviewing mobile health applications. *Health Affairs, 36*(2), 383–384. doi:10.1377/hlthaff.2017.0023

Huston, C. (2013). The impact of emerging technology on nursing care: Warp speed ahead. *The Online Journal of Issues in Nursing, 18*(2), Manuscript 1. doi:10.3912/OJIN.Vol18No02Man01

Institute of Medicine. (2012). *An integrated framework for assessing the value of community-based prevention.* Washington, DC: The National Academies Press.

Kaakinen, J., & Webb, J. (2016). Working with families in the community for healthy outcomes. In M. Stanhope & J. Lancaster (Eds.), *Public health nursing: Population-centered health care in the community* (pp. 594–621). St Louis, MO: Elsevier, Inc.

Kanner, A., Coyne, J., Schaefer, C., & Lazarus, R. (1981). Comparison of two modes of stress measurement: Daily hassles and uplifts versus major life events. *Journal of Behavioral Medicine, 4*(1), 1–39.

Kelli, H., Witbrodt, B., & Shah, A. (2017). The future of mobile health applications and devices in cardiovascular health. *European Medical Journal of Innovation, 1*(1), 92–97.

Kreps, G., & Neuhauser, L. (2010). New directions in eHealth communication: Opportunities and challenges. *Patient Education and Counseling, 78*(3), 329–336. doi:10.1016/j.pec.2010.01.013

Kressin, N., Manze, M., Russell, S., Katz, R., Claudio, C., Green, B., & Wang, M. (2010). Self-reported willingness to have cancer screening and the effects of sociodemographic factors. *Journal of the National Medical Association, 102*(3), 219–227. doi:10.1016/S0027-9684(15)30528-9

Leventhal, R. (2016). *Report: Majority of mHealth apps contain critical security vulnerabilities.* Healthcare Informatics. Retrieved from https://www.health-care-informatics.com/news-item/report-major-ity-mhealth-apps-contain-critical-security-vul-nerabilities

Li, C., Friedman, B., Conwell, Y., & Fiscella, K. (2007). Validity of the Patient Health Questionnaire 2 (PHQ-2) in identifying major depression in older people. *Journal of the American Geriatrics Society, 55*(4), 596–602. doi:10.1111/j.1532-5415.2007.01103.x

Lin, K. W., & Gostin, L. O. (2016). A public health framework for screening mammography: Evidence-based vs politically mandated care. *Journal of the American Medical Association, 315*(10), 977–978. doi:10.1001/jama.2016.0322

Litwinczuk, K., & Groh, C. (2007). The relationship between spirituality, purpose in life, and well-being in HIV-positive persons. *Journal of the Association of Nurses in AIDS Care, 18*(3), 13–22. doi:10.1016/j.jana.2007.03.004

Minthorn, C., & Lunney, M. (2012). Participant action research with bedside nurses to identify NANDA-International, Nursing Interventions Classification, and Nursing Outcomes Classification categories for hospitalized persons with diabetes. *Applied Nursing Research, 25*(2), 75–80. doi10.1016/j.apnr.2010.08.001

Misra, S. (2015). *New report finds more than 165,000 mobile health apps now available, takes close look at characteristics & use.* Retrieved on March 1, 2017, from http://www.imedicalapps.com

Monod, S., Rochat, E., Bula, C., & Spencer, B. (2010). The spiritual needs model: Spirituality assessment in the geriatric hospital setting. *Journal of Religion, Spirituality & Aging, 22*(4), 271–282. doi:10.1080/15528030.2010.509987

Moorhead, S., Johnson, M., Maas, M., & Swanson, E. (Eds.). (2013). *Nursing Outcomes Classification (NOC)* (5th ed.). St. Louis, MO: Elsevier, Inc.

National Academies of Science, Engineering, and Medicine. (2016). *Assessing progress on the Institute of Medicine Report The Future of Nursing.* Washington, DC: The National Academies Press.

Nishida, T., & Sakakibara, H. (2010). Association between underweight and low lymphocyte count as an indicator of malnutrition in Japanese women. *Journal of Women's Health, 19*(7), 1377–1383. doi:10.1089/jwh.2009.1857

Office of Minority Health, U.S. Department of Health and Human Services. (2013). *Think cultural health.* Retrieved on March 3, 2017, from http://aspe.hhs./gov/sp/reports/2010

Office of Minority Health, U.S. Department of Health and Human Services. (2017). *Cultural competency.* Retrieved on March 4, 2017, from http://aspe.hhs./hhs./gov

Office of the Assistant Secretary for Planning and Evaluation, U.S. Department of Health and Human Services. (2009). *Evaluation of the personal health record pilot for Medicare fee-for service enrollees from South Carolina.* Retrieved from http://aspe.hhs.gov/sp/reports/2010/phrpilot/index.shtml

Office of the National Coordinator for Health IT. (2017). More than 80 percent of docs use EHRs. *Health Care IT News.* Retrieved on February 16, 2017, from http://www.healthcarenews.com/news/more-80-percent-docs-use-ehrs

Olsen, J., Thorson, D., Baisch, M., & Monsen, K. (2017). Using Omaha System documentation to understand physical activity among rural women. *Public Health Nursing, 34*(1), 31–41. doi:10.1111/phn.12264

Patrick, K., Hekler, E., Estrin D., Mohr, D., Riper, H., Crane, D., . . . Riley, W. (2016). The pace of technologic change: Implications for digital health behavior intervention research. *American Journal of Preventive Medicine, 51*(5), 816–824. doi:10.1016/j.amepre.2016.05.001

Pierce, G., Sarason, I., & Sarason, B. (1991). General and relationship-based perceptions of social support: Are two constructs better than one? *Journal of Personality and Social Psychology, 61*(6), 1028–1039. doi:10.1037/0022-3514.61.6.1028

Qin, X., Tangka, F., Guy, G. P., & Howard, D. H. (2017). Mammography rates after the 2009 revision to the United States Preventive Services Task Force breast cancer screening recommendation. *Cancer Causes & Control, 28*(1), 41–48. doi:10.1007/s10552-016-0835-1

Renner, B., Klusmann, V., & Sproesser, G. (2015). Health behaviors, assessment of. In J. D. Wright (Ed.), *International encyclopedia of the social & behavioral sciences* (2nd ed., Vol. 10, pp. 588–593). New York, NY: Elsevier.

Report to Congress. (2016). *Health IT progress: Examining the HITECH era and the future of health IT.* Retrieved on February 17, 2017, from http://healthit.gov

Robert Wood Johnson Foundation. (2009). *Personal health records.* Retrieved from http://www.rwjf.org/en/search-results

Rosenbaum, S. (2013). *Principles to consider for the implementation of a community process.* Washington, DC: The George Washington University.

Sarason, I., Sarason, B., Shearin, E., & Pierce, G. (1987). A brief measure of social support: Practical and theoretical implications. *Journal of Social and Personal Relations, 4*(4), 497–510. doi:10.1177/0265407587044007

Sechrist, K., Walker, S., & Pender, N.(1987). Development and psychometric evaluation of the Exercise Benefits/Barriers Scale. *Research in Nursing & Health, 10*(6), 357–365. doi:10.1002/nur.4770100603

Seidell, J. (2010). Waist circumference and waist/hip ratio in relation to all-cause mortality, cancer and sleep apnea. *European Journal of Clinical Nutrition, 64*(1), 35–41. doi:10.1038/ejcn.2009.71

Sharma, R. K., Astrow, A. B., Texeira, K., & Sulmasy, D. P. (2012). The Spiritual Needs Assessment for Patients (SNAP): Development and validation of a comprehensive instrument to assess unmet spiritual needs. *Journal of Pain and Symptom Management, 44*(1), 44–51. doi:10.1016/j.jpainsymman.2011.07.008

Silva, B., Rodrigues, J., de la Torre Diez, I., & Lopez-Coronado, M. (2015). Mobile-health: A review of current state in 2015. *Journal of Biomedical Informatics, 56*, 265–272. doi:101016/j.jbi.2015.06.003

Spielberger, C., Gorsuch, R., Lushene, R., & Vagg, P. (1983). *Manual for State–Trait Anxiety Inventory.* Palo Alto, CA: Consulting Psychologists Press, Inc.

Stanhope, M., & Lancaster, J. (2016). *Public health nursing: Population-centered health care in the community.* St. Louis, MO: Elsevier, Inc.

Taylor, E., Mamier, I., Ricci-Allegra, P., & Foith, J. (2017). Self-reported frequency of nurse-provided spiritual care. *Applied Nursing Research, 35*, 30–35. doi:10.1016/j.apnr.2017.02.019

U.S. Census Bureau. (2013). *American Community Survey.* Retrieved from https://www.census.gov/history/pdf/2013computeruse.pdf

U.S. Centers for Disease Control and Prevention. (2013). *Community health assessment for population health improvement: Resource of most frequently recommended health outcomes and determinants.* Atlanta, GA: Office of Surveillance, Epidemiology, and Laboratory Services.

U.S. Department of Agriculture. (2017). *ChooseMyPlate.* Washington, DC: Author.

U.S. Preventive Services Task Force. (2014). *Guide to clinical preventive services*. Washington, DC: Agency for Healthcare Research and Quality.

Wright, L., & Leahey, M. (2012). *Nurses and families: A guide to family assessment and intervention*. Philadelphia, PA: F.A. Davis Company.

Wright, M., Creed, P., & Zimmer-Gembeck, M. (2010). The development and initial validation of a brief daily hassles scale suitable for use with adolescents. *European Journal of Psychological Assessment, 26*(3), 220–226. doi:10.1027/1015-5759/a000029

Developing a Health Promotion–Prevention Plan

OBJECTIVES

This chapter will enable the reader to:

1. Identify nine steps in a health planning process.
2. Discuss barriers to overcome in developing health plans for individuals, families, and communities including low-literacy, diverse populations.
3. Describe strategies to increase the client's "ownership" of a behavior change plan.
4. Discuss strategies to ensure that health planning is an interdisciplinary process.
5. Discuss barriers that hinder effective individual, family, and community health behavior changes.
6. Describe how community-level plans and interventions influence individual and family health plans.

Clients must be active participants in planning and interpreting assessment data. Collaboration between the nurse, client, and other health providers promotes positive perceptions of worth and affirms the ability of individuals, families, and communities to function collaboratively to create conditions supportive of healthy lifestyles.

The nurse assists clients with *planning* rather than *controlling* the process and together they develop a mutual understanding of the client's health, including the following:

1. Health status
2. Current health behavior patterns
3. Attitudes and beliefs that affect health and health-related behaviors

4. Expectations of important referent groups
5. Available behavioral options
6. Social–ethnic–cultural–racial background
7. Potential or actual barriers to health behavior change
8. Existing support systems for health-promoting behaviors

Developing a systematic plan for behavior change provides the client an opportunity to express purposeful ways to increase wellness and enhance life satisfaction.

Health planning is a dynamic process. Flexibility is critical to meet the client's changing needs. The health promotion–prevention plan systematically lends direction but does not dictate goals or behaviors. The plan should be reasonable in terms of both demands on the client and the time period allocated to accomplish desired health or health-related goals.

Literacy, problem-solving skills, basic technology skills, and strengths of the client are critical factors in the planning process. Identification of strategies to overcome deficiencies related to any of these factors is a priority. Capitalizing on current positive health practices creates a sense of competence or efficacy essential to successful behavior change. Together, the nurse and the client should identify behaviors the client wishes to adapt, eliminate, or modify. Individual, social, and environmental factors require exploration in order to tailor a plan for sustainable health behavior change.

The client and nurse can then discuss strategies for change that are likely to be most effective and conducive to long-term health behavior change. Factors influencing lifestyle behavior changes include beliefs, knowledge, costs, attitudes, and social networks (Murray et al., 2013). Initial response to changes is often encouraging followed by diminished enthusiasm and a reversal to old behaviors. For example, most participants in weight loss programs are successful initially, but regain weight gradually over time and return to their baseline weight in 3–5 years (Middleton, Anton, & Perri, 2013). Revisions in the plan may be necessary to make behavior change a positive experience. The ultimate goal of health planning and implementation is to integrate health promotion and prevention into the lives of individuals, families, and communities.

Innovative developments in information technology increasingly personalize health promotion planning to the unique characteristics and needs of clients. In addition, electronic health records enable clients to share health promotion plans with multiple health care professionals. As nurses work with clients to develop and implement health promotion plans, they must be aware of and knowledgeable about the increasingly significant role of technology in health assessments, such as fitness applications (apps) for smartphones and tablets, as well as Web-based technology for health behavior interventions (Alkhaldi et al., 2016). In a study of midlife and older adults who were new to smartphone technology, they improved their physical activity level in response to three daily reminders from their mobile apps (King et al., 2013). Mobile connectivity appears to facilitate improvement in adoption and adherence of positive health behaviors. Health coaching, with or without access to mobile technologies, also contributes significant benefits in planning for health behavior change, especially for low-literacy, diverse populations (Wayne, Perez, Kaplan, & Ritvo, 2015).

HEALTH PLANNING PROCESS

The process for developing a health promotion–prevention plan includes nine steps that actively involve both the client and nurse. The nine steps include the following:

1. Review and summarize data from assessment.
2. Emphasize strengths and competencies of the client.
3. Identify health goals and related behavioral change options.
4. Identify desired behavioral health outcomes.
5. Develop a behavior change plan based on the client's preferences and on the "state-of-the-science" knowledge about effective intervention strategies.
6. Reinforce benefits of change and identify incentives for change from the client's perspective.
7. Address environmental and interpersonal facilitators and barriers to behavior change.
8. Determine a time frame for implementation of plan.
9. Formalize a commitment to behavior change goals and provide support to accomplish goals.

Review and Summarize Assessment Data

During assessment, the nurse gathers a wealth of information from the client. As described in Chapter 4, the desired outcome of assessment activities is information displayed in a useful format in the following domains as a basis for planning and action:

1. Physical health status
2. Functional health patterns
3. Physical fitness
4. Nutritional status
5. Life stressors
6. Spirituality
7. Social support
8. Personal health behaviors
9. Family health practices
10. Environmental and community supports or constraints for health behaviors

During one or more face-to-face meetings or wireless contacts, including the use of tele-health, the nurse and client review the assessment summary. Both should retain a copy (paper or electronic) for continuing reference during the health planning process. See Chapter 4 for a discussion of assessment tools and activities.

Emphasize Strengths and Competencies of the Client

Clients bring unique strengths to the health planning task. Identifying, acknowledging, and reinforcing these strengths are critical. Cultural beliefs, preferences, and current level of knowledge and skills, including technology skills, influence the choice of health behavior strategies. It is important to integrate existing cultural practices into the overall health plan to reinforce the client's culture and ethnicity. The nurse and client should seek consensus on areas in which the client is already making informed and responsible health decisions as well as on areas for further development. Health practices outside the mainstream health care system are often compatible with standard practices. For example, Native Americans often use tribal "medicine elders," or "medicine men," to prescribe "natural" or alternative treatments. The surge of health and health-related apps also opens the door for clients to explore issues and treatments outside the traditional health care system. Both traditional and nontraditional health care practices and providers have important roles in the health of clients. When traditional and nontraditional health care providers collaborate, the client's belief system and cultural practices are valued, and the client often has positive outcomes.

The nurse promotes existing competencies to enhance health practices through teaching, guidance, and coaching. Plans tailored to an individual's preferences, interests, and readiness for change are effective with diverse populations (e.g., different racial/ethnic and socioeconomic groups) and majority populations as well. Strategies that produce changes, enhance maintenance, and prevent relapse include self-reward, positive feedback, and incorporating new and existing social networks (Centers for Disease Control and Prevention, 2011). See Chapter 2 for a discussion on additional behavioral change strategies.

Personal health responsibilities and resources vary according to the client's age, gender, developmental stage, socioeconomic and educational levels, and health status (Halbert et al., 2017). Although clients differ in their self-care competencies, it is important to emphasize each person's responsibility for self-care. Promoting individual responsibility for health does not negate the importance of changing the larger social infrastructure and providing environmental resources to make health-promoting options more available to groups and communities. Both personal change and social change are essential for effective health promotion and prevention.

Identify Health Goals and Related Behavior Change Options

The next step in the planning process is to identify and prioritize personal or family health goals and review related behavior change options. Systematically reviewing the range of strategies that are possible to achieve health goals assists clients in deciding the behavioral changes on which they will initially focus. Providing relevant options also enables the client to prioritize behavior change strategies. Clients should not feel guilty about their current health practices but be encouraged to focus on their behavior change plan. During health coaching sessions, the nurse creates enthusiasm and excitement about growth in positive directions and the benefits of new health-related experiences.

Many clients initially place high priority on preventive behaviors for which the threat of illness is tangible and easily understood. Decreasing risk for specific chronic health problems fits the medical model orientation of most Americans. Preventive behaviors often lead to health-promoting behaviors, as the client experiences positive changes. Tailoring, based on the client's readiness or interest level in reducing risk of a specific disease, indicates that prevention is likely the most meaningful area for emphasis in early health planning. For example, a smoker may be concerned about lung cancer and seek assistance to help quit. Mastery of specific preventive measures often motivates clients to consider making additional lifestyle changes directed toward health promotion to experience a higher level of health and well-being (Jerant et al., 2013). The rapid growth of health-related information technology (IT) has initiated a shift from a disease-centered approach to a healthy lifestyle/health promotion approach. Regardless of the many challenges confronting health-related technology, health providers are accepting and using technology to educate and involve clients in managing their own health (Nimkar, 2016).

Clients often give important emotional cues about the behaviors they wish to change. Examples of such cues include the following:

"I hate myself when I gorge on fattening foods!"

"I get mad at myself for being so uptight!"

"The only time our family is together is in front of the television."

"We need to stop eating so much fast-food."

"We are very critical of each other."

"We don't participate in physical activities together."

"Teenagers in the family spend too much time on social networking sites."

The more open an individual or family is in discussing health concerns, the greater the probability of developing a meaningful health promotion–prevention plan. Areas that clients are most reluctant to discuss—such as marital relationships, human sexuality, spirituality, mental health, and family cohesiveness—are often the most crucial ones for behavior change. A "safe" climate ensures that personal health issues are open for discussion with assurance of confidentiality.

Identify Desired Health Behavior Outcomes

The nurse and the client mutually decide on the desired health behavior outcomes of the health promotion–prevention plan. Clear identification of outcomes energizes and guides the client in changing or establishing new health behaviors. The client's desired outcomes should guide goal development and implementation of the plan. "Have I reached my goal or made significant progress toward it?" is a critical question the client must ask periodically to evaluate the relevance of the health promotion–prevention goal.

Evidenced-based interventions should be the basis of a plan. Integrating strategies known to increase the likelihood of maintaining a healthy diet into the plan of persons wishing to address nutritional issues increases the probability of success. Identifying smartphone and tablet apps on nutrition/diet, directing clients to interactive websites, or offering printed information are potential strategies for clients interested in technology in changing behaviors. Clients often need assistance in setting realistic outcomes. For example, a behavioral goal of eating only at meal times may be easier to attain than a goal of losing a certain number of pounds. Weight reduction is more likely to occur if the plan is realistic, with tangible behaviors reinforced and managed by the client.

Develop a Behavior Change Plan

A successful plan results when the client takes "ownership" of desired behavior changes. Client engagement signifies the involvement of the client in the process of integrating health information, professional advice, and their own needs, preferences, and abilities to improve their health. Engagement requires a health culture that welcomes open communication, shared decision-making, and transparency in sharing information. Asking clients where they access "outside information" and checking health-related websites with clients to find useful and accurate online information demonstrate collaboration (Marin & Delaney, 2017). Behaviors that are appealing are more likely to be implemented. The client's priorities for behavior change will reflect:

1. Personal values
2. Activity preferences
3. Cognitive, psychomotor, and technological skills
4. Affective responses to various behavioral options
5. Expectations for success
6. Ease with which the selected behaviors are integrated into one's daily lifestyle

Significant value–behavior inconsistencies may be exposed. Alternative actions that are both healthful and enjoyable should substitute for behaviors that are inconsistent with personal values. Many individuals and families prefer or value the American "lifestyle" diet (high-fat, high-sodium, high-calorie foods). To address this "unhealthy" preference, clarifying the value and meaning of health prior to developing the behavior change plan may influence the client's willingness to consider other options.

Information technology profoundly influences health promotion strategies and interventions to facilitate individual behavior change. Social networking sites (SNSs) claim over 1.5 billion users worldwide (Naslund, Aschbrenner, Marsch, & Bartels, 2016) and the number of users is growing very rapidly. This platform reaches traditional and alternative health and health-related sites. These sites provide opportunities to adopt healthier behaviors through a large network of social support, sharing of personal health experiences, and eliciting others' perspectives on specific health problems. With expertise in health promotion and health-related technology, the nurse assists clients in assessing the credibility of the sites and gaining the behavior change skills needed to adopt and maintain positive health behaviors.

DEVELOP A BEHAVIOR CHANGE PLAN FOR LOW-LITERACY, CULTURALLY DIVERSE POPULATIONS

In addition to the strategies outlined above, low-literacy (educational, technological), culturally diverse, and lower socioeconomic status (SES) populations require additional planning that is tailored to meet their unique needs. Rural, minority, low literacy, and low SES populations have disproportionately high rates of chronic health problems and less access to health-promoting resources, such as grocery stores and safe walking environments (Agency for Healthcare Research and Quality, 2016). Social network analysis (Hindhede & Aagaard-Hansen, 2017), health coaching (Wayne et al., 2015), and goal setting (Ries et al., 2014) have been shown to be effective strategies that lead to significant health benefits for these groups.

Nurses need to use literacy techniques such as having clients explain back to them what they have been told (teach-back method), asking clients what they think caused the health problem, questioning them about what outcome is expected, and understanding the level of family involvement in health decisions (cultural influences) (Agency for Healthcare Research and Quality, 2016). Attention to these cultural and literacy strategies encourages individual engagement in health care planning. Figure 5–1 presents a sample individual health promotion–prevention plan and Figure 5–2 presents a family health promotion–prevention plan. In both plans, emphasis is on client strengths.

Designed for: ___James Moore_____

Home Address: ___714 George Street_____

Home Telephone Number: ___222–3333_____

Occupation (if employed): ___Building Services Supervisor_____

Work Telephone Number: ___445-6666_____

Cultural Identification: ___African-American_____

Birth Date: ___3/14/68___ Date of Initial Plan: ___1/15/2018_____

Client strengths:	Satisfactory peer relationships, spiritual strength, adequate sleep pattern
Major risk factors:	Elevated cholesterol, mild obesity, sedentary lifestyle, moderate life change, multiple daily hassles, few reported uplifts
Nursing diagnoses: (derived from assessment of functional health patterns)	Diversional activity deficit; altered nutrition: more than body requirements; caregiver role strain (elderly mother)
Medical diagnoses: (if any)	Mild hypertension
Age-specific screening recommendations: (derived from *Guide to Clinical Preventive Services*)	Blood pressure, cholesterol, fecal occult blood, malignant skin lesions, depression
Desired behavioral and health outcomes:	Become a regular exerciser (3 times/week), lower my blood pressure, weigh 165 lb.

FIGURE 5–1   Example of an Individual Health Promotion–Prevention Plan

Personal Health Goals (1 = highest priority)	Selected Behaviors to Accomplish Goals	Stage of Change	Strategies/ Interventions for Change
1. Achieve desired body weight	Begin a progressive walking program	Planning	Counter-conditioning Reinforcement management Client contracting
	Decrease caloric intake while maintaining good nutrition	Action (eating 2 fruits and 2 vegetables daily; using low-fat dairy products for last 2 months)	Stimulus control Cognitive restructuring
2. Decrease risk for hypertension-related disorders	Change from high- to low-sodium snacks	Contemplation	Consciousness raising Learning facilitation
3. Learn to manage stress effectively	Attend relaxation classes and use home relaxation tapes	Contemplation	Consciousness raising Self-reevaluation Simple relaxation therapy
4. Increase leisure-time activities	Join a local walking group	Contemplation	Support system enhancement

FIGURE 5–1 Continued

Identify Stage of Change and Reinforce Benefits of New Behavior

The cycle of change seen in Figure 5–3 identifies the stages to move from precontempla-tion (no intention of changing) to maintenance (sustained new behavior). Long-term adaptation of new health behaviors is challenging, and relapse or return of the old behavior is common. The concept of *upward spiral* is that with each relapse, the person learns from the experience and the relapse time frame is shorter and less frequent. Rein-forcements and reminders of the positive benefits of the desired health behavior change provide support for the client. A list of benefits, kept in highly visible places such as the

Designed for (family name): ___The Marshals___

Home Address: ___1718 Green Street___

Home Telephone Number: ___777-4444___

Occupations of Employed
Members of Household: ___Mother—Dental assistant___

Work Telephone Number: ___883-7777___

Family Form: ___One-parent family___

Cultural Identification: ___White non-Hispanic___

Family Members: Position in Family	Birth Date	Occupation/Student/Retired
Joan (Mother)	9/1981	Dental Assistant
Dana (Daughter)	4/2001	Student
Tiffany (Daughter)	7/2004	Student
Eric (Son)	1/2006	Student

Date of Initial Plan: ___1/15/2018___

Family strengths:	Open communication patterns, positive family cooperation, healthy snacks consumed at home
Major risk factors:	Mother recently divorced, oldest daughter has driver's license, high life change for family, minimal family physical activity
Nursing diagnoses:	Family coping: potential for growth
Medical diagnoses for family members:	None
Desired behavioral and health outcomes:	Active family outings, avoidance of early sexual activity and binge drinking among adolescent family members, injury prevention for children, adjustment to new family form

FIGURE 5–2   Example of a Family Health Promotion–Prevention Plan

refrigerator door, the bathroom mirror, the dashboard of the car, the computer, or smartphone, serves as a reminder to the client to stay on target. Keeping lists of health goals in very visible places reminds the client that the desired outcomes in the health promotion–prevention plan are personally worthwhile and directed toward improving health and quality of life.

The benefits of change include both health-related and non-health-related outcomes. Sensitivity to non-health-related benefits of change such as increased self-concept

Family Health Goals (1 = highest priority)	Selected Behaviors to Accomplish Goals	Stages of Change	Strategies/ Interventions for Change
1. Positive adjustment to single-parent family status	Realign family responsibilities	Action (divorced 3 months)	Social liberation Family process maintenance Caregiver support
	Increase spiritual resources	Contemplation	Spiritual support Helping relationships
	Discuss life goals	Planning	Self-reevaluation Self-esteem enhancement
2. Develop more active family lifestyles	Plan active family outings (biking, recreation center)	Planning	Exercise promotion Environmental reevaluation
3. Foster healthy sexuality among preadolescent and adolescents	Provide age-appropriate information	Action	Parent education
	Enhance self-esteem through praise, expression of affection, and assistance with skill development	Maintenance	Self-esteem enhancement Helping relationships

FIGURE 5–2 Continued

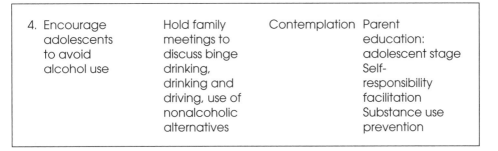

| 4. Encourage adolescents to avoid alcohol use | Hold family meetings to discuss binge drinking, drinking and driving, use of nonalcoholic alternatives | Contemplation | Parent education: adolescent stage Self-responsibility facilitation Substance use prevention |

FIGURE 5–2   Continued

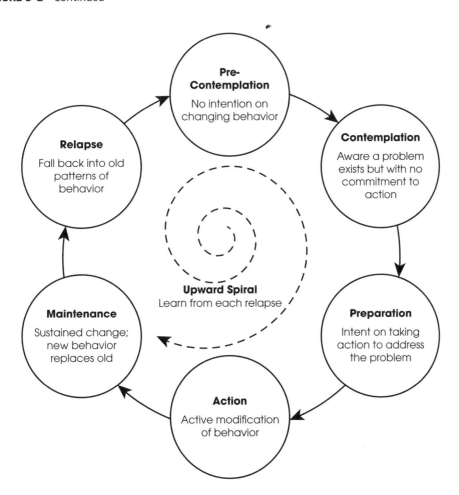

FIGURE 5–3   The Cycle of Change

Source: Prochaska, J. and DiClemente, C. as cited by Pacheco, I., Social Work Tech (2012). The Stages of Change: Prochaska and DiClemente. Retrieved from socialworktech.com on 17 July 2017.

or new friendships is important, as these may be central to the client's motivation to engage in and sustain new health behaviors.

Address Environmental and Interpersonal Facilitators and Barriers to Change

Multilevel strategies for change include the structured community and the economic environment in which people live and work. Positive features of the physical/economic environment and supportive interpersonal relationships bolster efforts to modify lifestyle. For example, social networks help counter barriers to change. Encouragement from family and friends helps the client persist when change efforts are difficult, or other demands or preferences compete for attention. Lack of community and economic resources serve as barriers to change. The nurse works with individuals and families as well as decision makers in communities to help bring about community changes to facilitate health.

Barriers to effective health behavior may arise from clients' internal conflicts, significant others, or the environment. Family members may impose considerable barriers if they encourage continuation of health-damaging behaviors, or if they actively discourage or sabotage attempts at behavior change.

Environmental barriers that inhibit positive changes include unsafe neighborhoods, such as heavy traffic or high crime rate; lack of facilities to support positive behaviors, such as access to parks, healthy foods, and sidewalks; and inclement weather. The nurse assists both the client and the community to address environmental barriers, as they are major challenges confronting individual and family behavior change.

Determine a Time Frame for Implementation

Integrating and stabilizing healthier behaviors into one's lifestyle is a time-consuming process. Attempting to change or initiate multiple new behaviors simultaneously may result in confusion, discouragement, and even abandonment of the health promotion–prevention plan. Whether the client is attempting to reduce risk for chronic disease or enhance health, gradual change is desirable. Just as education for self-care must proceed at the pace of the learner, changes in behavior, sequenced in reasonable steps appropriate for the client, will serve as a motivator to change. A review of interventions using apps found that multicomponent interventions (multiple strategies for behavior change) are more effective than single-component interventions. However, the actual number and combination of strategies and the optimal number of contacts needed with clients remain to be determined (Schoeppe et al., 2016).

The plan must allow time for the client to master the specific knowledge and skills necessary before implementing the new behavior. For example, if clients are not aware of how to initiate a physical activity program, they may begin an exercise routine before doing the warm-up. The period for developing a particular behavior may be several weeks or several months. Many online programs and smartphone apps include reminders and data recorders. They are easy to use and can be shared with the nurse and other supportive persons.

Accomplishing short-term goals is important and needs positive reinforcement, as this provides encouragement to continue pursuit of long-term goals and desired outcomes. A meaningful plan requires that deadlines be set for accomplishing specific goals. Adherence to deadlines should be encouraged, with the time shortened or lengthened *only* to make the plan more conducive to permanent behavior change.

Formalize Commitment to Behavior Change Plan

The client may be more motivated to follow through with selected actions if a formalized commitment follows one of these options:

1. Nurse–client contract agreements
2. Self-contracts
3. Public announcements to family members and friends of intentions to engage in new behaviors
4. Integration of new health behaviors into a written or online daily or weekly calendar
5. Purchase of necessary supplies (healthy foods, exercise videos, music, audiotapes) and equipment (exercise bike, walking shoes)

Behavioral contracts contain specific information about

1. The change to be made
2. How the change will be accomplished
3. The individual or family members who are to engage in the change
4. The time frame for behavior change
5. The consequences of meeting or not meeting the terms of the agreement

A *nurse–client contract* provides direction through the identification of mutual objectives and the responsibilities of each party. Contracts allow clients to participate actively by choosing goals that they want to accomplish realistically. Generally, the client is responsible for carrying out change behaviors, whereas the nurse is responsible for providing information, training, counseling, coaching, and/or specific reinforcement rewards. The nurse bears the additional responsibility of providing helpful input and continuing feedback about the adequacy of performance of activities identified in the contract. It is critical that the nurse be consistent and conscientious in managing the reinforcement–reward contingencies of the contract. Failure to fulfill this commitment will alter the trust and confidence placed in the nurse. Reinforcements/rewards may include an email to praise the increase in daily exercise, text messages to encourage family members to increase daily consumption of vegetables and fruits, and other rewards identified by the client.

In a nurse–family contract, the agreement may encourage family members to walk, jog, or bicycle together two to three times each week, or to modify their nutritional practices, such as increasing vegetables at family meals. Engaged family members serve as important sources of encouragement, reinforcement, and reward for one another due to their continuing contact and emotional bonding.

Answers to the following questions determine the effectiveness of the contract:

• Are the goals met fully, partially, or not at all?
• If failure occurred, what were the reasons?
• Is the client willing to rewrite or renegotiate the contract to increase the probability of success, or will the client terminate the contract?

Careful analysis of the contracting process and evaluation of subsequent outcomes enable the nurse and client to adjust the contract to move the client toward the desired health goals.

With a *self-contract*, the client is responsible for the behavioral commitment, monitoring, and reinforcement of identified behaviors. Self-contracting is an effective approach to enhancing control over behavior, thus creating a sense of independence, competence, and autonomy. The client does not become overly dependent on the nurse for reinforcements/rewards. Instead, individuals choose extrinsic sources for rewards such as tangible objects (new music app, cosmetics) or experiences (visit a friend, shopping, dinner with a friend), or intrinsic sources (self-praise, feelings of pride and success). Rewards must be highly desirable to have reinforcement value.

Success in fulfilling contracts enhances the client's self-esteem and problem-solving abilities. The client gains increased confidence in meeting future health needs. The client learns to manage a self-reward system to support new positive health practices.

Publicly announcing intentions to engage in a new behavior to family members and close friends is another way to increase commitment to a particular course of action. The positive expectations of family members or friends often enhance motivation to change behavior. Social media sites, including Facebook, blogs, and other online platforms, may also provide motivation and encouragement.

Integrating new behaviors into one's calendar is another important strategy to incorporate behaviors into daily routines, for example, exercise time scheduled during the lunch hour. The exercise appointment takes on importance, just as a lunch appointment with a friend or coworker. Lack of time is a frequent excuse for being unable to follow through with newly adopted behaviors, especially in workers in low-income jobs. Nurses need to work closely with these workers and their families to schedule time to accomplish health behaviors. Purchasing necessary supplies and equipment is another strategy to help make a commitment to behavior change. Clients are more likely to follow through with the desired behavior if they make a monetary investment. For example, people who have exercise equipment and videos in their homes are more likely to engage in physical activity than persons who do not have these resources. Nurses can work with low-income clients to help find resources in the community that might be available, such as community centers.

REVISED HEALTH PROMOTION–PREVENTION PLAN

An established schedule for periodic review of the health promotion–prevention plan ensures the client of the importance of the plan. Evaluation and resulting revisions made during office visits, coaching sessions via FaceTime, or other nonvisit contacts contribute to the process and increase commitment to the plan.

Impetus for changes in the plan may result from mastery of target behaviors, changes in client's values and priorities, or awareness of new options available to the client. Outdated plans fail to provide motivation or direction for change and become uninteresting and meaningless to the client. Periodic revisions and updates provide a systematic approach to assist the client in moving toward more positive health behaviors and a higher level of health.

COMMUNITY-LEVEL HEALTH PROMOTION–PREVENTION PLAN

Community-level planning and interventions may be the most effective way to engage members in improving their health. Important health concerns such as youth and family violence, substance abuse, unintended pregnancy in adolescents, and unintentional

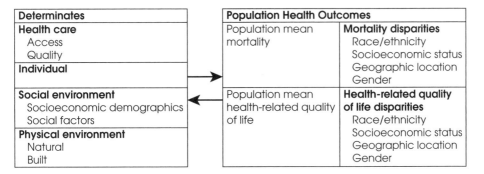

Determinates	Population Health Outcomes	
Health care Access Quality **Individual**	Population mean mortality	**Mortality disparities** Race/ethnicity Socioeconomic status Geographic location Gender
Social environment Socioeconomic demographics Social factors **Physical environment** Natural Built	Population mean health-related quality of life	**Health-related quality of life disparities** Race/ethnicity Socioeconomic status Geographic location Gender

FIGURE 5–4   Framework for Population Health Planning

Sources: Modified from Kindig and Brooke (2008); U.S. Centers for Disease Control and Prevention (2013). *Community health assessment for population health improvement.*

injuries require broad-based planning and intervention. Evidence has validated the influence of the community's social and physical environments on the health of its members (see Figure 5–4).

Financial resources, access to and quality of health services, social inequity, race, ethnicity, and culture are critical factors in developing a community plan for behavior change. Low-income families and minority populations often live in communities lacking the resources needed to focus on health promotion behaviors. However, it is now widely accepted that individuals cannot be separated from their communities and both need attention in achieving health. See Chapter 3 for a discussion on social capital and social-ecological models for multilevel behavior change. The nurse in her role as advocate consults with decision makers in communities and governmental institutions to improve the health of all citizens within the community.

CONSIDERATIONS FOR PRACTICE IN HEALTH PLANNING

Developing a plan to counsel clients about their health behaviors is a major responsibility of nurses in health promotion practice. The nurse must possess the skills necessary to enable clients to actively participate in developing a realistic, positive plan. Nurses with a working knowledge of current research evidence will ensure that accurate, timely information is incorporated into the plan.

An interdisciplinary approach often is more effective in interpreting the assessment data and recommending appropriate goals. Support is critical during the change process, so the nurse must learn to identify family members and other support systems for the client and to develop creative strategies to incorporate their support into the plan. The plan must be adapted to life span issues, gender, and cultural and socioeconomic differences.

Knowledge of a client's culture is important to the design of a culturally sensitive, age- and gender-appropriate plan. Whenever possible, technology is also an important resource to incorporate in developing the plan. Interactive software that provides feedback on achieving outcomes increases motivation, as immediate results are available. Developing a health promotion–prevention plan is straightforward, but complex. Nurses must continually update their skills to assist clients in this important process.

OPPORTUNITIES FOR RESEARCH IN THE PLANNING PROCESS

Nurses are in a pivotal position to address questions about planning for health promotion and prevention and to create new knowledge about the behavior change planning process. Answers to the following questions will enhance the behavior change process:

1. What is the effectiveness of combining face-to-face and computerized feedback from the health assessment in optimizing a client's level of motivation for health promotion planning?
2. Which technology apps are most effective in promoting clients' active participation in the health planning process?
3. What are the most effective family strategies to promote their participation in health planning for a family member?
4. What are the most effective criteria to evaluate health apps?
5. What are the major barriers to health planning for low-income, culturally diverse populations?

Summary

The health promotion–prevention plan provides individuals and families with a systematic approach to improve health practices and lifestyle. Clients are active participants and should receive a paper or electronic health portfolio that summarizes the health assessment, the health promotion–prevention plan, and other relevant information needed to implement the new behavior. It is essential that clients have all the information and planning documents needed to help reinforce their desired behavior changes. Focusing on outcomes desired by the client will energize and direct implementation of the plan. Evaluating and adjusting the plan as needed ensures client success. Community-level plans that address broad-based health concerns are complex and mandate broad support at multiple levels.

Learning Activities

1. Select a partner and develop an individual health plan using the nine-step planning process. Evaluate your experiences and outcomes.
2. Develop a health plan for a family with teenagers using the nine-step planning process.

Write a two-page summary of your experiences and outcomes.
3. Write a one-page summary of how community factors influence the individual and family planning processes you developed in Learning Activities 1 and 2.

References

Agency for Healthcare Research and Quality. (2016). *National healthcare quality and disparities report and 5th anniversary update on the national quality strategy.* Rockville, MD: Author. Retrieved from https://www.ahrq.gov

Alkhaldi, G., Hamilton, F., Lau, R., Webster, R., Michie, S., & Murray, E. (2016). The effectiveness of prompts to promote engagement with digital interventions: A systematic review. *Journal of Medical Internet Research, 18*(1), e6. doi:10.2106/jmir.4790

Centers for Disease Control and Prevention. (2011). *Strategies to prevent obesity and other chronic diseases: The CDC guide to strategies to increase physical activity in the community.* Atlanta, GA: U.S. Department of Health and Human Services.

Halbert, C., Bellamy, S., Briggs, V., Delmoor, E., Purnell, J., Rogers, R., . . . Johnson, J. (2017). A comparative effectiveness education trial for lifestyle health behavior change in African Americans. *Health Education Research, 32*(3), 207–218. doi:10.1093/her/cyx039

Hindhede, A., & Aagaard-Hansen, J. (2017). Using social network analysis as a method to assess and strengthen participation in health promotion programs in vulnerable areas. *Health Promotion Practice, 18*(2), 175–183. doi:10.1177/1524839916686029

Jerant, A., Kravitz, R., Fiscella, K., Sohler, N., Romero, R., Parnes, B., . . . Franks, P. (2013). Effects of tailored knowledge enhancement on colorectal cancer screening preference across ethic and language groups. *Patient Education and Counseling, 90*(1), 103–110. doi:10.1016/j.pec.2012.08.017

Kindig, D. A., & Brooke, B. (2008). A population health framework for setting national and state health goals. *Journal of the American Medical Association, 299*(17), 2081–2083.

King, A., Hekler, E., Grieco, L., Winter, S., Sheats, J., Buman, M., . . . Cirimele, J. (2013). Harnessing different motivational frames via mobile phones to promote daily physical activity and reduce sedentary behavior in aging adults. *PLoS One, 8*(4), e62613. doi:10.1371/journal.pone.0062613

Marin, H., & Delaney, C. (2017). Patient engagement and digital health communities. In H. Marin, E. Massad, M. A. Gutierrez, R. J. Rodriguez, & D. Sigulem (Eds.), *Global health informatics: How information technology can change our lives in a globalized world* (pp. 218–231). St. Louis, MO: Elsevier, Inc.

Middleton, K., Anton, S., & Perri, M. (2013). Long-term adherence to health behavior change. *American Journal of Lifestyle Medicine, 7*(6), 395–404. doi:10.1177/1559827613488867

Murray, J., Fenton, G., Honey, S., Bara, A., Hill, K., & House, A. (2013). A qualitative synthesis of factors influencing maintenance of lifestyle behavior changes in individuals with high cardiovascular risk. *BMC Cardiovascular Disorders, 13*, 48. doi:10.1186/1471-2261-13-48

Naslund, J., Aschbrenner, K., Marsch, L., & Bartels, S. (2016). Feasibility and acceptability of Facebook for health promotion among people with serious mental illness. *Digital Health, 2*, 1–10. doi:10.1177/2055207616654822

Nimkar, S. (2016). Promoting individual health using information technology: Trends in the US health system. *Health Education Journal, 75*(6), 744–752. doi:10.1177/0017896916632790

Prochaska, J. O., & DiClemente, C. C. (1983). Stages and processes of self-change of smoking: Toward an integrative model of change. *Journal of Consulting and Clinical Psychology, 51*, 390–395.

Ries, A., Blackman, L., Page, R., Gizlice, Z., Benedict, S., Barnes, K., . . . Carter-Edwards, L. (2014). Goal setting for health behavior change: Evidence from an obesity intervention for rural low-income women. *Rural and Remote Health, 14*, 2682.

Schoeppe, S., Alley, S., Van Lippevelde, W., Bray, N., Williams, S., Duncan, M., & Vandelanotte, C. (2016). Efficacy of interventions that use apps to improve diet, physical activity and sedentary behavior: A systematic review. *International Journal of Behavioral Nutrition and Physical Activity, 13*, 127. doi:10.1186/s12966-016-0454-y

Wayne, N., Perez, D., Kaplan, D., & Ritvo, P. (2015). Health coaching reduces HbA1c in type 2 diabetic patients from a lower-socioeconomic status community: A randomized controlled trial. *Journal of Medical Internet Research, 17*(10), e224. doi:10.2196/jmir.4871

PART 3

Interventions for Health Promotion and Prevention

CHAPTER 6

Physical Activity and Health Promotion

OBJECTIVES

This chapter will enable the reader to:

1. List the benefits and risks of physical activity.
2. Describe strategies to develop a physically active lifestyle across the life span.
3. Describe the application of the social-ecological model to promote physical activity.
4. Describe the relationship of built environments and active lifestyles in communities.
5. List the pros and cons of community interventions including digitalized technologies to promote physical activity.
6. Examine strategies for developing and implementing culturally appropriate physical activity interventions.

Regular physical activity is essential for healthy, energetic, and productive living. Automobiles, televisions, computers, mobile devices, video games, other sedentary activities, and low levels of physical activity in school and work environments necessitate a commitment of significant leisure time to physical activity. Changes are needed at all levels to reverse the growing sedentary lifestyle and increasing obesity across the life span by integrating physical activity into everyday life.

Physical activity, body movement produced by skeletal muscles, results in expenditure of energy and includes occupational, leisure-time, and routine daily activities. *Lifestyle physical activities*, carried out in the course of everyday life, contribute to energy expenditure, such as climbing the stairs instead of taking the elevator. *Exercise*, a subcategory of physical activity, aims to improve or maintain physical fitness or health through planned, structured, repetitive activities performed during leisure time. *Physical fitness* is a measure of a person's ability to perform physical activities that require endurance, strength, or flexibility, and is determined by a combination of cardiorespiratory endurance (aerobic power), flexibility, balance, and body composition (U.S. Department of Health and Human Services, 2008). In this chapter, the term physical activity encompasses a broad range of activities that, if performed regularly, will improve health.

Maintenance of regular physical activity is dependent on personal and social motivation within the day-to-day environment. Family, peers, and the community play a powerful role in encouraging active lifestyles. Many individuals rely on the school or work environments to create programs to help them achieve their physical activity goals. Others cycle through periods of activity and inactivity, never establishing regular physical activity patterns.

While the increase in the rate of obesity has slowed in recent years, obesity is one of the most serious and prevalent health problems in the United States (National Academies of Sciences, Engineering, and Medicine, 2016). The prevalence of overweight and obesity among children, adolescents, and adults is due to genetic influences, high-stress situations, environmental influences, and primarily dietary and physical activity behaviors (Centers for Disease Control and Prevention retrieved March 15, 2017, from https://www.cdc.gov/obesity/; Rauner, Mess, & Woll, 2013). Despite the abundance of evidence that physical inactivity and weight gain are associated, a significant proportion of the U.S. population remains sedentary. Because of the central role of physical activity in health, this chapter focuses on strategies to increase physical activity for clients of all ages, and racial, ethnic, cultural, and socioeconomic groups.

HEALTH BENEFITS OF PHYSICAL ACTIVITY

Regular physical activity contributes to physiological stability and high-level functioning. Research demonstrates the health benefits of participating in regular physical activity. For example, the U.S. Department of Health and Human Services (USDHHS) Physical Activity Guidelines Advisory Committee rated the evidence of health benefits as strong, moderate, or weak for children, adolescents, adults, and older adults. Type, number, and quality of published research, as well as consistency of findings across studies, determined the rating system. Current research is under review by the agency to update the 2008 Physical Activity Guidelines, which are expected to be released to the public in 2018. See the USDHHS website (www.hhs.gov) for more information.

Table 6–1 lists the rated health benefits of physical activity in all ages and all ethnic and racial groups. Scientific evidence documents the role of physical activity in (a) reducing the risk of premature death, (b) managing chronic health problems, (c) improving cardiorespiratory and metabolic health, (d) decreasing the risks for overweight and obesity, and (e) preserving bone, joint, and muscle health.

In addition, regular physical activity improves or maintains physical function, lowers the risk for colon and breast cancer, lessens the risk for depression and cognitive decline, and results in healthier skin, vibrancy, and sense of well-being. Millions of Americans are at risk for a wide range of common mental health problems that might well be prevented or modified by active lifestyles. Regular physical activity improves mental health, reduces stress, increases one's ability to do everyday tasks better, and serves as adjunct treatment in mental health disorders (National Academies of Sciences, Engineering, and Medicine, 2016; Smith, Potter, McLaren, & Blumenthal, 2013; VanKim & Nelson, 2013).

TABLE 6–1 Health Benefits Associated with Regular Physical Activity

Children and Adolescents

Strong evidence
- Improved cardiorespiratory and muscular fitness
- Improved bone health
- Improved cardiovascular and metabolic health biomarkers
- Favorable body composition

Moderate evidence
- Reduced symptoms of depression

Adults and Older Adults

Strong evidence
- Lower risk of early death
- Lower risk of coronary heart disease
- Lower risk of stroke
- Lower risk of high blood pressure
- Lower risk of adverse blood lipid profile
- Lower risk of type 2 diabetes
- Lower risk of metabolic syndrome
- Lower risk of colon cancer
- Lower risk of breast cancer
- Prevention of weight gain
- Weight loss, particularly when combined with reduced calorie intake
- Improved cardiorespiratory and muscular fitness
- Prevention of falls
- Reduced depression
- Better cognitive function (for older adults)

Moderate to strong evidence
- Better functional health (for older adults)
- Reduced abdominal obesity

Moderate evidence
- Lower risk of hip fracture
- Lower risk of lung cancer
- Lower risk of endometrial cancer
- Weight maintenance after weight loss
- Increased bone density
- Improved sleep quality

Source: U.S. Department of Health and Human Services. (2008). *Physical activity guidelines for Americans.* Retrieved July 17, 2009, from http://www.health.gov/paguidelines

Among children and adolescents, weight-bearing exercise is essential for normal skeletal development and attainment of peak bone mass. Regular physical activity increases strength and agility across all age groups, prevents falls among older adults, and increases independence in activities of daily living in older adults and persons with disabilities. Physical activity maintains and enhances quality of life for all age groups (Chen & Lee, 2013; Maher, Pincus, Ram, & Conroy, 2015).

POTENTIAL RISKS OF PHYSICAL ACTIVITY

Moderate-intensity physical activity is associated with very low risk for adverse events. A vigorous-intensity approach to physical activity may exaggerate existing health conditions and put individuals, particularly older adults, at risk for untoward effects. See the "Prescribing Physical Activity to Achieve Health Benefits" section later in this chapter for definitions of moderate and intensive physical activity. If an individual has an undiagnosed heart condition and is habitually sedentary, strenuous physical activity may create arrhythmias or precipitate a cardiac arrest or myocardial infarction, although adverse events are not common. Individuals over 50 years of age, or with an existing chronic illness such as obesity, diabetes, or cardiovascular disease, require a medical evaluation before starting regular physical activity. Persons with cardiovascular disease or other chronic conditions should avoid activity at levels that are physiologically untenable or result in untoward symptoms. Recommendations for pre-exercise evaluation in older adults with diagnosed chronic cardiovascular disease include an exercise stress test, health history, physical examination, and behavioral counseling (Lanier, Bury, & Richardson, 2016). Overstressing muscles and joints will result in muscle soreness and joint pain. The risk of musculoskeletal injury increases with the total amount of physical activity. A program of gradually increasing physical activity with an emphasis on moderate activity for older adults produces benefits that far outweigh the potential risks.

Proper warm-up and cool-down are important for any physical activity. Before physical activity, warming up is important to increase blood flow to the heart and skeletal muscles, enhance oxygenation of tissues, and increase flexibility of muscles. The warm-up period allows the heart rate and body temperature to increase gradually and the joints to become more flexible prior to initiating physical activity. Warm-up includes activities such as slow walking, arm circles, leg exercises, or wall push-ups. The warm-up period should last about 7–10 minutes and be followed immediately by moderate or vigorous physical activity. A cooling-down period is essential after physical activity. It is important to take time to cool down for 5–10 minutes following physical activity because physical activity raises heart rate, blood pressure, body temperature, and lactic acid in the muscles. Cooling down allows the heart rate to decrease gradually and prevents pooling of blood in muscles that can cause lightheadedness. During the cool-down period, it is important to keep the lower extremities moving in activities such as slow walking, jogging, or cycling. Warm-up and cool-down periods may include stretching after muscles are warm from activity. At the end of the cooling-down period, the client's resting heart rate should be lower than 100 beats per minute.

GENETICS, ENVIRONMENT, AND PHYSICAL ACTIVITY

Although exercise genetics and genomics research has been ongoing for several years, it is still in its infancy. However, there is consistent evidence showing that a genetic susceptibility to obesity and hypertriglyceridemia is reduced with physical activity versus inactivity (Loos et al., 2015). In other words, factors in the environment (physical activity behavior) modify the genetic risk, or the effect of the environmental exposure varies with the individual's genetic background. Shared family factors (household and environmental) as well as genetics play a role in individual differences in responses to exercise. Geographic differences in the incidence of disease, as well as differences in disease in immigrant populations, also support the idea of a role for environmental influences, which includes lifestyles (Cheek & Howington, 2017).

Studies of twins have also shed light on the gene–environment interaction in physical activity. In one twin study, genetics was found to contribute to differences in body composition, ranging from none to 21%, and to cardiorespiratory fitness differences ranging from 22 to 57% (Zadro et al., 2017). Gender differences in genetic variations were also reported. As research continues, these types of finding will have implications for predicting who will respond more positively to physical activity.

PRESCRIBING PHYSICAL ACTIVITY TO ACHIEVE HEALTH BENEFITS

To achieve health benefits, medium and high levels of regular physical activity are essential. Baseline activities are the light-intensity activities of daily life, such as climbing one flight of stairs, standing, or carrying lightweight objects. These are not health-enhancing physical activities. Health-enhancing physical activities produce benefits that increase quality of life.

The 2008 Physical Activity Guidelines describe four levels of physical activity for adults: inactive, low, medium, and high (U.S. Department of Health and Human Services, 2008). Low levels of physical activity amount to activity less than 150 minutes (2 hours and 30 minutes) per week. Medium physical activity refers to a range of 150–300 minutes of moderate-intensity physical activity a week, or 75–150 minutes of vigorous-intensity physical activity to obtain substantial benefits. A high level of physical activity is more than 300 minutes of moderate-intensity activity a week.

The American College of Sports Medicine includes frequency and duration—as well as intensity—in its guidelines and recommends 30 minutes of moderate-intensity activity five days a week, or a minimum of 20 minutes of high-intensity activity three days a week (Garber et al., 2011). Intensity (how hard), frequency (how often), and duration (how long) all make up the exercise prescription. However, for health benefits, the total amount of activity (minutes of moderate-intensity physical activity) is more important than any one component (U.S. Department of Health and Human Services, 2008).

A daily 30-minute structured exercise routine accumulated in 10-minute bouts has been shown to be as effective as 30 consecutive minutes of structured exercise in reducing cardiovascular disease risk factors. The 10-minute bout approach may be more appealing because adults are more likely to adopt and maintain an active lifestyle that is more in line with their natural interests and tendencies than to commit to a structured exercise program (Lee, Emerson, & Williams, 2016). The cost effectiveness of the active lifestyle approach compared to a structured exercise program is also an important consideration (Loprinzi & Cardinal, 2013).

Advanced practice nurses routinely counsel clients about physical activity and may be involved in developing exercise prescriptions and, therefore, should be knowledgeable about metabolic equivalent of task (MET). Likewise, nurses working in outpatient settings may be involved in helping explain MET equivalents to clients. Nurses report knowledge and confidence in some level of physical activity, but many acknowledge the need for additional education to prescribe exercise programs (Grimstvedt et al., 2012). A MET is the ratio of the rate of energy expenditure during an activity compared to the rate of energy expenditure at rest. One MET is the rate of energy expenditure at rest. Because the public is not familiar with METs, clients are more likely to understand activity recommendations in number of minutes needed per week and level of intensity. Additional information on MET equivalents is available on the Web.

The required minimum number and range of minutes per week for activities of moderate intensity is straightforward. Adults should participate in at least 30 minutes of moderate-intensity activity on a minimum of five days a week for a total of at least 150 minutes per week. A moderate-intensity activity can be explained as a level of effort of 5 or 6 on a scale of 0 to 10, where 0 is the effort level when sitting and 10 is all-out maximal effort. This effort produces noticeable changes in heart rate and breathing. A vigorous-intensity activity is 7 or 8 on a 10-point scale, which produces large increases in heart rate and breathing. The general rule of thumb is that one minute of vigorous-intensity activity is equivalent to two minutes of moderate-intensity activity. A person doing moderate-intensity activity is able to talk but not sing during the activity, and a person who is doing vigorous-intensity physical activity is only able to say a few words before pausing for a breath.

Most studies and measures define physical activity as leisure-time activity based on self-reported participation in "moderate" or "vigorous" physical activity in the past week or month. Recall bias and differences in interpreting the terms "moderate" and "vigorous" are factors that help explain inconsistencies between self-report and actual physical activity behaviors. In addition, education and literacy levels in understanding the terms may play a role, pointing to the need to ask about specific activities, including leisure and work-related activities (Saffer, Dave, Grossman, & Leung, 2013).

Another recommendation for daily physical activity is to walk 10,000 steps per day. Walking less than 5,000 steps is considered a sedentary activity behavior pattern (Tudor-Locke, 2014). Research has also shown that moderate-intensity activity is equivalent to walking 3,000 steps in 30 minutes for five days a week or three daily bouts of 1,000 steps in 10 minutes for five days each week. Moderate-intensity activity is considered equivalent to a minimum of 100 steps per minute. These guidelines point to the need to consider both number of steps taken daily and the intensity of the activity to achieve health benefits (Marshall et al., 2009; Matthews, Hagstromer, Pober, & Bowles, 2012; Tudor-Locke et al., 2011).

Pedometers have been used to self-monitor steps for many years. Early devices only counted steps, and have expanded to provide additional information about distance walked, total number of minutes spent walking, and number of minutes spent in aerobic walking. Pedometers have evolved to tracking devices and other electronic tracking monitors incorporated into applications (apps) in smartphones as well as wearable technology. These devices work as pedometers and interface with mobile apps to provide tailored, ongoing feedback (Bice, Ball, & McClaran, 2016). All forms of tracking devices have the potential to increase motivation to be physically active through tailored messages, continuous feedback, and self-monitoring.

PROMOTING PHYSICAL ACTIVITY ACROSS THE LIFE SPAN

The realization that many risk factors for cardiovascular disease, including obesity, hypertension, and elevated cholesterol, are evident in early childhood has increased interest in life span patterns of physical activity (Ogden, Carroll, Kit, & Flegal, 2014). Furthermore, of the major modifiable risk factors for coronary heart disease (elevated cholesterol, smoking, hypertension, and inactivity), physical inactivity is most prevalent across the life span. Despite the evidence of health benefits, more than half of Americans are not active enough to gain the physical and mental health benefits of physical activity (National Academies of Sciences, Engineering, and Medicine, 2016).

Patterns of physical activity that begin early in life are likely to persist over time. It is easier to develop positive physical activity patterns early in life than to change unhealthy behaviors after they are established habits. Lifestyle activities provide flexibility for increasing energy expenditure by altering daily patterns. Activities such as parking at a distance from your destination, taking stairs instead of elevators and escalators, walking to and from work or school, and walking during lunchtime or after school or work are ways to integrate physical activities into daily life (see Figure 6–1).

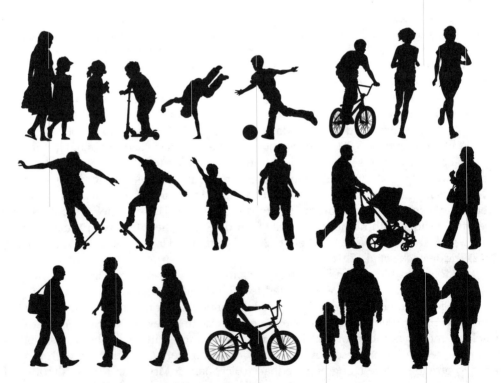

FIGURE 6–1   Fun Leisure-Time Physical Activities Reduce Stress and Encourage Adherence to Exercise Plan

PROMOTING PHYSICAL ACTIVITY IN CHILDREN AND ADOLESCENTS

Regular physical activity has many immediate and long-term health benefits for children and adolescents. It improves cardiovascular fitness, increases bone mass, and enhances mental well-being. It is also associated with less obesity, hypertension, and cigarette smoking, which prevent the development of cardiovascular disease, diabetes, and other chronic diseases in adulthood (Ogden et al., 2014).

Unfortunately, a significant number of children and adolescents do not participate in the level of regular activity needed to achieve health benefits. In addition, the rise in childhood and adolescent obesity is alarming. In the past 30 years, the prevalence of obesity has more than doubled among children and more than tripled in adolescents (Ogden et al., 2014). Although evidence indicates the trend is beginning to level off in children of college-educated parents, the large number of obese children and adolescents across all socioeconomic levels warrants strategies for lifestyle change. Studies consistently show that only about a third of high school adolescents and about two-thirds of children 9–13 years of age achieve the recommended amount of daily physical activity. Adolescent males are more physically active than adolescent girls, and Whites are more physically active than Hispanics or African Americans. Gender and type of physical activity influence motivation to exercise and are essential to consider in planning programs during adolescence (U.S. Department of Health and Human Services, 2008).

Social networking sites (SNSs), frequented by 91% of teens, have the potential to engage adolescents in achieving and maintaining physical activity goals (Laranjo, 2016). For example, many gamers play Pokémon Go (digital app) on smartphones, where players identify a virtual figure on their phone camera and walk to real-world locations to "catch" it. One study showed that Pokémon Go players added 2,000 steps a day to their step count and were more likely to walk 10,000 steps a day than they did before playing the game (Xu & Goldberg, 2017). However, maintaining the increased steps after the player loses interest in the game is not likely unless the player values the additional exercise or substitutes a similar physical activity app. There are risks associated with use of SNSs by adolescents. The questionable quality and validity of SNSs require adult supervision to monitor adolescents' use of information on these sites.

Gender and Physical Activity in Children and Adolescents

Physical activity patterns and related influences vary by gender. Gender differences start in adolescence. Boys report greater physical activity than girls in the preteen years and have been shown to increase their level of physical activity until about 11 years of age, plateau, and then decrease beginning about 13 years of age. Adolescent girls increase their activity until 12 or 13 years and then decrease, similar to boys. The Gates Millennium Study, a longitudinal cohort study with 8 years follow-up, found no evidence that physical activity decline was greater in girls than in boys. Physical activity level declined in both genders beginning at 7 years of age (Farooq et al., 2017). Specific factors associated with a decline in physical activity for boys and girls include increased screen time, changes in attitude toward physical education, perceived parental attitude about body shape and fitness, self-esteem, perceived attitude of peers about physical activity, and increase in risky behaviors, that is, binge drinking, recreational drug use, and smoking.

Implementing Guidelines for Physical Activity in Children and Adolescents

The physical activity recommendation for children and adolescents is a minimum of 60 minutes or more of moderate or vigorous physical activity every day (U.S. Department of Health and Human Services, 2008). Children and adolescents should participate in vigorous-intensity activities at least three days per week. Three types of activity are important: *aerobic*, *muscle-strengthening*, and *bone-strengthening activities* (see Chapter 4). *Aerobic* activities, such as running, hopping, skipping, jumping rope, swimming, dancing, and bicycling, increase cardiorespiratory fitness. *Muscle-strengthening* activities in this age group are usually unstructured, such as climbing on playground equipment. Structured *muscle-strengthening activities* for adolescents may include weight lifting. Activities that promote *bone growth* and *strength* include running, basketball, hopscotch, and jumping rope. Adolescents are more likely to engage in structured programs or play sports that provide aerobic benefits than unstructured activities, the opposite of what adults prefer. Examples of aerobic, muscle-strengthening, and bone-strengthening activities are provided in Table 6–2.

Physical activity should be age appropriate and enjoyable and should include a variety of activities. Sedentary and obese children may have difficulty performing physical activity for 60 minutes, so exercise should begin gradually and increase at regular intervals until the children are active for one hour. Developmentally appropriate activities are those that are suitable for the child's physical and cognitive development. A range of noncompetitive and competitive activities, age and ability appropriate, is necessary to achieve physical activity goals.

Interventions aimed at decreasing sedentary behavior, such as limiting screen time to two hours daily, including sitting-based social media and online chatting, are more likely to promote physical activity. Television is of particular concern due to the associated unhealthy eating habits that often accompany watching television, such as chips and sodas. A review of studies showed that the involvement of families, parental modeling, healthy eating at home, behavioral interventions, and electronic physical activity monitoring devices were effective strategies, especially for children under 11 years of age (Barkin et al., 2017; Biddle, Petrolini, & Pearson, 2014; Jackson et al., 2017).

The physical *inactivity* level of preschoolers has followed the pattern for primary, secondary, and high school students. In a seven-county study of preschoolers, only 54% of the children were sufficiently physically active (Espana-Romero, Mitchell, Dowda, O'Neill, & Pate, 2013). The amount of time spent in daycare with limited physical activity, increase in screen viewing (television, video games, computers, and wireless devices), greater parental safety concerns, and constraints in places to play have resulted in a dramatic increase in preschoolers' sedentary behavior.

Physical activity habits begin to develop in preschool years, so this age group needs interventions to increase physical activity. The national physical activity guidelines do not include preschool children, ages 3–5 years. However, the National Association for Sports and Physical Education recommends 60 minutes of structured physical activity and at least 60 minutes of unstructured physical activity daily for preschoolers (American Heart Association, 2016).

Preschools are an important place to implement interventions because more than half of the children in the United States attend preschool. Studies show that when the

TABLE 6–2   Aerobic and Muscle- and Bone-Strengthening Activities

Type of Physical Activity	Age Group	
	Children	**Adolescents**
Moderate-intensity aerobic	• Active recreation such as hiking, skateboarding, and rollerblading • Bicycle riding • Walking to school	• Active recreation such as canoeing, hiking, cross-country skiing, skateboarding, and rollerblading • Brisk walking • Bicycle riding (stationary or road bike) • House and yard work such as sweeping or pushing a lawn mower • Playing games that require catching and throwing, such as baseball, softball, basketball, and volleyball
Vigorous aerobic	• Active games involving running and chasing, such as tag • Bicycle riding • Jumping rope • Martial arts such as karate • Running • Sports such as ice or field hockey, basketball, swimming, tennis, or gymnastics	• Active games involving running and chasing, such as flag football, soccer • Bicycle riding • Jumping rope • Martial arts such as karate • Running • Sports such as tennis, ice or field hockey, basketball, and swimming • Vigorous dancing • Aerobics • Cheerleading or gymnastics
Muscle-strengthening	• Games such as tug of war • Modified push-ups (with knees on the floor) • Resistance exercises using body weight or resistance bands • Rope or tree climbing • Sit-ups • Swinging on playground equipment/bars • Gymnastics	• Games such as tug of war • Push-ups • Resistance exercises with exercise bands, weight machines, handheld weights • Rock climbing • Sit-ups • Cheerleading or gymnastics
Bone-strengthening	• Games such as hop-scotch • Hopping, skipping, jumping • Jumping rope • Running • Sports such as gymnastics, basketball, volleyball, and tennis	• Hopping, skipping, jumping • Jumping rope • Running • Sports such as gymnastics, basketball, volleyball, and tennis

Source: Centers for Disease Control and Prevention. Retrieved July 17, 2009, from http://www.cdc.gov/physicalactivity/everyone/guidelines/what_counts.html

preschooler, teacher, and parent are involved in interventions, positive changes result (Barkin et al., 2017). In addition, activity-friendly playgrounds that include balls, hoops, tricycles, movable equipment, and structured activities tend to increase physical activity in this age group.

PROMOTING PHYSICAL ACTIVITY IN FAMILIES

Family-based activities are important in promoting healthy lifestyles in children, adolescents, and adults. Parents' lifestyles influence their children's risk of developing active or inactive lifestyles as young adults. For example, parental obesity places male and female adolescents at greater risk for being overweight as adults. Parents influence their children's physical behavior by being directly involved in activities with their children, offering encouragement and support, and providing opportunities and resources to engage in recreational sports and programs (Biddle et al., 2014).

Family-based programs encourage parents to be active with their children in relationship-building experiences. For example, bike outings and aerobic and recreational activities create opportunities for parents to be role models for active lifestyles. Although the physical environment is important in the decision to walk to school, parental support for walking or cycling is associated with increases in physical activity, especially among younger children. Interventions to increase physical activity behaviors in children and adolescents should target the entire family.

Family-based programs are often a major challenge, as parents may be difficult to reach and recruit due to family/work commitments. Contacting families during organized activities is more effective than sending written materials home with the child. Telephone and wireless device interventions with family members also show promise. The intensity of the physical activity needs to be high enough to produce an effect, as intensive intervention programs result in greater behavior change. Programs that involve parent(s)/guardians in physical activities are successful in increasing time spent in physical activity by both children and adults. Childhood and adolescence are ideal periods to cultivate regular physical activity that can reap positive health benefits throughout life.

PROMOTING PHYSICAL ACTIVITY IN SCHOOLS

Schools play a major role in promoting involvement of children in recreational activities that they can enjoy for a lifetime. By promoting physical activity on a daily basis, teaching the personal value of regular activity, and encouraging continuing involvement in moderate-to-vigorous activities both at school and at home, schools contribute to the goal of an "active" generation.

In 2014, the U.S. Department of Health and Human Services developed strategies to increase physical activity among young people. The strategies highlight interventions that increase physical activity in youth across a variety of settings, including schools. Schools are an ideal setting for promotion of physical activities because they:

1. Have intense and continuous contact with most children ages 5–16 years
2. Employ teachers who have an interest in health promotion

3. Have appropriate facilities (gymnasium, sports equipment, and playground)
4. Have structured blocks of time (recess, lunch)
5. Have the capacity to interact with community-based activity providers

School strategies focus on increasing time allotted to physical education classes taught by well-prepared teachers and include moderate-to-vigorous physical activity; promoting short bouts of physical activity during classroom breaks; planning physical activities before and after school; providing space and equipment for after-school activities; and building individual student behavioral skills. The times allotted for recess and lunch are ideal for offering structured physical activities. Many elementary schools offer supervised after-school running programs for boys and girls. Efforts to encourage parents or community volunteers to walk/bike to school with students or support the "walking school bus" concept build community and provide positive role models for students. Multicomponent school-based programs are effective in increasing levels of physical activity, physical fitness, aerobic capacity, and time spent in moderate-to-vigorous activities. Based on the consistently positive results, the *Healthy People 2020* Steering Committee of the Midcourse Report recommends that these programs be adapted for all elementary, middle, and high school students (Centers for Disease Control and Prevention, Office of Disease Prevention and Health Promotion, 2014).

PROMOTING PHYSICAL ACTIVITY IN ADULTS AND OLDER ADULTS

Physical inactivity is associated with the risk of developing the major chronic diseases, including cardiovascular diseases, type 2 diabetes, and cancer. Sedentary (sitting) time, for example, screen time at home and work, travel time, and watching sports, accounts for the majority of an adult's waking hours. Sitting behaviors are receiving increasing attention as a potential risk factor for chronic diseases. Adults who meet the 30-minute recommended physical activity for most days of the week yet are sedentary (sitting) for the remaining hours may risk serious adverse health consequences. The 30-minute physical activity recommendation is not likely to be protective for those who spend their remaining hours in sedentary behaviors (Owen, 2012). In a systematic review of the relationship between sedentary behaviors and risks for diabetes and cardiovascular disease, results showed that sedentary behavior is associated with type 2 diabetes and cardiovascular disease risk, with greater sitting time associated with greater risk (Dempsey, Owen, Biddle, & Dunstan, 2014). Time spent in sedentary activities has also been associated with waist circumference as well as cardiovascular risk (Tigbe, Granat, Sattar, & Lean, 2017). These findings are associations only and support the need for more research with this potential risk factor (Mansoubi, Pearson, Biddle, & Clemes, 2014; Schoenborn, Adams, & Peregoy, 2013) (see Figure 6–2).

Regular physical activity prevents or reduces the risk for cardiovascular diseases, as well as improves quality of life in adults and older adults. Physical activity in older adults protects against loss of mobility and increases functional independence, flexibility and balance through improved muscle mass, increased bone density, and cardiovascular fitness (Ahn, Smith, & Ory, 2012; World Health Organization, 2011).

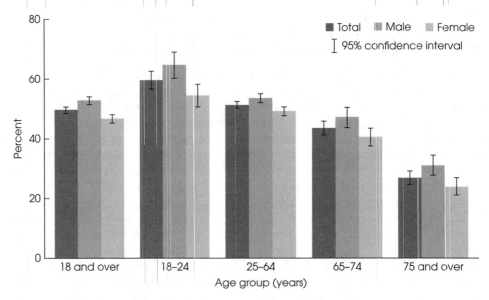

FIGURE 6-2   Percentage of Adults Aged 18 and Over Who Met 2008 Federal Physical Activity Guidelines for Aerobic Activity through Leisure-Time Aerobic Activity, by Age Group and Sex: United States, January–September 2015

Source: Clarke, Ward, Freeman, & Schiller (2016).

Racial and Gender Differences in Physical Activity in Adults and Older Adults

Physical activity varies across race and gender. Leisure-time physical activity is significantly lower among Asians, Blacks, Hispanics, and Native Americans compared to Whites (see Figure 6–3).

Work-related physical activity has been reported to be lowest among Whites and people with higher education and highest in blue-collar and minority groups. Work-related physical activity compares to leisure-time physical activity only when the work is strenuous, that is, physically demanding jobs in construction, manufacturing, and agriculture, and meets the intensity and duration of physical activity guidelines. Recreational (non-work) physical activity is related to positive physical and mental health outcomes. However, the ability to access recreational activity depends on factors such as living environment, working hours, education, and socioeconomic status. Time and money scarcities are major barriers to leisure-time physical activity. Attention to these findings will help reduce the disparities among race, ethnicity, and gender (Saffer et al., 2013; Venn & Strazdins, 2017).

Women report less leisure-time physical activity than do men, as they spend more time in paid and unpaid working roles. Multiple family obligations decrease women's time for physical activity. Unmarried women generally are more active than married women with children at home. Role changes in women's lives, including parenthood, employment, children leaving home, parental caregiving, and retirement, influence leisure-time physical activity.

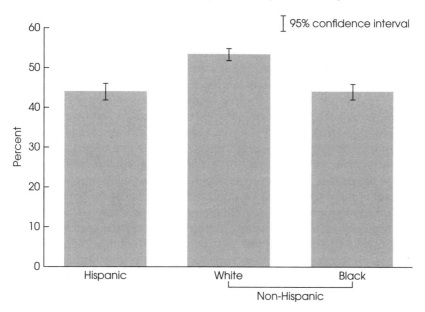

FIGURE 6–3   Age–Sex-Adjusted Percentage of Adults Aged 18 and Over Who Met 2008 Federal Physical Activity Guidelines for Aerobic Activity through Leisure-Time Aerobic Activity, by Race/Ethnicity: United States, January–September 2015

Source: Clarke et al. (2016).

Implementing Physical Activity Guidelines for Adults and Older Adults

The 2008 Guidelines recommend that adults under age 65 need to participate in at least 150 minutes each week of moderate-intensity aerobic activity or 75 minutes of vigorous-intensity physical activity each week. These levels of physical activity offer substantial benefits for lowering one's risk of heart disease and stroke, type 2 diabetes, and depression (U.S. Department of Health and Human Services, 2008). As stated previously, the benefits are dose-related, so that 300 minutes per week result in additional benefits, which include lower risk for colon and breast cancer and prevention of weight gain.

Also recommended are muscle-strengthening activities to increase muscle fitness and bone strength. Muscle-strengthening activities include weight lifting, resistance bands, calisthenics, carrying heavy loads, and gardening. Major muscle groups worked at moderate-to-high intensity levels for at least two days a week meet the requirement.

Inactive adults need to *begin slowly* and *gradually* increase the activity over a period of weeks to months. For example, they may begin with five minutes of slow walking several times a day and slowly increase each session. Initially, muscle-strengthening activities, performed one day a week at a light- or moderate-intensity effort, are then increased to exceed the minimum level.

Structured programs have been successful with both adults and older adults. Sedentary behavior increases with age, and older adults (65 years and older) are the most sedentary group. However, aerobic and strength-building activities are essential for healthy aging, and older adults should be encouraged to develop or continue healthy lifestyle habits. The guidelines for younger adults also apply to individuals 65 years and older: a minimum of 150 minutes of moderate-intensity physical activity, or 75 minutes of vigorous-intensity physical activity each week, or a combination of the two. All types of activities count, including walking the dog and taking an exercise class. Supervision may be initially required for older adults to ensure a moderate level of effort, especially for adults with low fitness levels.

Older adults also benefit from muscle strengthening. They should perform 8–10 exercises using resistance, such as weights, at 10–15 repetitions for each exercise, a minimum of two days a week. These exercises, performed at the same level of intensity as aerobic activities: 5 to 6 on a 10-point scale for moderate intensity and 7 to 8 for vigorous intensity, contribute to stamina and strength. Vigorous-intensity activities performed under supervision or by a physically fit adult are safe.

Older adults at risk for falls also need to perform balance training three days a week. Examples of exercises in a balance program include walking backward, walking sideways, heel and toe walking, and standing from a sitting position. Pilates and yoga strengthen the core muscles, and tai chi training improves balance and strength in older adults.

Adherence to home-structured exercise programs to prevent falls in persons over 60 years is low. Most adults enjoy the socialization associated with structured programs and place less emphasis on follow-up at home. Adherence improves in interventions where there is technological support and face-to-face contact (Simek, McPhate, & Haines, 2012).

Older adults consist of the young old (65–74 years), middle old (75–84 years), and very old (over 85 years). The ability to be physically active varies over this age spectrum. Getting older adults to engage in an active lifestyle is particularly challenging, as evidenced by the fact that only 14% of adults ages 65 to 74 years exercise and only 7% of those over 75 years exercise regularly (Anderson-Hanley et al., 2012).

Barriers to physical activity are important considerations for the elderly. Although work and family demands may lessen with age, convenience of facilities, cost, opportunities for interacting with others, fear of resultant illness or injury, disability, and sensory impairment become more important. Concerns about existing medical conditions may be a further deterrent to an active lifestyle. Environmental barriers such as weather (extreme temperatures, precipitation), presence or quality of sidewalks, and lack of places to sit and rest while walking are concerns of older adults.

Many older adults also have misconceptions about physical activity, believing that it can be unhealthy. Addressing barriers by including an educational component with physical activity programs may increase participation. Emphasis should be on reducing sedentary activity and increasing moderate activity; vigorous activities should be limited to select older adults with appropriate fitness levels. A stepwise program (additive approach) decreases the risks of injury and allows participants to gain experience and self-confidence in performing the activity. Table 6-3 describes strategies for all adults to overcome the major barriers to physical activity.

Inactive adults and adults with chronic conditions should consult with their health care provider who will assess their ability and recommend the level of participation in physical activity. Inactive adults should begin very slowly and increase activity gradually over a period of months. If an older adult who has a chronic condition is unable to meet the target goal of 150 minutes a week, even 60 minutes of moderate-intensity activity will produce some health benefits. Warm-up and cool-down activities are extremely important.

Tailored programs to increase physical activity in adults include attention to their interests, preferences, and readiness to change. *The CDC Guide to Increase Physical*

TABLE 6–3   Strategies for Overcoming Barriers to Physical Activity

Barrier	Strategies
Lack of time	Identify available time slots. Monitor your daily activities for one week. Identify at least three 30-minute time slots you could use for physical activity.
	Add physical activity to your daily routine. For example, walk or ride your bike to work or shopping, organize school activities around physical activity, walk the dog, exercise while you watch TV, park farther away from your destination, etc.
	Select activities requiring minimal time, such as walking, jogging, or stair climbing.
Social influence	Explain your interest in physical activity to friends and family. Ask them to support your efforts.
	Invite friends and family members to exercise with you. Plan social activities involving exercise.
	Develop new friendships with physically active people. Join a group, such as the YMCA or a hiking club.
Lack of energy	Schedule physical activity for times in the day or week when you feel energetic.
	Convince yourself that if you give it a chance, physical activity will increase your energy level, and then, try it.
Lack of motivation	Plan ahead. Make physical activity a regular part of your daily or weekly schedule and write it on your calendar.
	Invite a friend to exercise with you on a regular basis and write it on both your calendars.
	Join an exercise group or class.
Fear of injury	Learn how to warm up and cool down to prevent injury.
	Learn how to exercise appropriately considering your age, fitness level, skill level, and health status.
	Choose activities involving minimum risk.
Lack of skill	Select activities requiring no new skills, such as walking, climbing stairs, or jogging.
	Take a class to develop new skills.
Lack of resources	Select activities that require minimal facilities or equipment, such as walking, jogging, jumping rope, or calisthenics.
	Identify inexpensive, convenient resources available in your community (community education programs, park and recreation programs, worksite programs, etc.).
Weather conditions	Develop a set of regular activities that are always available regardless of weather (indoor cycling, aerobic dance, indoor swimming, calisthenics, stair climbing, rope skipping, mall walking, dancing, gymnasium games, etc.).

(Continued)

TABLE 6–3   Strategies for Overcoming Barriers to Physical Activity (Continued)

Barrier	Strategies
Travel	Put a jump rope in your suitcase and jump rope.
	Walk the halls and climb the stairs in hotels.
	Stay in places with swimming pools or exercise facilities.
	Join the YMCA or YWCA (ask about reciprocal membership agreement).
	Visit the local shopping mall and walk for half an hour or more.
	Bring your mp3 player with your favorite aerobic exercise music.
Family obligations	Trade babysitting time with a friend, neighbor, or family member who also has small children.
	Exercise with the kids: go for a walk together, play tag or other running games, get an aerobic dance or exercise tape for kids (there are several on the market) and exercise together. You can spend time together and still get your exercise.
	Jump rope, do calisthenics, ride a stationary bicycle, or use other home gymnasium equipment while the kids are busy playing or sleeping.
	Try to exercise when the kids are not around (e.g., during school hours or their nap time).
Retirement years	Look upon your retirement as an opportunity to become more active instead of less. Spend more time gardening, walking the dog, and playing with your grandchildren. Children with short legs and grandparents with slower gaits are often great walking partners.
	Learn a new skill that you have always been interested in, such as ballroom dancing, square dancing, or swimming.
	Now that you have the time, make regular physical activity a part of every day. Go for a walk every morning or every evening before dinner. Treat yourself to an exercycle and ride every day while reading a favorite book or magazine.

Source: Centers for Disease Control and Prevention. Retrieved July 20, 2009, from http://www.cdc.gov/physicalactivity/everyone/getactive/barriers.html

Activity in the Community (2011) recommends that programs teach behavioral skills needed to make leisure-time physical activity a daily habit. Other components of successful programs are:

1. Setting goals for physical activity and monitoring progress
2. Building social support
3. Incorporating self-rewards for the new behaviors
4. Learning to problem solve to maintain change and prevent relapse

Social support interventions have been successful, as they build, strengthen, and maintain social networks to promote physical activity (Kassavou, Turner, & French, 2013). These programs establish buddy systems and contracts or form walking groups. Group members or "buddies" provide motivational support, as well as companionship and encouragement to engage in regular leisure-time physical activities. Group facilitators provide encouragement and formal discussions to address barriers and other issues related to behavior change. Phone calls, e-mails, and text messages to provide encouragement and monitor progress are also useful.

Promoting Physical Activity in the Workplace

An increasingly sedentary workplace, an aging workforce, and a rising rate of preventable chronic diseases make health promotion workplace programming a priority. Worksites are ideal places to promote healthy changes, as large numbers of employees are available for an extended period. Employers have multiple tools and resources with which to engage employees, such as department meetings, communication systems such as phones, computers, and wireless devices, signage on bulletin boards, and the ability to make policy and health benefit changes. The workplace has been found to be a suitable environment for making changes in physical activity level, but evidence that these changes are long term requires further study (Hutchinson & Wilson, 2012).

In any workplace, it is necessary to make a "business" case for health promotion programs. Business leaders want to know that they will garner a positive return on their investment for a particular intervention. The following workplace characteristics effect the successful development of health promotion programs:

1. Health culture in the workplace
2. Incentives and communications
3. Evidence-based program offerings
4. Availability of onsite or offsite programs
5. Secure and relevant social connections and networks
6. Positive program outcomes (Pronk, 2010)

Wellness programs that focus on nutrition and physical activity have been associated with a decrease in absenteeism and medical costs. Get Moving, a website developed by the American Heart Association to promote physical activity in sedentary employees, demonstrated improved physical activity in those participating in the program. Employees visited the website regularly to develop a personalized physical activity plan and to seek information and support. Technology continues to play a major role in improving the health of employees and has the potential to become the primary health promotion format in the workplace (Irvine et al., 2011).

Worksite wellness program research has found that employees who lowered their BMI also reported increased feelings of calmness, improved ability to cope with stress, and increased physical energy (Merrill, Aldana, Garrett, & Ross, 2011). In general, physical activity programs report positive findings; however, there continue to be health-promoting barriers in the workplace environment. Successful programs incorporate a social-ecological approach, targeting the individual as well as the work environment, and engaging the organization (Kahn-Marshall & Gallant, 2012).

PROMOTING PHYSICAL ACTIVITY IN PERSONS WITH DISABILITIES

Physical inactivity is particularly prevalent in persons with disabilities. Physical activity can improve functional capacity; reduce secondary conditions such as obesity, hypertension, and pressure sores; provide opportunities for leisure enjoyment; and improve the overall quality of life for persons with disabilities. The aim of physical activity in this population is to emphasize the importance of carrying out daily activities with a minimum of assistance. Young people with disabilities are often not fully included in health promotion school programs; yet they are often more inactive and overweight than children without disabilities. Physical activity recommendations for persons with disabilities are available at the National Center on Health, Physical Activity and Disability and Guidelines for Disability Inclusion in Physical Activity, Nutrition, and Obesity Program Initiatives websites.

COMMUNITY PROGRAMS TO PROMOTE PHYSICAL ACTIVITY

Community programs to promote physical activity take place in schools, worksites, churches, and other community organizations, reaching much larger groups than one-on-one interventions. Community-level interventions focus on the entire population through mass media campaigns or by changing the physical or built environment.

Community programs use participatory planning to develop strategies at the individual, social, environmental, and legislative levels. Although individual factors, such as motivation, are important, community programs require multiple components, targeting the social and physical community environments as well (Williams, 2016).

The Guide to Community Preventive Services summarized findings to increase physical activity in communities. The findings and recommendations are:

1. Campaigns and informational approaches, that is, TV and radio spots
2. Behavioral and social approaches, including:
   a. *Individual health promotion programs* tailored to individual needs and interests
   b. *Social support interventions* such as organizing a buddy system, walking groups, or dances
   c. *Enhanced school-based physical education* to increase in-school and after-school physical activities
3. Environmental and policy initiatives, including:
   a. *Community-scale design and land use* to increase access to parks, safe streets, and sidewalks
   b. *Street-scale design and land use* to increase places for physical activities
   c. *Improving access* to physical activity places and equipment
   d. *Point-of-decision prompts* such as signage placed at stairwells to prompt people to use stairs instead of elevators or escalators (The Community Preventive Services Task Force, 2013).

Community-based interventions to increase physical activity are complex and require financial and human resources and time to implement. Walking and biking trails are the most **cost-effective** community-based interventions, while trails, pedometers, and school health education programs are the most **efficient** community interventions (Laine et al., 2014). Ongoing monitoring and evaluation of community-based interventions using multiple data sources are essential. Determining cost effectiveness of community-based interventions is an extremely important component of the evaluation process.

A review and assessment of the effectiveness of community-based physical activity clinical trial interventions among women ages 18 to 65 years between 2000 and 2013 found insufficient evidence to support community interventions for enhancing physical activity in women. The authors recommend implementation of high-quality, randomized community clinical trials to determine whether community-based programs increase and sustain physical activity among women, and to determine what type of interventions are most effective (Farahani et al., 2015).

The National Physical Activity Plan Alliance is a roadmap for community change to promote achievement of the physical activity guidelines. Health care professionals are encouraged to work with institutions to develop statewide plans for its citizens to be physically active across their life span (health.gov).

The Built Environment and Physical Activity

The most place-dependent health behavior is physical activity. Physical activity environments are a subset of physical environments, which encompass natural and built environments. Places hinder or facilitate physical activity based on the presence or absence of a supportive infrastructure; in other words, some places are physical activity friendly, and others are physical activity unfriendly.

Built environments include all spaces, buildings, and objects created or modified by people, such as homes, schools, workplaces, parks, and transportation systems. The regulations and policies that govern built environments also hinder or facilitate physical activity. For example, policy reform may need to occur to implement and maintain walking paths or recreational parks. In the Institute of Medicine's report, *Accelerating Progress in Obesity Prevention*, sustainable strategies for creating and/or enhancing access to green areas, rethinking community design, and increasing places and opportunities for physical activity are proposed to enhance the physical and built environments of our cities and towns (Institute of Medicine, 2012).

Neighborhood built environments influence physical activity behaviors. In a study of the association of neighborhood environments on rural and urban middle school youth, significantly lower moderate to vigorous physical activity was reported in rural youth compared to urban youth. Urban youth had physical supports for activity, for example, basketball courts, ball fields, and skateboard areas, compared to rural youth (Moore, Brinkley, Crawford, Evenson, & Brownson, 2013).

Moderate physical activity is higher in high-walkability neighborhoods compared to low-walkability neighborhoods. *Walkability* refers to the ability of individuals to walk to nearby destinations. Walking has been associated with access to aesthetically pleasing neighborhoods, convenient facilities, safe neighborhoods, and limited traffic. Neighborhood environmental variables that increase physical activity include single-family houses or housing type, shops within walking distance, transit stop 10–15 minutes from home, sidewalks, bicycle facilities in or near neighborhoods, low-cost recreation facilities, and low crime rate. A significant predictor of physical activity is sidewalks on most streets in a neighborhood. In contrast, unsafe neighborhoods are barriers to physical activity.

Research supports the need to design activity-friendly communities to provide opportunities and facilities for families with children to participate in leisure-time physical activity. Playability looks at the relationship of neighborhood built and social environments in shaping children's play. Evidence supports an association between neighborhood walking/cycling infrastructure and pedestrian safety. The indicators of activity-friendly communities need further refinement to design friendly physical activity environments including parks and playgrounds (Timperio, Reid, & Veitch, 2015).

Multiple sectors in the community play a role in promoting physical activity in the community. Concerns about crime and safety involve law enforcement. Urban planners play a major role in designing activity-friendly communities, and the transportation sector plays a role in building pedestrian and bicycle paths for walking/biking to school or work, or for leisure activities. Parks and recreation departments are also involved to facilitate access to recreational facilities and playgrounds for all.

Researchers, practitioners, and policy makers see the value of paying attention to factors in the social and physical environments that influence lifestyle behaviors and have implemented approaches, such as social-ecological models, to guide health promotion interventions and policy initiatives. Ecological models have proven useful for guiding physical activity interventions. Rigorous evaluation of these community-level models across the multiple levels is complex, but necessary to understand the usefulness of multilevel interventions. Figure 6–4 is an example of an ecological model that describes the relationship among multiple levels of a community, including the

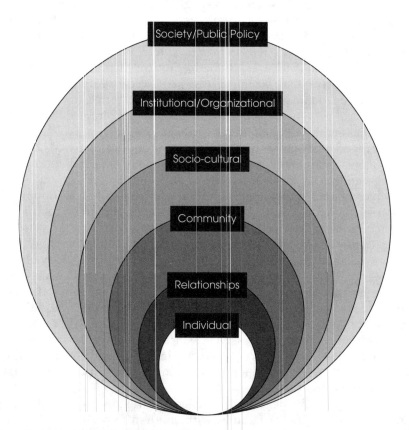

FIGURE 6–4 Social-Ecological Model

Sources: Adapted from the Centers for Disease Control and Prevention, http://www.cdc.gov/ violenceprevention/overview/social-ecologicalmodel.html; Mehtala et al. (2014).

individual level (age, education, income), the **relationship level** (influence of peers, partners, and family), the **community level** including the physical environment (residences and workplaces), the **sociocultural level** (health practices, economics), the **institutional/organizational level** (workplace, schools), and the **society or public policy level** (educational and social policy). These factors determine an activity-friendly community. Although the model needs additional testing, it shows promise in evaluating interventions for physical activity in which multiple levels of change are implemented (Mehtala, Saakslahti, Inkinen, & Poskiparta, 2014).

PHYSICAL ACTIVITY INTERVENTIONS FOR DIVERSE POPULATIONS

Some minority populations and people of lower socioeconomic status report the lowest levels of regular physical activity and are most vulnerable to chronic conditions, such as cardiovascular disease and diabetes (Havranek, et.al, 2015; Mezuk, Concha, Perrin, & Green, 2017). In addition, inequity in environments influences the ability of these groups to meet physical activity guidelines. People of color and those with low SES have less leisure time and energy to exercise, limited access to safe and affordable places to exercise, less support for regular physical activity, and are exposed to more stressful living conditions. Living in impoverished neighborhoods is associated with depression, anxiety, anger, and apathy, which lead to increased stress and physical inactivity (Greitemeyer, & Sagioglou, C. 2016; Smith & Huo, 2014).

The built environment has a negative influence on physical activity in low-income communities. Low-income neighborhoods have fewer recreational facilities, and those available may be of lower quality and poorly maintained. Fewer parks and open spaces are available in low-income communities of color than in affluent areas.

The amount of commute time is also a factor in leisure-time physical activity, especially for those who use public transportation. Long commute times leave little time or energy for social interaction and physical activity after work. The process of changing environmental conditions in these communities is a challenge for individuals, local governments, and policy makers.

Cultural factors influence physical activity in diverse populations. Cultures are not homogeneous, and subgroup variations in language, income, education, and acculturation exist. Gender socialization and role expectations also differ across cultures. Cultural beliefs and practices contribute to different patterns of activity across groups. Cultural attitudes influence physical activity as well. Ownership of automobiles and televisions, indicators of sufficient income, may promote inactivity. Some groups view physical activity as work and resort to sedentary activities during leisure time.

Considerations in designing culturally appropriate programs for diverse populations include exploring the community's history, cultural values, and potential cultural barriers to physical activity. Knowing which cultural values are critical to incorporate in a physical activity intervention will affect the success of the intervention. Barriers may be environmental, interpersonal, financial, or legal. For example, transportation may not be available to reach safe walking paths. Engaging members of the target community in the initial planning stage of community activities is essential. The integration of cultural values and strategies will minimize barriers in the activity plan and emphasize the community's strengths and resources to maximize their assets. Activities need to be tailored to the diversity of cultural patterns and practices, including the group's history, beliefs, and preferences.

Differences among underserved groups in physical activity examples are available in the literature. African Americans often value the collectivist versus the individualist approach. Because African Americans generally value faith-based communities, they are more likely to participate in physical activities organized by religious communities.

Physical activity programs are likely more successful when:

1. Faith-based messages present a positive ethnic identity
2. Physical activity participation is rewarded
3. Role models are prominent African Americans

Latino interventions are more successful when strategies focus on changing Latino female perceptions of activity, including all family members in the activity, and linking group physical activity to traditional celebrations and intergenerational activities. In a randomized trial, Mexican-origin parents and their children increased their physical activity when provided family health history-based risk information and family encouragement (de Heer et al., 2017). Latinos value family engagement and respond to interventions that emphasize family ties.

Native American Indians share several cultural concepts, including:

1. Oral tradition
2. Intergenerational activities
3. Use of ceremonies for sharing health information

Native Americans also have norms about not telling others what to do, and supporting different strategies to increase physical activities. Incorporating music and dances in Native American fitness programs makes the activity a source of motivation and pride (Duncan et al., 2014).

Asians and Pacific Islanders value

1. Collectivism
2. Intergenerational living
3. Respect for elders

Group physical activity participation, such as dance and martial arts, is a potential intervention for this population.

In summary, physical activity programs that respect the cultural practices of diverse populations are more likely to blend into community activities without changing social norms and community values. Also recommended are intergenerational approaches, which include children as well as elders. When community preferences are incorporated into programs, personal and group assets are emphasized. Programs should be flexible in accommodating the culture, offering choices to the extent possible. These steps empower diverse communities to take an active role in promoting the physical activity of their members to promote health.

Recommendations to address the built environment in low-income diverse communities include identifying the most critical environmental needs and integrating social and cultural variables in meeting the needs. Next, determine which environmental factors can be modified, and last, ensure adequate representation of community members using community-based participatory methods.

Stakeholders should be community members as well as members of organizations in the community that may be helpful in promoting the change. Involve stakeholders in all phases of development, implementation, and evaluation. Following these steps will enable changes to be implemented to increase physical activity in low-income communities.

TECHNOLOGY AND THE PROMOTION OF PHYSICAL ACTIVITY

The availability of health and fitness apps for mobile technology, including physical activity apps, continues to increase. Physical activity apps are incorporated into mobile devices, including smartphones, tablets, and wearable tracking devices, to motivate individuals to become physically active. They have multiple advantages, including continual self-monitoring and feedback, and standardized activity protocols. They also overcome the barriers of costs and access to physical activity programs. Mobile phone apps can also be used to set goals and daily reminders to be physically active.

Persuasive technology is increasingly being used in mobile apps for physical activity to motivate users to exercise (Matthews, Win, Oinas-Kukkonen, & Freeman, 2016). Self-monitoring is a basic feature of this technology, which also includes tailoring positive feedback, reminders, social support, and social comparison. The principles of persuasive technology have tremendous potential to increase behavior change, when they are incorporated into mobile technologies.

Physical activity can be promoted in children and adolescents with active play video games that provide enjoyable ways to exercise (Chaddha, Jackson, Richardson, & Franklin, 2017). These games include goal setting, feedback, and positive reinforcement to increase adherence. Exergames can be played indoors and include both children and adult family members to make physical activity a daily family routine.

The use of technology to increase physical activity has shown promising results. Several meta-analyses indicate that smartphone mobile apps have a positive effect on physical activity (Lewis, Napolitano, Buman, Williams, & Nigg, 2017). Studies of wearable technology have also shown positive effects on physical activity. However, most of the studies have limitations and point to the need for large, randomized controlled trials (Lewis et al., 2017). In addition, the physical activity apps need ongoing quality assessment.

NURSES AS ROLE MODELS OF PHYSICAL ACTIVITY BEHAVIOR

Nurses, the largest segment of the health professions, are educated professionals who are valued by the public and colleagues across the spectrum. They have the knowledge and skills required to advance health-promoting activities for their clients and themselves. Nurses are on the front line and in the public view and while the majority of Americans are not meeting physical activity guidelines, it is important for nurses to serve as role models for healthy behaviors (i.e., leisure-time physical activities and healthy eating patterns). Professional nursing organizations have taken a leadership role in emphasizing the health status of practicing nurses. Nurses often take better care of their patients than they do themselves. Nurses' health is important for quality patient care. In this regard, the American Nurses Association (ANA) designated 2017 as the Year of the Healthy Nurse. This emphasis encourages nurses to take better care of their own physical and mental health, to set goals and implement action plans to improve their health, and to encourage each other. Together nurses can improve their own health and support each other to meet the health-promoting physical activity guidelines for themselves as well as their clients.

CONSIDERATIONS FOR PRACTICE TO PROMOTE PHYSICAL ACTIVITY

The chapter emphasizes approaches the nurse can implement to increase physical activity and strategies to overcome barriers to physical activity. This information can guide nurses in counseling persons of all ages to adopt regular physical activity.

Motivation to change habits and engage in healthy behaviors requires commitment and a desire to live a healthier life. Within any given age, gender, or cultural group, nurses start by assessing the client's level of physical activity. For example, when working with children the nurse assesses patterns of physical activity; preferred activities; perceptions of barriers to being active; perceptions of self-efficacy; intentions to be active; availability of active parents, siblings, and friends; access to safe recreational facilities; and time spent outdoors. Inactive and sedentary clients need to be taught to change their definition of exercise and physical activity and build activity into their work and leisure behaviors. An example would be counseling them to take the stairs instead of the elevator or to park at a distance from work and shopping. Teaching small changes can make a big difference and serve as motivators for larger behaviors, such as walking 15 minutes a day.

Counseling assists children and adolescents to select activities they enjoy, not focusing solely on competitive sports. Children who are engaged in activities that are fun are likely to incorporate them into their daily life year-round and carry them into adulthood. By offering simple recommendations to children and parents/guardians, nurses play a key role in promoting lifelong physical activity.

Clients should be counseled to perform physical activities that are medically safe, enjoyable, convenient, realistic, and are structured to achieve self-selected goals. Routine monitoring, follow-up, and booster sessions are encouraged to assist clients in maintaining their exercise programs.

The nurse is more successful in promoting behavior change when the activities are tailored to individuals or groups. Home exercise programs may work for some adults, while others may prefer structured programs offered at worksites or convenient community locations. Group activities may be particularly appealing to adults who prefer the social support and comradeship of group programs. For older adults, current health status, existing medical conditions, disabilities, fear of injury, and preferences guide their choices.

Nurses can use existing computer-based and mobile apps to tailor programs for clients to optimize physical activity. Assessment and counseling followed with mail, e-mail, text messages, or phone calls at periodic intervals encourage client's adherence to their plan. Facebook and other SNSs may be used to disseminate reminders, encouragement, and health tips. Contracts should focus on appropriate strategies to increase or maintain activity and overcome any encountered barriers to being active. The barriers and strategies outlined in Table 6–3 encourage clients to identify specific barriers to increasing their physical activity level and commit to trying strategies to overcome them. Mobile apps are available to record data and set reminders. It is important to review contracts on a regular basis and adjust as needed.

Collaboration with health care teams and health care systems is important to establish systems that facilitate regular physical activity counseling for all clients. When health care teams and agencies integrate counseling protocols, physical activity counseling is much more likely to be an integral part of care by all health professionals.

OPPORTUNITIES FOR RESEARCH IN PHYSICAL ACTIVITY

Research is vital to tailoring exercise programs to meet the needs of diverse populations. Developing and testing interventions for very young children to accept physical activity as enjoyable and rewarding is critical. Interventions to prevent decreases in physical activity that occur before and during adolescence also need further study. Focusing on development of healthy behaviors rather than behavior change in later life is easier, as behaviors established in youth are highly resistant to change.

Additional suggestions for research include the following:

1. Describe family and environmental influences during early childhood that promote or inhibit the development of physically active lifestyles.
2. Test multiple levels of the social-ecological model to promote physical activity in low-income communities.
3. Test the effects of changing the built environment in rural communities on physical activity in older adults.
4. Develop and test strategies to promote the adoption and maintenance of physical activity for low-income sedentary women.
5. Test the long-term effectiveness of family interventions to increase physical activity for both children and parents.
6. Test the effectiveness of changing national policies to promote physical activity on the health of communities.

Summary

Nurses, as key health professionals, use evidence-based knowledge to assist clients in developing lifelong physical activity habits. Physical activity is integral to everyday life in order to have optimum effects on health. "Something is better than nothing" needs to be emphasized across the age spectrum. Research findings promote focusing on multiple levels in the environment, as well as on individual behaviors, to promote leisure-time physical activity. The application of mobile technology can make maintaining physical fitness enjoyable and rewarding for persons of all ages and contribute to improving quality of life.

Learning Activities

1. Conduct a self-assessment and design a physical activity plan for yourself. Identify barriers and strategies (refer to Table 6–3) you are likely to experience. Implement your plan for two weeks. Describe your successes and failures in a one-page summary.
2. Review the guidelines for promoting physical activity in children. Develop a plan that includes video games for a healthy child, 8 years of age. Tailor the plan to a sedentary child and describe steps and activities needed to reach the recommended activity guidelines.
3. Develop a physical activity program for a low-income cultural group of your choice. Outline how you would ensure that the program is sensitive to gender, age (persons age 65 years and over), and the cultural values of the group.
4. Develop a plan to promote physical activity for workers employed by a company with 50 to 100 employees. Describe worksite and leisure-time strategies to enable them to meet the national physical activity guidelines.
5. Find the percentage and estimated cost of obesity for all racial/ethnic groups in your region.

References

Ahn, A., Smith, M., & Ory, M. (2012). Physicians' discussions about body weight, healthy diet, and physical activity with overweight or obese elderly patients. *Journal of Aging and Health, 24*(7), 1179. doi:10.1177/0898264312454573

American Heart Association. (2016). *The American Heart Association recommendations for physical activity in kids.* Dallas, TX: Author. Retrieved April 15, 2017, from http://www.heart.org/idc/groups/heart-public/@wcm/@fc/documents/downloadable/ucm_469558.pdf

Anderson-Hanley, C., Arciero, P., Brickman, A., Nimon, J., Okuma, N., Westen, S., . . . Zimmerman, E. (2012). Exergaming and older adult cognition: A cluster randomized clinical trial. *American Journal of Preventive Medicine, 42*(2), 109–119. doi:10.1016/j.amepre.2011.10.016

Barkin, S., Larmichhane, A., Banda, J., JaKa, M., Buchowski, M., Evenson, K., . . ., Stevens, J. (2017). Parent's physical activity associated with preschooler activity in underserved populations. *American Journal of Preventive Medicine, 52*(4), 424–432. doi:10.1016/j.amepre.2016.11.017

Bice, M., Ball, J., & McClaran, S. (2016). Technology and physical activity motivation. *International Journal of Sport and Exercise Psychology, 14*(4), 295–304. doi:10.1080/1612197X.2015.1025811

Biddle, S., Petrolini, I., & Pearson, N. (2014). Interventions designed to reduce sedentary behaviors in young people: A review of reviews. *British Journal of Sports Medicine, 48*(3), 182–186. doi:10:1136/bjsports-2013-093078

Centers for Disease Control and Prevention. (2011). *Strategies to prevent obesity and other chronic diseases: The CDC guide to increase physical activity in the community.* Atlanta, GA: U.S. Department of Health and Human Services. Retrieved from https://www.cdc.gov/obesity/downloads

Centers for Disease Control and Prevention, Office of Disease Prevention and Health Promotion. (2014). *Physical activity guidelines for American Midcourse Report: Executive summary and key messages.* U.S. Department of Health and Human Services. Retrieved from www.cdc.gov/nchs/healthy_people/hp2020

Chaddha, A., Jackson, E., Richardson, C., & Franklin, B. (2017). Technology to help promote physical activity. *American Journal of Cardiology, 119*(1), 149–152. doi:10.1016/j.amjcard.2016.09.025

Cheek, D., & Howington, L. (2017). Patient care in the dawn of the genomic age. *American Nurse Today, 12*(3), 16–22.

Chen, J., & Lee, Y. (2013). Physical activity for health: Evidence, theory, and practice. *Journal of Preventive Medicine and Public Health, 46*(Suppl 1), S1–S2. doi:10.3961/jpmph.2013.46.S.S1

Clarke, T. C., Ward, B. W., Freeman, G., & Schiller, J. S. (2016). *Early release of selected estimates based on data from the January–September 2015 National Health Interview Survey.* National Center for Health Statistics. Available from http://www.cdc.gov/nchs/nhis.htm

Community Preventive Services Task Force (2013). The community guide to increase physical activity. https://www.thecommunityguide.org/topic/physical-activity?field_recommendation_tid=All&items_per_page=5&page=2

de Heer, H., de la Haye, K., Skapinsky, K., Goergen, A., Wilkinson, A., & Koehly, L. (2017). Let's move together: A randomized trial of the impact of family health history on encouragement and co-engagement in physical activity of Mexican-origin parents and their children. *Health Education & Behavior, 44*(1), 141–152. doi:10.1177/1090198116644703

Dempsey, P., Owen, N., Biddle, S., & Dunstan, D. (2014). Managing sedentary behavior to reduce the risk of diabetes and cardiovascular disease. *Current Diabetic Reports, 42*, 522. doi:10.1007/s11892-014-0522-0

Duncan, G., McDougall, C., Dansie, E., Garroutte, E., Buchwald, D., & Henderson, J. (2014). Association of American Indian cultural identity with physical activity. *Ethnicity & Disease, 24*(1), 1–7.

Espana-Romero, V., Mitchell, J., Dowda, M., O'Neill, J., & Pate, R. (2013). Objectively measured sedentary time, physical activity and markers of body fat in preschool children. *Pediatric Exercise Science, 25*(1), 154–163. doi:10.1123/pes.25.1.154

Farahani, A., Asadi-Lari, M., Mohammadi, E., Parvizy, S., Haghdoost, A., & Taghizadeh, Z. (2015). Community-based physical activity interventions among women: A systematic review. *British Medicine Journal Open, 5*, e007210. doi:10.1136/bmjopen-2014-007210

Farooq, M., Parkinson, K., Adamson, A., Pearce, M., Reilly, J., Hughes, A., . . . Reilly, J. (2017). Timing of the decline in physical activity in childhood and adolescence: Gateshead Millennium Cohort Study. *British Journal of Sports Medicine.* doi:10.1136/bjsports-2016-096933

Garber, C. E., Blissmer, B., Deschenes, M. R., Franklin, B. A., Lamonte, M. J., Lee, I., . . . Swain, D. P. (2011). Quantity and quality of exercise for developing and maintaining cardiorespiratory, musculoskeletal, and neuromotor fitness in apparently healthy adults: Guidance for prescribing exercise. *Medicine & Science in Sports & Medicine, 43*(7), 1334–1359. doi:10.1249/MSS.0b013e318213fefb

Greitemeyer, T. & Sagioglu, C. (2016). Subjective socioeconomic status causes aggression: A test of the theory of social deprivation. *Journal of Personality and social Psychology, 111*(2), 178.

Grimstvedt, M., Ananian, C., Keller, C., Woolf, K., Sebren, A., & Ainsworth, B. (2012). Nurse practitioner and physician assistant physical activity counseling knowledge, confidence and practice. *Preventive Medicine, 54*(5), 306–308. doi:10.1016/j.ypmed.2012.02.003

Havranek, E., Mujahid, M., Barr, D., Blair, I., Cohen, M., Cruz-Flores, S., . . . & Rosal, D. (2015). Social determinants of risks and outcomes for cardiovascular disease: a scientific statement from the American Heart Association. *Circulation, 132*(9), 873–898. doi:10.1161/CIR.0000000000000228.

Hutchinson, A., & Wilson, C. (2012). Improving nutrition and physical activity in the workplace: A meta-analysis of intervention studies. *Health Promotion International, 27*(2), 238–249. doi:10.1093/heapro/dar035

Institute of Medicine. (2012). *Accelerating progress in obesity prevention: Solving the weight of the nation.* Washington, DC: National Academies Press.

Irvine, A., Philips, L., Seeley, J., Wyant, S., Duncan, S., & Moore, R. (2011). Get Moving: A web site that increases physical activity of sedentary employees. *American Journal of Health Promotion, 25*(3), 199–206. doi:10.4278/ajhp.04121736

Jackson, J., Smit, E., Branscum, A., Gunter, K., Harvey, M., Manore, M., & John, D. (2017). The family home environment, food insecurity, and body mass index in rural children. *Health Education & Behavior, 44*(4), 648–657. doi:10.1177/1090198116684757

Kahn-Marshall, J., & Gallant, M. (2012). Making healthy behaviors the easy choice for employees: A review of the literature on environmental and policy changes in worksite health promotion. *Health Education & Behavior, 39*(6), 752–776. doi:10.1177/1090198111434153

Kassavou, A., Turner, A., & French, D. (2013). Do interventions to promote walking in groups increase physical activity? A meta-analysis. *International Journal of Behavioral Nutrition and Physical Activity, 10*(1), 18. doi:10.1186/1479-5868-10-18

Laine, J., Kuvaja-Kollner, V., Pietila, E., Koivuneva, M., Valtonen, H., & Kankaanpaa, E. (2014). Cost-effectiveness of population-level physical activity interventions: A systematic review. *American Journal of Health Promotion, 29*(2), 71–80. doi:10.4278/ajhp.131210-LIT-622

Lanier, J., Bury, D., & Richardson, S. (2016). Diet and physical activity for cardiovascular disease prevention. *American Family Physician, 93*(11), 919–924.

Laranjo, L. (2016). Social media and health behavior change. In S. Sayed-Abdul, E. Gabarron, & A. Lau (Eds.), *Participatory health in social media* (pp. 83–111). New York, NY: Elsevier.

Lee, H., Emerson, J., & Williams, D. (2016). The exercise–affect–adherence pathway: An evolutionary perspective. *Frontiers in Psychology, 7*, 1285. doi:10.3389/fpsyg.2016.01285

Lewis, B., Napolitano, M., Buman, M., Williams, D., & Nigg, C. (2017). Future directions in physical activity intervention research: Expanding our focus to sedentary behaviors, technology, and dissemination. *Journal of Behavioral Medicine, 40*(1), 112–126. doi:10.1007/s10865-016-9797-8

Loos, R. J., Hagberg, J. M., Pérusse, L., Roth, S. M., Sarzynski, M. A., Wolfarth, B., . . . Bouchard, C. (2015). Advances in exercise, fitness, and performance genomics in 2014. *Medicine & Science in Sports & Exercise, 47*(6), 1105–1112. doi:10.1249/MSS.0000000000000645

Loprinzi, P., & Cardinal, B. (2013). Association between biologic outcomes and objectively measured physical activity accumulated in ≥ 10-minute bouts and < 10-minute bouts. *American Journal of Health Promotion, 27*(3), 143–151. doi:10.4278/ajhp.110916-QUAN-348

Maher, J., Pincus, A., Ram, N., & Conroy, D. (2015). Daily physical activity and life satisfaction across adulthood. *Developmental Psychology, 51*(10), 1407–1419. doi:10.1037/dev0000037

Mansoubi, M., Pearson, N., Biddle, S., & Clemes, S. (2014). The relationship between sedentary behavior and physical activity in adults: A systematic review. *Preventive Medicine, 69*, 28–35. doi:10.1016/j.ypmed.2014.08.028

Marshall, S. J., Levy, S. S., Tudor-Locke, C. E., Kolkhorst, F. W., Wooten, K. M., Ji, M., . . . Ainsworth, B. (2009). Translating physical activity recommendations into a pedometer-based step goal: 3000 steps in 30 minutes. *American Journal of Preventive Medicine, 36*(5), 410–415. doi:10.1016/j.amepre.2009.01.021

Matthews, C., Hagstromer, M., Pober, D., & Bowles, H. (2012). Best practices for using physical activity monitors in population-based research. *Medicine & Science in Sports & Exercise, 44* (1 Suppl 1), S68–S76. doi:10.1249/MSS.0b013e3182399e5b

Matthews, J., Win, K., Oinas-Kukkonen, H., & Freeman, M. (2016). Persuasive technology in mobile applications promoting physical activity: A systematic review. *Journal of Medical Systems, 40*, 72. doi:10.1007/s10916-015-0425-x

Mehtala, M., Saakslahti, A., Inkinen, M., & Poskiparta, M. (2014). A socio-ecological approach to physical activity interventions in childcare: A systematic review. *International Journal of Behavioral Nutrition and Physical Activity, 11*, 22. doi:10.1186/1479-5868-11-22

Merrill, R., Aldana, S., Garrett, J., & Ross, C. (2011). Effectiveness of a workplace wellness program for maintaining health and promoting healthy behaviors. *Journal of Occupational and Environmental Medicine, 53*(7), 782–787. doi:10.1097/JOM.0b013e318220c2f4

Mezuk, B., Concha, J., Perrin, P., & Green, T. (2017). Commentary: Reconsidering the role of context in diabetes prevention. *Ethnicity & Disease, 27*(1), 63–68. doi10.18865/ed.27.1.63

Moore, J., Brinkley, J., Crawford, T., Evenson, K., & Brownson, R. (2013). Association of the built environment with physical activity and adiposity in rural and urban youth. *Preventive Medicine, 56*(2), 145–148. doi:10.1016/j.ypmed.2012.11.019

National Academies of Sciences, Engineering, and Medicine. (2016). *Driving action and progress on obesity prevention and treatment: Proceedings of a workshop—In brief.* Washington, DC: The National Academies Press.

Ogden, C., Carroll, M., Kit, B., & Flegal, K. (2014). Prevalence of childhood and adult obesity in the United States, 2011–2012. *Journal of the American Medical Association, 311*(8), 806–814. doi:10.1001/jama.2014.732

Owen, N. (2012). Sedentary behavior: Understanding and influencing adults' prolonged sitting time. *Preventive Medicine, 55*(6), 535–539. doi:10.1016/j.ypmed.2012.08.024

Pronk, N. (2010). Six trends affecting the business case for worksite health promotion. *ACSM's Health & Fitness Journal, 14*(5), 41–43. doi:10.1249/FIT.0b013e3181ed5b2f

Rauner, A., Mess, F., & Woll, A. (2013). The relationship between physical activity, physical fitness and overweight in adolescents: A systematic review of studies published in or after 2000. *BMC Pediatrics, 13*, 19.

Saffer, H., Dave, D., Grossman, M., & Leung, L. (2013). Racial, ethnic, and gender differences in physical activity. *Journal of Human Capital, 7*(4), 378–410.

Schoenborn, C., Adams, P., & Peregoy, J. (2013). Health behaviors of adults: United States, 2008–2010. *Vital Health Statistics: Series 10, Data from the National Health Survey,* (257), 1–184.

Simek, E., McPhate, L., & Haines, T. (2012). Adherence to and efficacy of home exercise programs to prevent falls: A systematic review and meta-analysis of the impact of exercise program characteristics. *Preventive Medicine, 55*(4), 262–275. doi:10.1016/j.ypmed.2012.07.007

Smith, H. & Huo, Y. (2014). Relative deprivation: How subjective experiences of inequality influence social behavior and health. *Policy Insights from the Behavioral and Brain Sciences, 1*(1), 231–238. doi:10.1177/2372732214550165

Smith, P., Potter, G., McLaren, M., & Blumenthal, J. (2013). Impact of aerobic exercise on neurobehavioral outcomes. *Mental Health and Physical Activity, 6*(3), 139–153. doi:10.1016/j.mhpa.2013.06.008

Tigbe, W., Granat, M., Sattar, N., & Lean, M. (2017). Time spent in sedentary posture is associated with waist circumference and cardiovascular risk. *International Journal of Obesity, 1*, 8. doi:10.1038/ijo.2017.30

Timperio, A., Reid, J., & Veitch, J. (2015). Playability: Built and social environment features that promote physical activity within children. *Current Obesity Reports, 4*(4), 460–476. doi:10.1007/s13679-015-0178-3

Tudor-Locke, C. (2014). How many steps per day are too few? *Journal of Science and Medicine in Sport,* 18S, e108. doi:10.1016/j.jsams.2014.11.060

Tudor-Locke, C., Craig, C., Clemens, S., De Cocker, K., Giles-Corti, B., Hatano, Y., . . . Blair, S. (2011). How many steps are enough for adults? *International Journal of Behavioral Nutrition and Physical Activity, 8*(79), 1–17.

U.S. Department of Health and Human Services (2008). *2008 Physical Activity Guidelines for Americans.* Retrieved from http://www.health.gov/paguidelines

VanKim, N., & Nelson, T. (2013). Vigorous physical activity, mental health, perceived stress, and socializing among college students. *American Journal of Health Promotion, 28*(1), 7–15. doi:10.4278/ajhp.111101-QUAN-395

Venn, D., & Strazdins, L. (2017). Your money or your time? How both types of scarcity matter to physical activity and healthy eating. *Social Science & Medicine, 172,* 98–106. doi:10.1016/j.socscimed.2016.10.023

Williams, C. (2016). Community and prevention-oriented, population-focused practice: The foundation of specialization in public health nursing. In M. Stanhope & J. Lancaster (Eds.), *Public health nursing: Population-centered health care in the community* (6th ed., pp. 3–21). St Louis, MO: Elsevier, Inc.

World Health Organization (2011). Global recommendations on physical activity for health. www.who.int/dietphysicalactivity/physical-activity-recommendations-18-64years.pdf?ua=

Xu, H., & Goldberg, N. (2017). 'Pokemon Go' players add 2,000 steps a day. *Health Day.* https://medlineplus.gov/news/fullstory_163978.html

Zadro, J., Shirley, D., Andrade, T., Scurrah, K., Bauman, A., & Ferreira, P. (2017). The beneficial effects of physical activity: Is it down to your genes? A systematic review and meta-analysis of twin and family studies. *Sports Medicine, 3,* 4. doi:10.1186/s40798-016-0073-9

CHAPTER 7

Nutrition and Health Promotion

OBJECTIVES

This chapter will enable the reader to:

1. Discuss the current status of the nutritional health of Americans.
2. Evaluate the 2015–2020 U.S. Dietary Guidelines for promoting a healthy, nutritionally adequate diet.
3. Discuss the use and value of MyPlate in implementing the 2015–2020 Dietary Guidelines.
4. Summarize evidence-based factors that influence eating behaviors.
5. Describe the nutritional needs of infants and children, adolescents, adults, and older adults.
6. Examine factors related to overweight/obesity and intervention goals in weight loss.
7. Describe strategies to motivate individuals to change eating patterns and maintain a healthy weight.

Good nutrition is one of the primary determinants of health and contributes significantly to the reduction of chronic diseases. Major risk factors responsible for the global threat of noncommunicable chronic diseases (NCDs) are an unhealthy diet and sedentary behavior. Nutrition has transitioned from a focus primarily on nutrients necessary to feed populations to its role in promoting health and preventing disease. The global epidemic of obesity has resulted in nutrition being considered a lifestyle risk factor when accompanied by sedentary lifestyles, obesogenic environments, and the availability and affordability of poor nutritious, high calorie foods. Urbanization, an increase in availability of labor-saving devices, wireless technologies, and a decrease in total daily energy expenditure of most Americans have "engineered" energy expenditure out of people's daily lives, resulting in NCDs or "diseases of inactivity" (Hills, Street, & Byrne, 2015).

PROMOTING HEALTHY DIET AND NUTRITION

Noncommunicable chronic diseases, including cardiovascular disease, cancer, respiratory disease, diabetes, and obesity, account for 70% of deaths globally, an increase of 7% over 2008 (World Health Organization, 2017). NCD rates in low- and middle-income countries are more similar to developed countries due to a rapid "nutrition transition" associated with unhealthy dietary patterns and sedentary living. Undernutrition and overnutrition coexist in many low- and middle-income countries, underscoring the double burden placed on society's quest for healthy citizens.

Lifestyle factors account for a large percentage of NCDs. About 50% of American adults have one or more NCDs, and this rate continues to rise. In addition to increases in health risks, cost to the U.S. economy increases as well. In 2012, the cost of diagnosed diabetes alone was $176 billion including $69 billion in decreased productivity (U.S. Department of Health and Human Services & U.S. Department of Agriculture, 2015). Yearly medical costs for obese adults compared to adults of normal weight continue to increase.

Healthy nutrition for children and adolescents is critical as dietary patterns that develop during these years tend to persist throughout life. Activity levels, high in childhood and adolescence, tend to decline in adulthood, disrupting the balance of food intake and energy expenditure. Unhealthy nutrition practices and decreased physical activity lead to overweight and obesity.

Multiple complex factors influence food choices making successful promotion of optimal dietary patterns a challenge. Policy makers and health promotion experts acknowledge the need for population-based, multilevel changes based on transdisciplinary, culturally relevant approaches that target individuals, communities, the food environment, and the food industry (Scharf & DeBoer, 2016). In view of the enormity of the challenge, efforts directed toward improving the nutritional status of Americans are a priority.

Nutritional Health of Americans

Food preferences, portion and plate size, and sedentary behavior, as well as culture, socioeconomic status, advertising and marketing, and "obesogenic" environments, influence health outcomes (Hollands et al., 2015). The incidence of chronic disease in young people parallels the increase in obesity rates in this population. Approximately 17% (12.5 million) of those ages 2–19 years are obese. Adult obesity prevalence in 2015 in all 50 states was greater than 20% of the state population. Regional data show that the South has the highest prevalence of obesity (31.2%) with the Midwest reporting 30.7%, the Northeast 26.4%, and the West 25.2%. These percentages represent increases in obesity in all four regions compared to 2008 figures. Non-Hispanic black women have the highest obesity prevalence at 56.9%, and women overall have a higher prevalence of obesity than men. Among youth, no difference was reported in obesity between males and females (Centers for Disease Control and Prevention, 2017).

The increase in adult obesity has slowed since 2014 and stabilized for youth. However, the 2015 obesity prevalence for adults remained higher than the *Healthy People 2020* goal of 30.5%. Likewise, the prevalence of childhood obesity was 17% in 2015, higher than the *Healthy People 2020* goal of 14.5% (Centers for Disease Control and Prevention, 2017).

Americans rank prevention as the most important health reform priority. This shift has occurred over the past two decades. Prevention of obesity and reversal of the obesity epidemic, designated as key public health issues confronting America, require a coalition of health professionals, educators, policy makers, civic organizations, industry, schools, families, and private citizens committed to finding solutions and resources to solve this problem (Robert Wood Johnson Foundation & Trust for America's Health, 2017).

Dietary Guidelines for Americans

The *Dietary Guidelines for Americans*, published every five years by the U.S. Department of Health and Human Services (USDHHS) and the U.S. Department of Agriculture (USDA), contain nutritional and dietary information and guidelines and form the basis for federal nutritional policies. The guidelines are developed for professionals to assist Americans ages 2 years and older to establish and maintain good dietary habits. They also include recommendations to reduce risks for chronic disease. The *Dietary Guidelines for Americans 2015–2020* focus on:

- Encouraging a healthy eating pattern across the life span
- Consuming a variety of nutrient-dense foods in appropriate amounts
- Limiting calories from refined sugars and saturated fats and reducing sodium intake
- Choosing healthier foods and beverages
- Supporting healthy eating patterns for everyone
- Meeting the 2008 Physical Activity Guidelines for Americans (U.S. Department of Health and Human Services & U.S. Department of Agriculture, 2015)

A basic premise of the guidelines is that food is the primary source of nutrients an individual needs to be healthy. Although dietary supplements and fortified foods may be useful for one or two nutrients, they cannot replace a healthy diet. The 2015–2020 guidelines place greater emphasis on personal, cultural, and traditional preferences, eating patterns, and food and nutrient characteristics. Supporting individual choices that fit within budget considerations is also emphasized.

Guideline changes also include modification of restrictions on saturated fat, for example, butter and extra virgin olive oil, and the ban on eggs and cholesterol-containing foods. As medical science advances understanding of the underlying etiologies of cardiovascular disease, ongoing changes in the dietary guidelines are critical (Malhotra, Redberg, & Meier, 2017).

Americans need to be taught the essential relationship between diet and physical activity to balance caloric intake and energy expenditure. In a study of normal weight individuals, a threshold for energy balance of food intake and energy expenditure found that physical activity equivalent to 7,116 steps per day is necessary, an amount attainable by most adults (Shook et al., 2015). (See Chapter 6 for strategies to achieve the daily exercise requirement.) Reducing caloric intake is key to weight loss, while regular physical activity is essential for preventing weight gain and maintaining the desired weight after weight loss.

The Healthy U.S.-Style Food Pattern is designed to meet required nutritional needs without exceeding required caloric levels. It serves as the standard to compare with the average American diet (U.S. Department of Health and Human Services & U.S. Department of Agriculture, 2015). The typical American dietary pattern does not align with the Healthy U.S.-Style Food Pattern as shown in Figure 7–1. The comparison of the typical American dietary pattern with the Healthy U.S.-Style Food Pattern shows the following discrepancies:

- Three-fourths of the population eat a diet low in vegetables, fruits, dairy, and healthy oils.
- Over half of the population exceeds protein and total grain recommendations but does not meet the subgroup recommendations within these food groups.
- More than half of the population exceeds added sugars, saturated fats, and sodium recommendations (U.S. Department of Health and Human Services & U.S. Department of Agriculture, 2015).

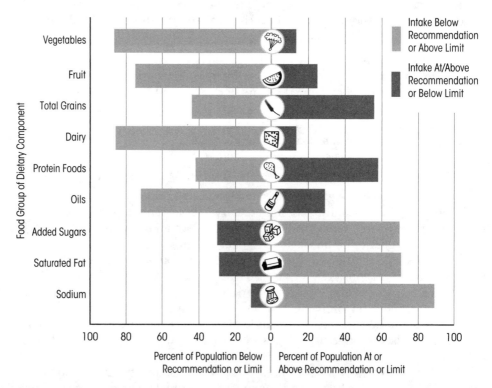

FIGURE 7–1   Dietary Intakes Compared to Recommendations. Percent of the U.S. Population Aged 1 Year and Older Who Are Below, At, or Above Each Dietary Goal or Limit

Source: U.S. Department of Health and Human Services & U.S. Department of Agriculture. (2015). *Dietary Guidelines for Americans 2015–2020* (8th ed.). Available at http://health.gov/dietaryguidelines/2015/guidelines/

Two examples of eating patterns that implement the 2015–2020 Dietary Guidelines are the Healthy Mediterranean-Style Eating Pattern and the Healthy Vegetarian Eating Pattern. Both plans require substitutions of some foods in subgroups of the 2015–2020 Dietary Guidelines. The substitutions are primarily differences in food group composition and amounts, reflect eating patterns associated with positive health outcomes. The Healthy Vegetarian Eating Pattern includes dietary choices recognized by self-identified vegetarians in the National Health and Nutrition Examination Survey (NHANES). Both the Mediterranean-Style and the Healthy Vegetarian Eating Patterns are available in Appendix 4 and Appendix 5, respectively, of the 2015–2020 Dietary Guidelines (U.S. Department of Health and Human Services & U.S. Department of Agriculture, 2015).

The dietary guidelines are used by health professionals and policy makers to develop educational material, and design and implement nutrition-related programs. Modifications are necessary to integrate food preferences of different ethnic and racial groups, vegetarians, and groups with specific cultural preferences. The guidelines, based on a 2,000-calorie diet, also present caloric options based on age, sex, and activity level. Following all or even some of the recommendations will improve nutritional outcomes.

Challenges to Dietary Guidelines

Some scientists have suggested that prior dietary guidelines share responsibility for the obesity epidemic in America. When the 2005 Dietary Guidelines recommended that people eat less dietary saturated fat, sugar consumption increased resulting in increased caloric intake and weight gain (Zhang, Roslin, & Chopra, 2017).

According to some experts, "good" saturated fatty acids, for example, nuts, extra virgin olive oil, and oily fish, reduce inflammation, an underlying cause of cardiovascular disease, and chronic elevation of insulin, a primary culprit in coronary disease (Malhotra et al., 2017). An intake of recommended levels of "good" fatty acids and a decrease in refined carbohydrates, sodium, and caloric intake significantly contribute to the reduction of coronary artery disease (CAD). The 2015–2020 Dietary Guidelines address all of these components and are an important strategy to share the best science-based information available to improve Americans' health.

MyPlate: A Visual Guide to Healthy Eating

The dietary guidelines have been translated into messages and resources that lay individuals, families, and communities understand. MyPlate, an illustration of a dinner plate, is a guide to healthy eating that professionals use to educate and support consumers in their efforts to implement the guidelines (see Figure 7–2).

The MyPlate illustration is a circle divided into four brightly colored wedges representing vegetables and fruits (50%), and proteins and grains (25% each) with a smaller circle for dairy products. *How to Build a Healthy Eating Pattern*, based on the 2015–2020 Dietary Guidelines, is a resource to share with clients to teach healthy eating patterns that fit their personal tastes and traditions (Centers for Disease Control and Prevention, 2017).

The MyPlate website offers interactive tools and personalized recommendations to help individuals improve their dietary intake. The website is also a teaching resource

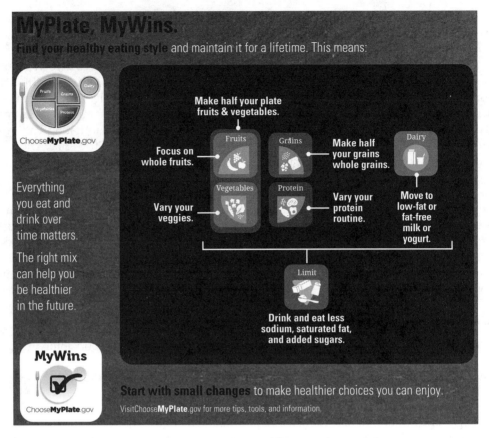

FIGURE 7–2   Implementation of the Dietary Guidelines through MyPlate

Source: U.S. Department of Health and Human Services & U.S. Department of Agriculture. (2015). *Dietary Guidelines for Americans 2015–2020* (8th ed.). Available at http://health.gov/dietaryguidelines/2015/guidelines/

for nurses and other health care professionals. It offers information to develop a personalized plan for preschoolers (2–5 years), children (6–11 years), and mothers. Information can also be downloaded to tablets and smartphones.

In 2016, the U.S. Food and Drug Administration (USFDA) revised the Nutrition Facts label found on prepackaged foods and beverages to help consumers make healthier choices (see Figure 7–3). The revised label better defines serving size and servings per container and includes information about added sugars. The first major revision to the Nutrition Facts label since 1996, the 2016 label more accurately reflects current nutrition science and facilitates implementation of the 2015–2020 Dietary Guidelines (Casavale, 2017).

Issues in Undernutrition

Although the major problem in America is overnutrition, undernutrition is a problem in some segments of the population. Undernutrition occurs more frequently in persons

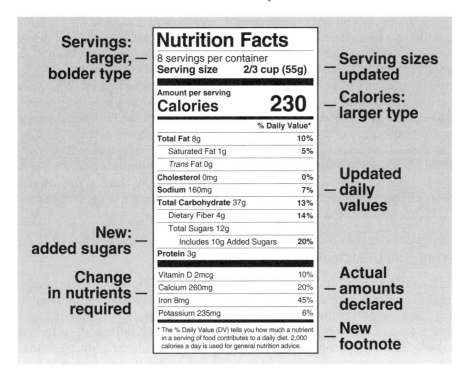

FIGURE 7–3 Highlights of What's Different on the New Nutrition Facts Label

Source: Changes to the Nutrition Facts label. U.S. Food and Drug Administration. Retrieved from https://www.fda.gov/downloads/Food/GuidanceRegulation/GuidanceDocumentsRegulatoryInformation/LabelingNutrition/UCM501643.pdf

living below the poverty line and in children, adolescents, and older adults. Iron deficiency, the world's most common nutritional deficiency, is associated with multiple health problems. Iron-deficiency anemia occurs most often when a diet is insufficient in iron. Chronic iron deficiency in childhood has an adverse effect on growth and development. The correction of an iron deficiency accompanied by anemia decreases the potential for developmental delays, impaired behavior, diminished intellectual functioning, and resistance to infection (Hassan et al., 2016; National Institutes of Health, 2014).

Bone mass reaches its peak in adolescents between the ages of 16 and 24 years. Although genetic factors play a major role in skeletal mass development, nutrition and physical activity also play critical roles. Calcium plays a key role in bone health, and vitamin D is necessary for its absorption. An inadequate calcium intake in the first two decades of life may result in failure to attain peak bone mass and lead to osteoporosis in later life (Bianchi, Sawyer, & Bachrach, 2016). Many of the physical complications of eating disorders are secondary to malnutrition, with osteoporosis and cardiac changes being significant problems (National Institutes of Health, 2014).

Eating disorders, such as anorexia nervosa and bulimia, are nutritional threats to the health of youth, primarily young White and Hispanic females. The prevalence of anorexia nervosa and bulimia is increasing, resulting in a significant proportion of midlife women experiencing eating disorders. Increased attention to this disorder in midlife women will mitigate some underlying chronic health problems likely to surface in this age group (Micali et al., 2017; Smink, van Hoeken, & Hoek, 2013).

Malnutrition is also a problem in older adults. In nursing homes, older adult residents experience weight loss due to multiple issues, including loss of appetite and a decreased ability to feed themselves. Malnutrition is an altered nutritional state resulting from a combination of inflammation and a negative nutrient balance (Soeters et al., 2017). Malnourished nursing home residents who have a BMI less than 20 kg/m^2 (kilograms per square meter) and weight loss greater than 10 pounds in one year require increased nutritional care supplements to prevent premature death (Wirth et al., 2016). Assessment of the nutritional status of older adults is necessary to prevent or treat deficiencies before they become serious issues.

FACTORS INFLUENCING EATING BEHAVIOR

A healthy eating pattern is the cornerstone of good health. However, factors underlying eating behaviors make healthy changes in eating patterns challenging, as eating behaviors are an integral part of the lifestyle of individuals, families, and communities. Factors influencing eating behaviors include **genetic–biological**, **psychological**, **socioeconomic**, **cultural–ethnic**, **environmental**, and **health policy issues**. Effective strategies to change eating patterns require an understanding and management of these factors.

Genetic–Biological Factors

Food intake and energy expenditure are controlled and kept in balance by complex neural systems. Humans have the ability to store a tremendous energy supply (fat) for later use, which has resulted in obesity in our modern society. The neural system has the ability to defend the lower limits of body weight by initiating external and internal nutrient-depletion signals, such as increased appetite, foraging, and stimulating the autonomic and endocrine systems to initiate an internal energy saving mode. There are numerous regulatory mechanisms in the body, and their redundancy speaks to the biological importance of body weight regulation and to the futility of managing obesity without considering the neuroregulatory determinants of energy balance.

Considerable research is underway to understand the genetic and cellular mechanisms that regulate energy balance and the events that converge and result in obesity. Eating behaviors are regulated by multiple specific hormones and genes. In the mid-1990s, the obesity gene was isolated from adipose tissue, and its protein product, leptin, was identified. This landmark discovery ushered in a new era in understanding the control of energy balance. The hormone, leptin, has been shown to play a role in regulating energy balance. Several possible mechanisms are under investigation, including leptin deficiency and leptin resistance (Crujeiras et al., 2015). Increased leptin sensitivity may protect against obesity, whereas loss of leptin sensitivity may predispose one to obesity, opening the door for potential pharmacological interventions (Quarta, Sanchez-Garrido, Tschop, & Clemmensen, 2016; Tung et al., 2015). However, evidence for leptin's role as an "anti-obesity" hormone is currently lacking until more animal and human research is conducted (Flier & Maratos-Flier, 2017).

Heredity is estimated to explain anywhere from 30% to 70% of the variation in susceptibility to obesity (van Dijk, Tellam, Morrison, Muhlausler, & Molloy, 2015). Researchers have identified at least 150 common genetic variants associated with body composition, although the individual influence of each one has been reported to be small (Romieu et al., 2017). A fat mass and obesity-associated protein gene (FTO) has been shown to be associated with lifestyle in obesity, but the relationship has also been found to be quite small. Individuals who inherit the FTO gene from each parent, compared with noncarriers, are about 6.5 pounds heavier. However, exposure to the modern food environment with the availability of fast-food, 24-hour takeout meals, and convenience foods increases susceptibility to selecting unhealthy foods in persons with the genetic risk (Claussnitzer et al., 2015; Graff, Church, & Lavie, 2017).

Epigenetics is the study of factors that change the way genes respond without changing the genetic code itself. There is some evidence that epigenetics influences the way methylation of genes occurs and may potentially serve as a biomarker of energy balance and gene–environmental interactions in obesity (Romieu et al., 2017). This relationship supports the role of the interaction of genetic and environmental factors in the eating patterns of overweight and obese individuals. More research is needed in this area (Huang & Hu, 2015; van Dijk et al., 2015).

The **biological** changes of aging have a marked effect on eating behavior. A progressive loss of taste buds on the anterior tongue occurs with age, resulting in decreased sensitivity to sweet and salty tastes. In contrast, taste buds sensitive to bitter and sour increase with age. This taste distortion may result in decreased enjoyment of food and decreased intake of necessary nutrients by older adults.

Changes in gastric secretions may result in limited absorption of iron, calcium, and vitamin B12 in older adults. Decreased gastric mobility augments the need for foods high in fiber, including fresh fruits, raw vegetables, whole-grain breads, and cereals (see Figure 7–4), and increases the importance of water consumption to promote regularity in bowel evacuation. A decrease in basal metabolic rate associated with aging often results in a decrease in caloric intake. Sensitivity to these changes will enable the nurse to improve the eating behaviors of older adults.

Psychological Factors

The most commonly performed human behaviors are eating and drinking, and making choices associated with these behaviors. These behaviors are determined by many factors, including individual psychological determinants. In selecting foods, Americans rate **taste** and **price** more important than whether food is healthy. Individual factors that influence eating, drinking, and food choices must be addressed if healthier nutritional practices are to become a reality.

Affective (depression, low self-esteem, and lack of personal control over life demands) and negative emotions (anger, frustration, fear, and insecurity) influence nutritional practices. Both can have a positive or negative effect on eating behavior resulting in decreased food intake in some individuals and increased intake in others. Increased food intake during an emotional period is comforting for many people. Recognizing the underlying emotion may help emotional eaters self-monitor food intake by increasing an awareness of eating behaviors and avoiding situations that support negative eating behaviors (Reed, Struwe, Bice, & Yates, 2017).

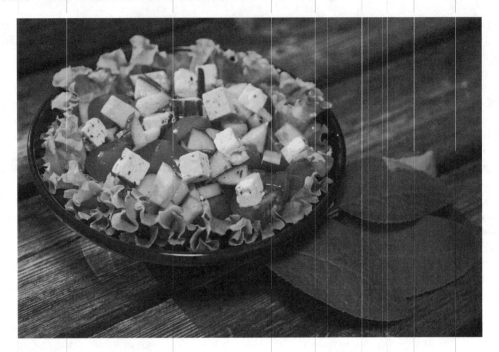

FIGURE 7–4   Raw Vegetables Are Good Sources of Fiber

Habits constitute another important determinant of eating behavior. A habit is a behavior that occurs often and performed automatically or with little conscious awareness. Habits are formed when a behavior has been consistently performed over and over. Cues within the environment serve as signals for the habitual behavior. People may become psychologically addicted to the consequences of habitual behaviors, such as the "energy spurt" experienced after the ingestion of highly refined sugars, for example, doughnuts, sweet rolls, and snack foods, or the "caffeine rush" after drinking sodas, coffee, and energy drinks (Barson, Morganstern, & Leibowitz, 2012). However, since habits are the result of the repetition of behaviors, new health habits, such as healthy eating, can be formed because eating behaviors are repetitive.

Socioeconomic and Cultural Factors

Socioeconomic and cultural factors play dominant roles in eating behaviors and nutrition. People exist within a social and cultural context that shapes their eating behaviors (see Figure 7–5). Within these groups, life circumstances that make it more difficult to manage weight and obesity include the following:

- Employment disadvantages
- Limited literacy skills
- Educational disparities
- Geographic disparities
- Stereotyping by news media

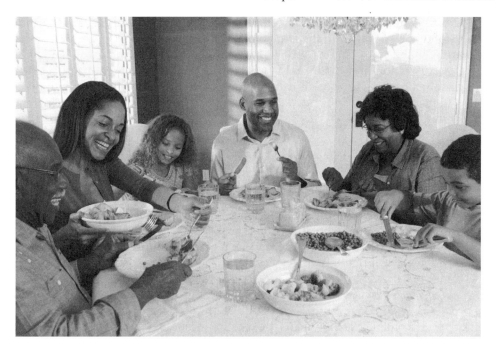

FIGURE 7–5   Family Enjoying Food and Sharing Stories

The relationship between *socioeconomic status* and consumption of fast-foods suggests a possible reason for higher levels of obesity among individuals of low socioeconomic status. For example, significant differences exist in knowledge of federal dietary guidance programs in racial and ethnic groups. Regardless of having greater knowledge about healthy food or having more disposable income, many Americans across the economic spectrum choose to eat fast-food. Research showed that 79% of participants of all economic levels consume fast-food at least once a week and almost one-fourth eat fast-food three or more times a week. The consumption of fast-food does not fluctuate based on changes in income. However, lack of free time and longer working hours influence fast-food habits (Dallas, 2017). People who feel rushed during food preparation are less likely to avoid packaged products that are high in sodium and carbohydrates, and more likely to eat at fast-food restaurants (Venn & Strazdins, 2017).

Ethnicity and culture also influence eating behavior. Food creates environments for social interaction and conveys symbolic meanings across cultures. Ethnic foods are a source of pride and identity and create a deep emotional association with the country of origin. In addition, particular foods may be associated with childhood memories.

Cultural factors contribute to patterns of obesity in childhood and youth in many minority populations. High-status and highly valued foods associated with success are often red meat, refined sugar, and fatty foods. Culture may also have differing attitudes about body size and shape. Larger body size has been associated with beauty, fertility, wealth, and power in some cultures. In others, overweight is neutral or positive unless linked with a health problem, especially for women.

Sensitivity to the difficulties that ethnic groups have in identifying the nutritional contents of foods packaged in the United States and understanding nutrition labels is imperative. Inability to obtain familiar foods and eating unfamiliar foods may be a source of frustration and distress. Language and confusing media messages about foods are often barriers to good nutrition. Nurses are challenged to work with diverse groups to increase their ability to access accurate information for making informed food choices.

Environmental Factors

Preference for unhealthy diets and large portions is influenced by advertising, the food environment, and other obesogenic factors. It is well known that food and nutrition environments contribute to obesity and chronic diseases. *Food environments* include available food sources, and what individuals are exposed to in the environment, such as healthy or unhealthy foods, food price, and food marketing. The *macro food environment* consists of food and agriculture policy, economics and pricing, and food marketing and advertising.

Obesogenic environments are all the surroundings, opportunities, and conditions that promote obesity in individuals and populations (Townshend & Lake, 2017). Social, political, and economic factors mediate exposure to obesogenic environments. *Obesogenic food environments* include home and out-of-home food sources, such as cafes, grocery stores, takeaways, and convenience stores.

The *neighborhood environment* often is a promoter of obesity. Obesogenic neighborhoods discourage physical activity due to an absence of urban parks and green space, lack of walking paths or sidewalks, fewer large retail markets and fresh food markets, and a higher concentration of small grocers, convenience stores, and fast-food restaurants. Neighborhoods with walking trails, well-maintained sidewalks, and affordable recreational facilities, as well as access to supermarkets and fresh food stores, promote healthy lifestyles. Neighborhood disparities and limited access to healthy food sources are of concern because of their potential influence on obesity. These factors reinforce the complexity of geography and eating behaviors.

Healthy food choices depend on healthy foods that are *accessible*, *available*, and *affordable*. The complexities of modern life make it difficult for many individuals to have consistent access to foods rich in required nutrients. "Food deserts" describe neighborhoods with inadequate supermarkets or other outlets for healthy food choices, while "food swamps" describe neighborhood with far greater fast-food and junk food places to eat than healthy places.

Research has shown that simply opening more supermarkets in food deserts does not change people's food purchasing and eating patterns (Cummins, Flint, & Matthews, 2014). Geographic distribution of supermarkets may be only one factor in healthy food purchasing, as socioeconomic characteristics, specifically income and education, influence the quality of food purchases (McDermot, Igoe, & Stahre, 2017). Food quality, affordability, cultural acceptability, personal preferences, and store hours influence where people shop. In addition, some people prefer to shop in small stores to minimize wait times and crowds. Improving fresh food options in small stores may help neighborhoods become healthier (Zenk, Mentz, Schulz, Johnson-Lawrence, & Gaines, 2016).

Food cost is a critical consideration for many families, given the increasing number of families living at or below the poverty level. The cost of complex carbohydrates (fruits, vegetables, and whole-wheat grains) often exceeds the cost of highly refined sugar and grain products, although other factors may also be operating (Venn & Strazdins, 2017). Even when low-cost healthy foods are available, if food preparation is time consuming, many choose convenience food over healthier choices. An important responsibility of nurses who provide nutritional guidance to diverse populations is to assist families in identifying low-cost, high-density options that are easy to prepare and within their budget.

Ease of preparation plays an important role in food selection for families across the economic spectrum. Quick preparation techniques appeal to families because of busy home/work schedules. In addition, attractiveness of prepared foods is an important consideration. Assisting clients in selecting nutritious foods that are quick to prepare and aesthetically appealing increases the likelihood of their sustaining healthy eating behaviors.

Health Policy Factors

As science advances, information sharing and marketing strategies to communicate new policies are critical. For example, beginning in 2006, the Food and Drug Administration (FDA) required the labeling of the amount of *"trans* fat" per food serving. The *Dietary Guidelines for Americans 2010* reflected this change. However, there was no coordinated effort to publicize the change, and the public only learned of the change through the mass media. Based on the sales immediately following the news coverage, the recommendations were heeded, as fewer products containing *trans* fats were purchased. However, this trend was short-lived, and after one week, sales of *trans* fat products reached pre-news levels (Niederdeppe & Frosch, 2009). *Trans* fat intake significantly decreased in 2012 as a result of (1) increased public awareness of its negative health effects, (2) required changes in the Nutrition Facts labels, (3) voluntary reformulation of foods by the food industry, and (4) state and local governments' restriction on *trans* fat in food service outlets (Doell, 2012). In 2015, the FDA announced that *trans* fats in processed foods are not safe and should be removed from all processed foods (U.S. Food and Drug Administration, 2015). This decision was largely based on results from the Nurses' Health Study that reported a 50% increase in cardiovascular heart disease (CHD) in nurses who consumed large quantities of *trans* fats (Curtis, Clapp, Goldstein, & Angell, 2016). The food industry was given three years to become compliant with the new ruling.

Supersized fast-foods including sodas and larger serving portions of food are under attack by some federal, state, and local governments and consumer groups. A lesson learned from the *trans* fat campaign was that a well-planned and ongoing public awareness campaign helps bring about sustained change. Individual responsibility for food selection and eating patterns balanced with science-based policies that are communicated to the public contribute to acceptance of evidence-based recommended changes.

The use of food additives retards spoilage and prevents deterioration of quality, improves nutritional value, enhances consumer acceptability, and facilitates preparation. Regulations require that many products list the manufacturer, packer, distributor, and the amount of each ingredient. Even with ingredients listed, information on the product is often insufficient to guide knowledgeable food selection. Not only are potentially carcinogenic additives used in the preparation of foods, such as nitrates in bacon and other processed meats, but unintentional food additives such as pesticides and other agricultural chemicals may also appear in foods. Unfortunately, some of the synergistic, cumulative, and long-term effects of many additives will be determined only after years of use and exposure within human populations.

NUTRITIONAL NEEDS ACROSS THE LIFE SPAN

Infants and Children (0 to 8 Years)

Adequate caloric and nutrient intake is critical to support proper growth and development. A healthy start for infants means encouraging mothers to breastfeed and/or use iron-rich infant formulas. Infants, whose diet is primarily mother's milk or infant formula, consume 40% or more of their calories from fat. When children reach two years of age, they need a diet lower in saturated and total fat to reduce risk of chronic diseases in later years. Children two years of age and older should limit saturated fats to 10% of calories and total fats to 30–35% of calories per day (American Heart Association, 2014).

Many Latino and African American children are overweight or obese. The home environment is a key contributor. A review of studies from 2005 to 2015 identified five factors within Latino homes associated with child obesity. These factors are:

- Parental feeding and modeling practices
- Screen time
- Physical activity level
- Socioeconomic status
- Child's sleep duration (Ochoa & Berge, 2017)

The dietary habits of young children are profoundly affected by family food preparation and eating behaviors. Parental beliefs about good nutrition for children may not match healthy recommendations and contribute to an unhealthy diet. Appropriate food choices and portions at home and when eating out are important to develop healthy eating patterns.

Food substitutions, for example, low-fat milk for whole milk and reduced-fat cheese for whole-milk cheese, markedly decrease total fat intake. However, consuming a balanced diet with appropriate portion sizes negates the need to use substitutions as the primary means to ensure a healthy diet for children. Children may find substitutions unacceptable and resist changes. Moderate changes in food consumption patterns and portions result in favorable dietary intake of most children.

Nutritional practices of day care and preschool providers and other caretakers also have significant influences on children. Organized day care is an important setting for teaching nutrition and healthy behaviors. Concerns about food costs should not interfere with the provision of nutritious meals. Parents should monitor food choices and insist that childcare facilities and providers follow healthy food guidelines.

Adolescents (9 to 19 Years)

Adolescence is a period of biological and social change. Body size, composition, and physical abilities are changing rapidly. Undernutrition slows height and weight growth and may delay puberty. Among adolescents, minimal dietary requirements are those that maintain an optimal rate of pubertal growth and development. Adolescents who are vigorously active have increased energy needs and need to consume diets providing more total nutrients than they consumed as young children. When caloric intake is too high, adolescent will gain weight, potentially leading to overweight and obesity. A caloric intake that is too low will result in loss of energy, weight loss, and, in the extreme, eating disorders that lead to health problems and even premature death.

In terms of fat intake, adolescents need to reduce total fat to less than 30% of calories per day with less animal fat and added sugars to lower risk factors for chronic disease. Because many adolescents consume fast-foods for lunch and during the evening hours, selecting healthy fast-food is a significant challenge. An example of a high-fat, fast-food meal is a double burger with sauce, milkshake, and French fries. Fat calories account for 46% of the total calories in this typical fast-food meal. Consumption of such meals day after day increases the risk for chronic diseases as early as adolescence. Consumption of added sugars found in sodas, cookies, dairy desserts, and candy also contributes to the risk. Accumulating evidence indicates that adolescent risk carries into adulthood (Centers for Disease Control and Prevention, 2015).

Adolescent girls in the United States typically begin menstruating around 12 years of age. Menstrual losses and increased physical activity increase the need for iron. Particular attention to adequate intake of iron in women's diets in general, and active young women in particular, minimizes the potential for iron-deficiency anemia. Calcium contributes to strong bones. An adequate intake of calcium throughout childhood to the age of 25 years reduces the risk of osteoporosis in later life. Young girls' food choices should ensure adequate calcium, iron, and vitamin D.

Young men are the biggest consumers of added sugars, with one-third of calories consumed from added sugars. Beverages are the main source of added sugars. Young men consume the majority of added sugars in cookies and sodas at home (U.S. Department of Health and Human Services & U.S. Department of Agriculture, 2015). Efforts to teach young people about the importance of reducing intake of sugars and other empty calories have not succeeded. The challenge is to make nutritious food options appealing to adolescents who may eat primarily for taste rather than for good nutrition or health. Peer support for healthy eating practices is critical during the adolescent years. Selecting low-fat fast-food options such as salads and wraps creates opportunities for adolescents to model good eating habits that may also influence their peers to make better food choices.

Pressure on fast-food establishments to offer healthier options creates a more supportive environment for healthier nutrition practices among adolescents. Schools are also a vehicle for early health promotion activities. School lunch programs are monitored more so than in the past. Children from families with incomes at or below the poverty level are currently eligible for subsidized or free breakfast and/or lunch, resulting in an improved nutritional status of most children.

A staged approach for weight management of overweight children and adolescents is recommended with behavioral interventions the first line of treatment. Pharmacological interventions have been restricted to severely overweight or obese adolescents due to the limited availability of safe drugs for this age group (Kumar & Kelly, 2017). Bariatric surgery has also been used in adolescents with severe obesity, but the long-term efficacy and safety are unknown.

Adults (20 to 50 Years)

The young and middle adult years are periods of rapid weight gain. The "Freshman 15" phenomenon highlights the average weight gain of young adults during their college years. This age group is exposed to a variety of highly processed foods and drinks in an "obesogenic" environment that includes eating out frequently at fast-food restaurants.

Many eating behaviors and patterns of young and middle adults are developed in childhood and adolescence. Caloric needs decrease when growth stops, so adults have less leeway for meeting nutritional requirements to maintain a healthy weight. Young and middle-aged adulthood brings the stresses of family, career, and life responsibilities. Maintaining or improving healthy eating behaviors is critical during adulthood, as the health decisions made during this period greatly influence quality of life in the later years.

Older Adults (51 Years and Older)

Research on the nutritional needs of older adults is expanding as Americans are living longer. While geographic location, economic, and lifestyle factors influence longevity, overall life expectancy increased for American men and women by 5.3 years between 1980 and 2014 (Mokdad & Hanen, 2017). However, considerable geographic disparities in longevity were reported in counties across the country, based on socioeconomic status and racial/ethnic groups.

Aging alters nutrition requirements for calories, protein, and other nutrients and brings about changes in lean body mass, physical activity, and intestinal absorption. Many older adults maintain healthy eating patterns, but for some, changing nutritional needs accompanied by deterioration in diet quality and quantity jeopardize nutritional status, quality of life, and functional independence (see Figure 7–6).

Many older adults skip meals and exclude whole categories of food from their diet because of reduced appetite, infrequent grocery shopping, lack of interest in cooking, and difficulties in chewing and swallowing. Self-medication may result in toxic levels of some multivitamin and mineral supplements. Many older adults take nutritional supplements; however, there is limited scientific support for their benefits. Nurses are encouraged to review current research findings about nutritional supplements to advise older adults about their safety.

For individuals ages 65 years and older, recommended eating patterns lower in total fat and higher in healthy fats help maintain desired body weight and lower the risk of cardiovascular heart disease (CHD). Daily physical activity, along with a healthy diet to maintain adequate weight, prevents premature mortality from CHD and maintains vigor into old age (Malhotra et al., 2017).

Essential components of the diets of older adults generally are complex carbohydrates and fiber. Many older adults have chewing and swallowing issues that make eating fruits and vegetables difficult. They also report less than half the recommended intake of 20 to 35 grams of daily fiber. The health benefits of fiber include proper bowel function, reduced risk of colon cancer, reduced serum cholesterol, and improved glucose response. Six servings of whole grain daily are the recommended minimum for older adults.

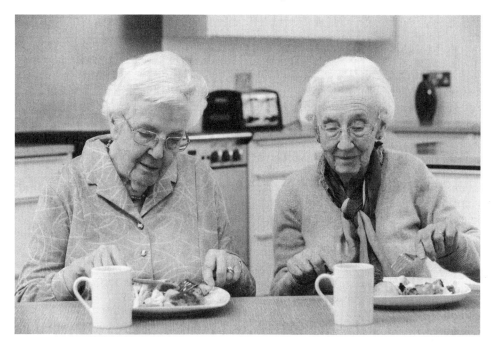

FIGURE 7–6   Healthy Eating Patterns Are Important for Older Adults

Energy requirements decline with reduction in body size, loss of lean body mass, decreased basal metabolism rate, and decreased physical activity. Physical activity maintains muscle mass, so it is highly desirable to be physically active in later years. Diets may also be deficient in protein and calories as the result of an inability to afford protein-rich foods. Older adults with limited incomes need assistance in selecting low-cost foods that are easy to chew, swallow, and meet recommended nutritional requirements. Nutrition is integral to quality of life, especially for the older adult, and thus, it is a primary focus for nurses who provide care for this age group.

STRATEGIES TO PROMOTE DIETARY CHANGE

Strategies for promoting changes in dietary patterns include the following:

- Increase access to nutrition information, education, counseling, and healthy foods in all settings and for all subpopulations.
- Strengthen the link between nutrition and physical activity in promoting healthy lives.

Nutrition education, the **food industry**, and **dietary consumption patterns** all contribute to better nutrition and healthier lives. Despite the gaps in current knowledge, cumulative research findings support the following five recommendations:

- Eat fewer calories
- Eat more vegetables, fruits, and whole grains

- Eat healthy fats, for example, walnuts, olive oil, avocadoes, and salmon
- Consume less refined sugar
- Move more

Information technology plays an increasingly important role in the delivery of **nutrition education**. Delivery methods include user-friendly applications (apps), interactive computer programs, videos, social media, blogs, and healthy nutrition instant messaging or combinations of these formats. Individual and small group sessions are also valuable, but are constrained by time and financial resources.

The **food industry** has been reluctant to recognize its role in moving Americans toward a healthier society. However, legislation and regulations on the production and availability of food options have influenced the industry by affecting cost and product development. Healthy food choices must have appeal in terms of taste and texture. Research in the food production industry has begun to focus on creating food options that are both consistent with dietary recommendations and acceptable to the public. Although marketing research plays an important role in determining what the American public chooses, food production research must also focus on how to provide more healthy food choices and motivate the public to choose healthier foods. Every facet of food production, from the grower to the processor, has a part to play in the nutritional health of Americans.

Dietary consumption patterns are the focus of the 2015–2020 Dietary Guidelines. Normal weight individuals, along with overweight and obese individuals, are likely to require changes to improve their eating patterns. The focus for normal weight individuals has shifted from reducing calories to managing food choices both within and across the food groups. Some shifts are minor and accomplished by making substitutions, and other shifts require a committed effort to make significant changes. The guidelines are easily accessible on the Web (U.S. Department of Health and Human Services & U.S. Department of Agriculture, 2015).

STRATEGIES FOR MAINTAINING RECOMMENDED WEIGHT

Weight maintenance is necessary throughout life to prevent or reduce health problems associated with overweight and obesity and contribute to a healthy life. The physical basis for excessive weight gain is relatively simple and straightforward, although the etiologies of these behaviors are complex. Overweight and obesity result from an imbalance in energy because of eating too many calories and performing too little physical activity. Weight management means balancing the number of calories consumed with the number of calories burned. Despite the multiple factors involved, diet and regular physical activity are the cornerstones to prevent overweight and obesity. Strategies to promote healthy eating habits and physical activity are available at the National Institute of Diabetes and Digestive and Kidney Diseases website. Strategies include the following:

- Choose foods that are lower in unhealthy fats
- Learn healthier ways to make favorite foods
- Learn to recognize and control environmental cues that increase the desire to eat

- Have a healthy snack an hour before a social gathering
- Engage in moderate-intensity physical activity for 30 minutes daily or 150 minutes per week
- Take a walk instead of watching television
- Do not eat meals in front of the television
- Keep records of food intake and physical activity
- Pay attention to why you are eating

STRATEGIES TO PROMOTE DIETARY CHANGES IN DIVERSE POPULATIONS

Promoting dietary changes in diverse populations requires an understanding of the influence of culture on eating patterns. Specific factors include the following:

- Understanding cultural beliefs about the relationship between food and health
- Recognizing how food consumption practices contribute to cultural identity
- Assessing the extent of acculturation to dominant-group nutritional behaviors
- Offering consultants who have similar ethnic backgrounds
- Recognizing nutritional attributes of ethnic foods
- Reinforcing positive ethnic nutritional practices
- Providing information on nutrient values of ethnic foods
- Working with ethnic restaurants to offer acceptable healthy choices
- Incorporating healthy ethnic food choices in work and school cafeterias

In all cultures, foods symbolize a group's heritage and identity and play important roles in celebrations, rites of passage, and religious practices. Dietary rules and preferences, food preparation, food taboos, and customs are unique to all racial and ethnic groups around the world. In addition, the definition of "healthy" or "unhealthy" foods may vary across cultures. Many food customs have been developed based on food availability and geographic location. An assessment of an individual's cultural food patterns and meanings is essential to understand dietary behaviors and to learn what changes may be needed to promote health. Engaging members of a culture who are responsible for food preparation in the assessment and planning process enables the nurse to incorporate cultural values and food preferences in the change process to facilitate realistic, feasible changes.

STRATEGIES FOR INITIATING A WEIGHT-REDUCTION PROGRAM

The most effective ways to lose weight are still debated. However, the primary focus of dietary changes for overweight and obese individuals is to modify dietary patterns to reduce weight. Counting calories to lose weight, based on one-pound equivalent to 3,500 calories, means cutting 500 calories per day to lose one pound a week. This calculation does not work for everyone. It may be too low for an active man and too high for a sedentary woman. One's baseline caloric intake (including food and beverages) should be calculated for one week using a food journal or online calorie counter. Most people underestimate their daily caloric intake, so an accurate baseline is needed to calculate the correct calorie target.

Another strategy is to focus on what *motivates* an individual to change unhealthy dietary patterns to healthy ones. Personal motivation plays a fundamental role in this effort. Persons who are ready, determined to change, and understand the need to change are more likely to incorporate new behaviors into their diet (Livia et al., 2016). Lack of continued personal commitment to a healthy diet is the major barrier to long-term success. Relapse is high in weight loss programs. **High motivation, self-efficacy, self-monitoring, positive body image**, and **eating restraint** are predictors of weight control and represent targets for interventions in overweight and obese populations (Teixeira et al., 2015).

Behavioral management strategies refer to specific techniques used to change an individual's behavior and lifestyle. Behavioral management strategies include **self-monitoring, stress management, stimulus control, problem solving, rewarding behavior changes, cognitive restructuring, social support, motivational interviewing,** and **relapse prevention training. Planning** and **self-monitoring** are two successful behavioral management strategies. Planning meals for healthy dietary intake, scheduling time for physical activity, and keeping personal daily paper dairies or using smartphone apps to assess progress give insight into personal behaviors. Additional helpful strategies include realistic **goal setting**, learning to **problem solve** difficult eating situations, and ongoing **feedback** and **support** from a professional (Heymsfield & Wadden, 2017). (See Chapter 2 for additional behavioral management strategies.)

Weight management is difficult and requires a lifelong commitment, making it a challenge for individuals and health care professionals. Individuals who are overweight or obese and desire to lose weight should consult a health care professional before starting an aggressive weight loss program. An assessment of current dietary habits, a personal health and family history, and physical examination are essential to develop an individualized, effective program.

The assessment should include the following questions:

- Is the person strongly motivated to lose weight?
- Is the person willing to commit the time and financial resources needed?
- Does the person believe he or she can be successful in a weight loss program?
- Does the person understand the possible risks of weight loss interventions?
- Are weight loss goals realistic?
- What is the person's attitude toward physical activity?
- Does the person have a support system to facilitate weight loss?
- What are the potential barriers to successful weight loss?
- Has the person had past success in weight loss? If so, what worked? What did not work?
- What factors caused the person to relapse in the past?

Caloric reduction with attention to portion size, while maintaining adequate nutrient levels, adequate vitamins and minerals, and adequate fiber, is the best way to achieve and maintain desired weight in conjunction with a regular physical activity program. It is important for clients to understand that even a modest weight loss is beneficial.

Making changes to eating patterns is often overwhelming. Emphasizing small changes or shifts in food choices within a meal, one day a week, for example, is an important step. Small changes may motivate an individual to progress to larger changes.

A simple choice of a green salad rather than French fries in one meal plan reduces calories and may encourage other shifts toward healthier eating patterns.

Strategies for long-term weight loss maintenance that have been successful include the following:

- Relapse prevention training to teach specific skills
- Prompts via wireless devices/phones to provide frequent contacts
- Peer/social support, face-to-face meetings, and social networks
- Cognitive behavioral therapy
- Collaboration among health care team members

INTERVENTIONS TO CHANGE EATING PATTERNS

Interventions that are based on research evidence add to nutrition knowledge and are more likely to be successful in changing eating patterns. Evidence-based interventions occur in settings such as homes, schools, organized childcare centers, and worksites. These interventions also target individuals and groups in community settings such as churches, schools, and worksite.

Interventions for Children and Adults

Effective strategies to change eating behaviors in children suffer from many barriers, including lack of family motivation and support, costs, and lack of time by parents to commit to changes in eating patterns and physical activity behaviors. Parental support is critical for behavior change, as parents purchase and plan meals, prepare the food, and role model healthy or unhealthy behaviors.

When planning dietary interventions for adults, important considerations include an individual's ability to incorporate dietary changes into the daily routine. Dietary options include low carbohydrate, low fat, high protein, low glycemic, high fiber, or a combination of plans. Commercial weight loss programs, such as Weight Watchers, and meal replacement programs have become popular and have reported weight loss outcomes (Thom & Lean, 2017). Very low-calorie diets are risky and should be avoided or undertaken only under close supervision.

Meal replacement diets are increasingly popular for adults who have time constraints, lack the inclination to prepare meals, and/or have difficulty controlling portion size. The results of implementing meal replacements have been favorable with sustained weight loss up to four years. However, when substitute meals are no longer used, individuals are likely to regain weight if they have not learned to manage portions and plan and implement a well-balanced diet. Although short-term weight loss is positive, a supportive approach with extended contacts is effective in maintaining behavior change (Livia et al., 2016).

The Mediterranean diet is based on the traditional diet in the Mediterranean area. It is considered a sociocultural eating style that emphasizes fruits and vegetables, olive oil, grains, nuts, beans, fish and seafood, and limited consumption of dairy and red meats. Advantages of the diet include moderation, pleasant taste, and familiarity. Research has well established the health benefits of the diet as well as its role in weight loss, particularly for persons who are at risk for cardiovascular disease (Katz & Meller, 2014; Thom & Lean, 2017).

Interventions for Worksites and Schools

The U.S. Community Preventive Services Task Force conducts ongoing systematic reviews of nutrition and physical activity to determine the effectiveness of worksite and school-based interventions in preventing overweight and obesity. School and worksite interventions are potentially more effective because children and adults spend most of their time in these respective sites and primarily rely on others to provide and prepare their food for a considerable part of the day. Health promotion in schools, workplaces, and communities is discussed in Chapter 13.

ROLE OF TECHNOLOGY IN DESIGNING INTERVENTIONS

As the number of health-related apps rapidly increases, interventions incorporating these apps are increasing as well. Wireless health apps and computers are promising tools to change and manage health behaviors. However, they only reach a portion of the population. More people across the world use smartphones than computers, but significant numbers of the population are not users of either technology, continuing the digital divide (Ernsting et al., 2017). The use of health apps usually reflects an individual's motivation to change a behavior. However, many health app users discontinue using the apps due to the time needed to input required data, lack of long-term appeal, and concerns about sharing personal data.

Nutrition, weight management, and physical activity apps are the most popular. These apps have the potential to reach large numbers of people, providing opportunities for diet monitoring with tailored information, tracking behaviors, self-monitoring, and the availability of a community of supporters and social networks. The most frequently used behavioral techniques are *goal setting, self-monitoring*, and *provision of feedback*. Apps that include communication with monitors or health care professionals are particularly appealing to users (Krebs & Duncan, 2015). Although some short-term benefits have been reported, the benefits of weight loss apps on long-term changes in nutritional behaviors are still unknown (Bardus, van Beurden, Smith, & Abraham, 2016).

The quality of apps available varies greatly. Behavior change theories should be incorporated into the development of mobile app interventions to ensure the efficacy of interventions (Schoeppe et al., 2016). Emerging technologies such as image recognition, artificial intelligence, and language processing will further enhance the quality of health-related apps and computer software (Franco, Fallaize, Lovegrove, & Hwang, 2016).

Evidence-based apps to improve diet show promise for adults but few apps have targeted children. Over 100,000 individuals used a smartphone app to self-monitor eating disorders over a two-year period. Over half of the users reported that they were not receiving clinical treatment and one-third reported that they had not shared their eating disorder with anyone (Tregarthen, Lock, & Darcy, 2015). Smartphone apps and computer software programs have the potential to reach large underserved populations. Regardless of the issues and challenges, the use of computers and wireless devices to deliver health information and services continues to grow and is fast becoming an essential component in health behavior change and maintenance (see Figure 7–7).

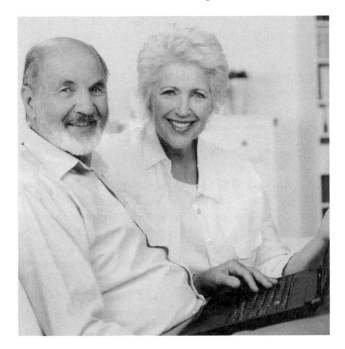

FIGURE 7–7   Family Members Using Computer to Seek Health Information

CONSIDERATIONS FOR PRACTICE IN NUTRITION AND HEALTH PROMOTION

Health professionals are role models for healthy eating and weight management. Role modeling recommended eating patterns, as well as managing issues that undermine maintenance of positive nutritional practices, indicates sincerity and commitment to good health practices. The public expects all health care professionals to be healthy and to model positive eating and exercise habits.

Monitoring the nutritional health of individuals, families, and the community is the shared responsibility of all members of the health care team. Dietary counseling and education should be a central component of nursing practice. Follow-up of at-risk clients who are overweight or obese must be a priority. Focusing on healthy eating patterns with preschoolers is a priority so that they develop and sustain positive eating habits throughout life.

Engaging clients in dialogue about their dietary practices creates teaching opportunities and promotes behavior change. Many nurses express lack of time and/or lack of knowledge to be able to discuss nutrition and diet with clients. Priority should be given to learning how to address these topics to assist clients adopt healthier eating patterns and meet their dietary goals. Nutrition websites are readily available for nurses to learn or update their knowledge about evidence-based interventions and dietary guidelines.

Nurses can also partner with school, business, and community leaders and policy makers to improve food choices in cafeterias and vending machines in schools and worksites. Participating in community and legislative activities to promote the nutritional health of all is a responsibility of all health care professionals.

OPPORTUNITIES FOR RESEARCH IN NUTRITION AND HEALTH PROMOTION

Preventing obesity and helping overweight individuals change unhealthy behaviors require new, innovative approaches. The emphasis should be on promoting health by preventing weight gain, especially in childhood and adolescence, rather than managing weight loss.

Novel strategies to reverse the health consequences of overweight and obesity need to be identified and tested. The underlying factors that prevent weight gain and/or sustain weight loss are unknown and need to be explored. Research that addresses the underlying genetic and epigenetic mechanisms of energy balance and weight offers exciting opportunities for many nurse researchers.

Physical activity and healthy eating patterns are both essential in preventing weight gain. Yet interventions that address both physical activity and healthy eating patterns with long-term success are limited. Additional interventions that incorporate technology are required to determine their joint and respective relationships in successful weight loss programs.

Individual dietary interventions have had limited success in sustaining weight loss. While multicomponent interventions are resource intensive and often difficult to implement, they are the most successful weight loss programs. In addition, family interventions to promote physical activity and encourage healthy food choices need to be developed and tested for long-term effectiveness. Community-level interventions that target the food and neighborhood environments in ethnic and low-income communities will also address a critical need.

It is no longer sufficient to focus solely on the individual to promote healthy food choices. The complexity of the multiple social and environmental factors involved necessitates a transdisciplinary approach and the involvement of government and health policy makers as well.

Summary

Lifelong healthy eating patterns decrease the risks of chronic health problems that occur in individuals who are overweight or obese. Individual, social, physical, and environmental barriers to healthy eating behaviors contribute to the significant problems associated with the increase in overweight and obese individuals. Good nutrition is a critical component in health promotion and prevention and an important dimension of competent self-care.

Cultural and ethnic backgrounds influence eating behavior and must be accounted for in changing eating patterns. The individual, family, and community must all participate in interventions to increase healthy eating behaviors. Research has substantiated the complexity of factors that determine eating behaviors. Ongoing research is essential to develop interventions that promote successful behavior change.

Learning Activities

1. Compare your personal diet with the *2015–2020 Dietary Guidelines for Americans* recommendations and identify two changes you are willing to make in your diet.
2. Use MyPlate to assist you in making the modifications you identified in Learning Activity 1.
3. Interview an adult from a cultural group different from your own to assess the role of culture in their food preferences and practices. Identify one culturally sensitive strategy to promote healthy eating in their culture based on your assessment.

4. Engage an adolescent and an older adult in discussions to assess their knowledge and understanding of their nutritional status. Assist them to develop a plan to overcome identified barriers to healthy eating.
5. Select a mobile app for weight management. Review the app to identify the behavior change techniques used by the app. Discuss the effectiveness of these techniques, and make suggestion for improving the app.

References

American Heart Association. (2014). *Dietary recommendations for healthy children*. AHA Scientific Position. Retrieved from http://www.heart.org/HEARTORG/HealthyLiving/Dietary-Recommendations-for-Healthy-Children_UCM_303886_Article.jsp#.WbwPZU2oupo

Bardus, M., van Beurden, S., Smith, J., & Abraham, C. (2016). A review and content analysis of engagement, functionality, aesthetics, information quality, and change techniques in the most popular commercial apps for weight management. *International Journal of Behavioral Nutrition and Physical Activity, 13*, 35. doi:10.1186/s12966-016-0359-9

Barson, J., Morganstern, I., & Leibowitz, S. (2012). Neurobiology of consummatory behavior: Mechanisms underlying overeating and drug use. *Institute for Laboratory Animal Research Journal, 53*(1), 35–38. doi:10.1093/ilar.53.1.35

Bianchi, M. L., Sawyer, A. J., & Bachrach, L. K. (2016). Rationale for bone health assessment in childhood and adolescence. In E. Fung, L. Bachrach, & A. Sayer (Eds.), *Bone health assessment in pediatrics* (pp. 1–21). Switzerland: Springer International.

Casavale, K. (2017). *Help your patients use the Nutrition Facts label to cut down on added sugars*. Food Facts: New and Improved Nutrition Facts Label. Retrieved from https://fda.gov/downloads/Food/IngredientsPackingLabeling/LabelingNutrition/

Centers for Disease Control and Prevention. (2015). *Adult obesity causes & consequences*. Retrieved from https://www.cdc.gov/obesity/adult/causes.html

Centers for Disease Control and Prevention. (2017). *Adult obesity prevalence maps*. Retrieved from https://www.cdc.gov/obesity/data/prevalence-maps.html

Claussnitzer, M., Dankel, S., Kim, K., Quon, G., Meuleman, W., Haugen, C., . . . Kellis, M. (2015). FTO obesity variant circuitry and adipocyte browning in humans. *New England Journal of Medicine, 373*(10), 895–907. doi:10.1056/NEJMoa1502214

Crujeiras, A., Carreira, M., Cabia, B., Andrade, S., Amil, M., & Casanueva, F. (2015). Leptin resistance in obesity: An epigenetic landscape. *Life Sciences, 140*, 57–63. doi:10.1016/j.lfs.2015.05.003

Cummins, S., Flint, E., & Matthews, A. (2014). New neighborhood grocery store increased awareness of food access but did not alter dietary habits or obesity. *Health Affairs, 33*(2), 283–291. doi:10.1377/hlthaff.2013.0512

Curtis, C., Clapp, J., Goldstein, G., & Angell, S. (2016). How the Nurses' Health Study helped Americans take the *trans* fat out. *American Journal of Public Health, 106*(9), 1537–1539.

Dallas, M. (2017). *America loves fast food*. National Institutes of Health/U.S. National Library of Medicine. Retrieved from https://Medlineplus.gov/news/fullstory_165511.html

Doell, D. (2012). *Trans fat intake by the U.S. population*. Office of Food Additive Safety. Retrieved from http://www.fda.gov

Ernsting, C., Dombrowski, S., Oedekoven, M., O'Sullivan, J., Kanzler, M., Kuhlmey, A., & Gellert, P. (2017). Using smartphones and health apps to change and manage health behaviors: A population-based survey. *Journal of Medical Internet Research, 19*(4), e101. doi:10.2196/jmir.6838

Flier, J., & Maratos-Flier, E. (2017). Leptin's physiological role: Does the emperor of energy balance have no clothes? *Cell Metabolism, 26*(1), 24–26. doi:10.1016/j.cmet.2017.05.013

Franco, R., Fallaize, R., Lovegrove, J., & Hwang, F. (2016). Popular nutrition-related mobile apps: A feature assessment. *Journal of Medical Internet Research, 4*(3), e85. doi:10.2196/mhealth.5846

Graff, M., Church, T., & Lavie, C. (2017). *No excuses: Exercise can overcome the 'obesity gene'.* National Institutes of Health/U.S. National Library of Medicine. Retrieved from https://medlineplus.gov/news/fullstory_164987.html

Hassan, T., Badr, M., Karam, N., Zkaria, M., Saadany, H., Rahman, D., . . . Selim, A. (2016). Impact of iron deficiency anemia on the function of the immune system in children. *Medicine (Baltimore), 95*(47), e5395. doi:10.1097/MD.0000000000005395

Heymsfield, S., & Wadden, T. (2017). Mechanisms, pathophysiology, and management of obesity. *New England Journal of Medicine, 376*(3), 254–266.

Hills, A., Street, S., & Byrne, N. (2015). Physical activity and health: "What is old is new again". In F. Toldra (Ed.), *Advances in food and nutrition research* (Vol. 75, pp. 77–95). St. Louis, MO: Elsevier, Inc.

Hollands, S., Shemilt, I., Marteau, T. M., Jebb, S. A., Lewis, H. B., Wei, Y., . . . Ogilvie, D. (2015). Portion, package or tableware size for changing selection and consumption of food, alcohol and tobacco. *Cochrane Database of Systemic Reviews,* (9), 1–393. doi:10.1002/14651858.CD011045.pub2

Huang, T., & Hu, F. (2015). Gene–environment interactions and obesity: Recent developments and future directions. *BMC Medical Genomics, 8*(Suppl 1), S2. doi:10.1186/1755-8794-8-S1-S2

Katz, D., & Meller, S. (2014). Can we say what diet is best for health? *Annual Review of Public Health, 35,* 83–103. doi:10.1146/annurev-publhealth-032013-182351

Krebs, P., & Duncan D. (2015). Health app use among US mobile phone owners: A national survey. *Journal of Medical Internet Research, 3*(4), e101. doi:10.2196/mhealth.4924

Kumar, S., & Kelly, A. (2017). Review of childhood obesity: From epidemiology, etiology, and comorbidities to clinical assessment and treatment. *Mayo Clinic Proceedings, 92*(2), 251–265. doi: 10.1016/j.mayocp.2016.09.017

Livia, B., Elisa, R., Claudia, R., Roberto, P., Cristina, A., Emilia, S., . . . Claudia, M. (2016). Stage of change and motivation to a healthier lifestyle before and after an intensive lifestyle intervention. *Journal of Obesity.* doi:10.1155/2016/6421265

Malhotra, A., Redberg, R., & Meier, P. (2017). Saturated fat does not clog the arteries: Coronary heart disease is a chronic inflammatory condition, the risk of which can be effectively reduced from healthy lifestyle interventions. *British Journal of Sports Medicine, 51*(15). doi:10.1136/bjsports-2016-097285

McDermot, D., Igoe, B., & Stahre, M. (2017). Assessment of healthy food availability in Washington State—Questioning the food desert paradigm. *Journal of Nutrition Education and Behavior, 49*(2), 130–136. doi:10.1016/j.jneb.2016.10.012

Micali, N., Martini, M., Thomas, J., Eddy, K., Kothari, R., Russell, E., . . . Treasure, J. (2017). Lifetime and 12-month prevalence of eating disorders amongst women in mid-life: A population-based study of diagnoses and risk factors. *BMC Medicine, 15,* 12. doi:10.1186/s12916-016-0766-4

Mokdad, A., & Hanen, L. (2017). Longevity in the U.S.: Location, location, location. *JAMA Internal Medicine.* Retrieved from https://medlineplus.gov/news/fullstory_165345.html

National Institutes of Health. (2014). *What is iron-deficiency anemia?* Heart, Lung, and Blood Institute Health Report. Retrieved from https://www.nhlbi.nih.gov/health-topics/topics/ida

Niederdeppe, J., & Frosch, D. (2009). News coverage and sales of products with trans fat: Effects before and after changes in federal labeling policy. *American Journal of Preventive Medicine, 36*(5), 395–401. doi:10.1016/j.amepre.2009.01.023

Ochoa, A., & Berge, J. (2017). Home environmental influences on childhood obesity in the Latino population: A decade review of literature. *Journal of Immigrant and Minority Health, 19*(2), 430–447. doi:10.1007/s10903-016-0539-3

Quarta, C., Sanchez-Garrido, M., Tschop, M., & Clemmensen, C. (2016). Renaissance of leptin for obesity therapy. *Diabetologia, 59*(5), 920–927. doi:10.1007/s00125-016-3906-7

Reed, J., Struwe, L., Bice, M., & Yates, B. (2017). The impact of self-monitoring food intake on motivation, physical activity and weight loss in rural adults. *Applied Nursing Research, 35,* 36–41. doi:10.1016/j.apnr.2017.02.008

Robert Wood Johnson Foundation & Trust for America's Health. (2017). *What is the state of obesity in America?* Better Policies for a Healthier America. Retrieved from http://www.rwjf.org/content/rwjf/en/search-results.html?k=policy&u&sp

Romieu, I., Dossus, L., Barquera, S., Blottière, H., Franks, P., Gunter, M., . . . Willett, W. C. (IARC Working Group on Energy Balance and Obesity). (2017). Energy balance and obesity: What are the main drivers? *Cancer Causes & Control, 28*(3), 247–258. doi:10.1007/s10552-017-0869-z

Scharf, R., & DeBoer, M. (2016). Sugar-sweetened beverages and children's health. *Annual Review of Public Health, 37,* 273–293. doi:10.1146/annurev-publhealth-032315-021528

Schoeppe, S., Alley, S., Van Lippevelde, W., Bray, N., Williams, S., Duncan, M., & Vandelanotte, C. (2016). Efficacy of interventions that use apps to improve diet, physical activity and sedentary behavior: A systematic review. *International Journal of Behavioral Nutrition and Physical Activity, 13*, 127. doi:10.1186/s12966-016-0454-y

Shook, R., Hand, G., Drenowatz, C., Hebert, J., Paluch, A., Blundell, J., . . . Blair, S. (2015). Low levels of physical activity are associated with dysregulation of energy intake and fat mass gain over 1 year. *American Journal of Clinical Nutrition, 102*(6), 1332–1338. doi:10.3945/ajcn.115.115360

Smink, F., van Hoeken, D., & Hoek, H. (2013). Epidemiology, course, and outcome of eating disorders. *Current Opinion in Psychiatry, 26*(6), 543–548. doi:10.1097/YCO.0b013e328365a24f

Soeters, P., Bozzetti, F., Cynober, L., Forbes, A., Shenkin, A., & Sobotka, L. (2017). Defining malnutrition: A plea to rethink. *Clinical Nutrition, 36*(3), 896–901. doi:10.1016/j.clnu.2016.09.032

Teixeira, P., Carraca, E., Marques, M., Rutter, H., Oppert, J., De Bourdeaudhuji, I., . . . Brug, J. (2015). Successful behavior change in obesity interventions in adults: A systematic review of self-regulation mediators. *BMC Medicine, 13*, 84. doi:10.1186/s12916-015-0323-6

Thom, G., & Lean, M. (2017). Is there an optimal diet for weight management and metabolic health? *Gastroenterology, 152*(7), 1739–1751. doi:10.1053/j.gastro.2017.01.056

Townshend, T., & Lake, A. (2017). Obesogenic environments: Current evidence of the built and food environments. *Perspectives in Public Health, 137*(1), 38–45. doi:10.1177/1757913916679860

Tregarthen, J., Lock, J., & Darcy, A. (2015). Development of a smartphone application for eating disorder and self-monitoring. *International Journal of Eating Disorders, 48*(7), 972–982. doi:10.1002/eat.22386

Tung, Y., Gulati, P., Liu, C., Rimmington, D., Dennis, R., Ma, M., . . . Yeo, G. (2015). FTO is necessary for the induction of leptin resistance by high-fat feeding. *Molecular Metabolism, 4*(4), 287–298. doi:10.1016/j.molmet.2015.01.011

U.S. Department of Health and Human Services & U.S. Department of Agriculture. (2015). *Dietary Guidelines for Americans 2015–2020* (8th ed.). Retrieved from https://health.gov/dietaryguidelines/2015/guidelines/

U.S. Food and Drug Administration. (2015). *Final determination regarding partially hydrogenated oils.* Retrieved June 23, 2017 from https://www.fda.gov/food/ingredientspackaginglabeling/foodadditivesingredients/ucm449162.htm

van Dijk, S., Tellam, R., Morrison, J., Muhlausler, B., & Molloy, P. (2015). Recent developments on the role of epigenetics in obesity and metabolic disease. *Clinical Epigenetics, 7*, 66. doi:10.1186/s13148-015-0101-5

Venn, D., & Strazdins, L. (2017). Your money or your time? How both types of scarcity matter to physical activity and healthy eating. *Social Science & Medicine, 172*, 98–106. doi:10.1016/j.socscimed.2016.10.023

Wirth, R., Streicher, M., Smoliner, C., Kolb, C., Hiesmayr, M., Thiem, U., . . . Volkert, D. (2016). The impact of weight loss and low BMI on mortality in nursing home residents—Results from the nutritionDay in nursing homes. *Clinical Nutrition, 35*(4), 900–906. doi:10.1016/j.clnu.2015.06.003

World Health Organization. (2017). *WHO Fact Sheet: Noncommunicable diseases.* Geneva, Switzerland: Author.

Zenk, S., Mentz, G., Schulz, A., Johnson-Lawrence, V., & Gaines, C. (2016). Longitudinal associations between observed and perceived neighborhood food availability and body mass index in a multiethnic urban sample. *Health Education & Behavior, 44*(1), 41–51. doi:10.1177/1090198116644150

Zhang, J., Roslin, M., & Chopra, R. (2017). Have Americans given up on losing weight? *Journal of American Medicine Association.*

CHAPTER 8

Stress Management and Health Promotion

OBJECTIVES

This chapter will enable the reader to:

1. Describe the relationship between stress and health.
2. Discuss the significance of workplace stress.
3. Describe ways to minimize the frequency of stress-inducing situations.
4. Discuss six strategies to increase resistance to stress.
5. Contrast complementary therapies to manage stress.
6. Examine the influence of technology on stress-reducing interventions.

Stress is a significant issue that needs to be addressed by all nurses and health care professionals. Early childhood stressors, including traumatic life events and poverty, have been associated with increased risk for depression and suicide (Sharma, Powers, Bradley, & Ressler, 2016; Steptoe & Kivimaki, 2013). In adults, heavy workloads, job insecurity, and poor socioeconomic circumstances have been associated with chronic stress disorders, such as depression and cardiovascular disease (Bot & Kuiper, 2017; Tawakol et al., 2017). The continuing increase in stress-related health problems highlights the importance for nurses to promote mental health by fostering resistance to stress-inducing situations among individuals and families. Nurses' personal approach to stress reduction and stress management practices contributes to their own mental health and enables them to promote healthy responses to stress in their clients.

THE STRESS RESPONSE

Stress is an inevitable, unavoidable, human experience in any society, more so in a society characterized by rapid and accelerating change. Over 80 years ago, Selye, a pioneer in stress research, defined stress as "a nonspecific response of the body to any demand." He described the "general adaptation syndrome (GAS)," or the "fight-or-flight" response, that resulted from central nervous system activation and release of hormones to respond to the threat (Selye, 1936). Research has greatly expanded our understanding of biological stress responses to psychological and physiological stressors, including identification of stress neural pathways with brain imaging and molecular genetics and epigenetics (Fink, 2016).

Individuals react differently to stress. Some are able to adapt to stress, while others see stress as a threat. These differing reactions to stress led to a re-evaluation of homeostasis, the process of maintaining an internal physiological balance through constancy. *Allostasis*, the process of adapting in the face of potentially stressful events, maintains stability through change. When exposed to a stressor, the body responds by turning on complex systems and processes to respond and adapt to the threat (McEwen, 2017a). If the stress continues over weeks and months, negative effects, described as allostatic load results (McEwen, 2017b).

A continued elevated stress response results in *allostatic load*, with resultant vulnerability and dysfunction. *Allostatic load* reflects the cumulative negative effects of prolonged environmental and psychosocial stressors such as poverty, adverse early life experiences, circadian disruptions, excess calorie intake, smoking, and alcohol use. In other words, how individuals cope with challenges over a lifetime influences allostasis, allostatic load, and resulting disease (McEwen, 2017a). Physiological indicators of allostatic load include (1) **hypertension**, (2) **increased high-density lipoproteins (HDLs)** and **total cholesterol**, (3) **increased glycosylated hemoglobin (HgbA1c) levels**, and (4) **immune suppression**. *Cumulative stress* has the potential to predict risk for many chronic diseases, such as diabetes, cardiovascular disease, and cancer (McEwen, 2017a, 2017b).

Stressors are environmental demands and conflicts that may or may not challenge a person's resources. Stressors may be viewed as challenging, stimulating, and exciting, or perceived as uncontrollable or emotionally distressing. Healthy individuals with support systems are resilient and are able to manage stressors successfully. Stress in modern society tends to stem primarily from psychological rather than physical threats (see Figure 8–1). However, the document *Stress in America: Coping with Change*, reported that more Americans were concerned about terrorism, police violence, and personal safety, than in previous years, evidence of growing concern about physical threats (American Psychological Association, 2017a).

Frequent excessive daily life stressors may also result in physiological responses. Individuals may respond to stress by experiencing digestive symptoms, headaches, irritability, sleeplessness, and depression (see Figure 8–2). If these stressors continue over time, they can contribute to serious health problems such as cardiovascular disease, hypertension, diabetes, and other illnesses (Steptoe & Kivimaki, 2013; Tawakol et al., 2017).

Coping strategies are learned and purposeful cognitive, emotional, and behavioral efforts to manage or reduce stressors by adapting to the environment or changing

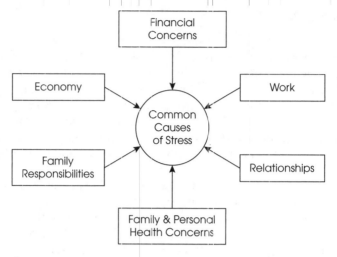

FIGURE 8-1 Causes of Psychological Stress

it (Lazarus, 1999). In the coping process, the ability to regulate emotions, behavior, and the environment is critical to successful outcomes. In other words, coping is behavior that uses one's available resources to manage stressful situations (Folkman, 2013).

Cognitive appraisal and coping constitute the stress-coping process. Cognitive appraisal consists of two phases. In *primary appraisal*, the person evaluates the stress to determine whether there is potential harm or benefit to one's health and well-being.

In *secondary appraisal*, the person evaluates available options or resources to address the threat. In other words, the individual evaluates what can be done, such as

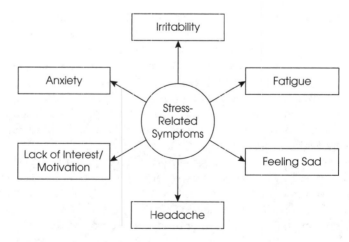

FIGURE 8-2 Symptoms of Stress

altering the situation, accepting it, seeking more information, and/or holding back from acting impulsively (Folkman, 2013; Lazarus & Folkman, 1984).

Coping strategies regulate stressful emotions (emotion-focused coping) and/ or alters the person–environment relationship that is causing the distress (problem-focused coping). Both forms of coping occur in stressful encounters. *Problem-focused coping* is likely to be dominant in encounters viewed as changeable, whereas *emotion-focused coping* often dominates in encounters viewed as unchangeable. Encounters involving threats to self-esteem are often the most difficult to resolve. These threats include the possibility of losing the affection of someone significant, losing self-respect or the respect of others, and appearing to be unethical or incompetent (Folkman, 2013).

Everyone experiences stress. Some people are able to cope with stress more effectively and recover from stressful events quickly. Of the many life events that affect individuals, none is more widespread than stress and stress-related health conditions.

STRESS AND HEALTH

In 2017, adults 18 years and older reported the first significant increase in overall stress level in America in 10 years. They also reported experiencing more physical and psychological stress symptoms leading to the possibility of long-term consequences (American Psychological Association, 2017a). Stress is associated with decreased life satisfaction, development of mental disorders, and other chronic diseases, including cardiovascular disease, gastrointestinal disorders, low back pain, headaches, and decreased immunological functioning. Stress induces negative risk behaviors such as smoking, physical inactivity, overeating, and drug and alcohol abuse (Stults-Kolehmainen & Sinha, 2014).

Exposure to stress and negative life experiences—loneliness, poverty, financial insecurity—can exact a toll and may result in poor health and disease. The nature of interpersonal relationships may also be detrimental to health. The quality of the relationship is the variant (Shapero et al., 2014).

Epigenetics, the study of developmental and environmental influences on the alteration of gene expression, is an attempt to describe how experiences such as stress, while not altering the DNA sequence, may modify DNA proteins, leading to enhanced or silenced expression of a specific gene. Using data from the VA Normative Aging Study, researchers tested the association between chronic cardiovascular disease and psychological factors (anxiety, depression, hostility, and life satisfaction) and DNA methylation of genes related to inflammatory system markers. Positive and negative psychological factors were associated with the DNA of selected genes. Research is ongoing to determine if epigenetic changes result in mediation of the effects of psychological factors on chronic cardiovascular disease (Kim et al., 2016). These initial results provide evidence of the person–environment connection. The challenge is to determine whether stress management interventions can block stress-induced damage caused by environmental and personal exposures, such as infections, toxins, and social interactions.

STRESS ACROSS THE LIFE SPAN

Children

Childhood is a critical period characterized by increased vulnerability to stressors. The prevalence of stress-related disorders in children appears to be increasing, although this increase may be due to increased access to health care resulting in more diagnoses, changes in public perception of mental illnesses, or changes in the definition of mental disorders. Physician office visits resulting in a diagnosis of psychological or developmental disorders have significantly increased, especially among male children (Olfson et al., 2014). The increase in office visits has been associated with an increase in the availability and prescribing of psychotropic drugs, raising potential safety issues due to possible adverse side effects.

Children experience stress and develop coping patterns early in life that often become lifelong coping patterns. Self-esteem, personality characteristics (temperament), gender, social support, parental child-rearing patterns, previous stressful experiences, and illness are some of the factors related to stress in children. Early life event experiences and parenting styles have been shown to result in either adaptive or maladaptive outcomes in later life (McEwen, 2017a).

Environmental and social stressors also place children at high risk. Stressors identified by children include (1) sickness, (2) idle time, (3) being alone, (4) frequent family conflict, (5) economic insecurity, (6) pressure to get good grades, (7) feeling left out, (8) bullying, and (9) violence (Ryan-Wenger, Wilson (Sharrer), & Broussard, 2012). Environmental and social stressors include the following:

- Personal safety concerns
- Community violence
- Prolonged poverty
- Increased availability of alcohol and drugs
- Homelessness

The majority of children have a resiliency that enables them to overcome adversity and function well in spite of major personal and environmental stressors. *Family protective factors,* such as warm, close, supportive relationships among its members, and *environmental protective factors,* such as satisfying peer and adult relationships, and safe neighborhoods, mediate the relationship between risk factors and healthy coping.

Resilience is a personal characteristic that decreases the negative effects of stress. Personal resilience factors within children include their cognitive abilities and problem-solving skills, prior experience in successfully managing stressful situations, an ability to adapt, and a positive self-image. One or more of these factors, along with family and environmental protective factors, contribute to the development of resilience in children (Ryan-Wenger et al., 2012).

Children who are affected by stressful situations need to learn constructive coping techniques to enhance their well-being and health. Untreated chronic stress in children often leads to mental health issues as well as chronic diseases. Children with chronic illnesses, compared with healthy children, are less confident in their ability to handle problems and more often use ineffective coping skills. Chronically ill children who use problem-focused coping are better able to suppress depression and anxiety. Recognizing the need to incorporate coping strategies into family and school interventions ensures optimal physical and mental health of all children (Gerber et al., 2017). Assessment measures of coping for children are widely available.

Adolescents

Adolescents experience many stressful situations. The most common stressors during the adolescent years are changes related to growth and development; family-related issues, such as arguments and neglect; peer relationships across early and mid-adolescence; and school performance concerns in high school-age youths (Tottenham & Galvan, 2016).

Higher stress in early adolescence is associated with a range of risk-taking behaviors such as smoking, alcohol misuse, and sexual experimentation. Warning signs of stress-related disorders may be subtle and require careful observation by parents, friends, and health professionals. Warning signs include excessive time spent alone, anger, loss of appetite, changes in sleep patterns, persistent irritability, changes in school performance, and excessive screen use to the exclusion of face-to-face, social contacts (Solecki & Fay-Hillier, 2015).

Adolescents can learn to apply effective stress-coping strategies to avoid risky behaviors. They need to be taught specific strategies, including the following:

- Gathering information about the risk behavior
- Using problem solving to make decisions
- Focusing on the positive to minimize stress
- Talking with an adult
- Learning mindfulness-based stress reduction and meditation (Boustani et al., 2015)

Chapter 4 discusses measures that can be used to assess adolescents' coping skills.

Young and Middle-Age Adults

Many coping strategies that are learned early in life do not change significantly from childhood to adolescence to adulthood. However, as young adults mature, they usually increase their use of problem-solving coping and decrease the use of avoidance coping compared with the preteen and adolescence years. The stresses often experienced in young adulthood relate to establishing careers and long-term relationships, starting families and raising children. Young adults aspire to create a sense of self-identity as an independent, yet interdependent adult (American Psychological Association, 2017a).

Middle-age adults spend much of their time managing their relationships with spouses, parents, siblings, children, and friends and the stressors generated by these relationships. Divorce is a major stressor in this age group. Couples were more than twice as likely to divorce in 2010 than in 1990 (Stepler, 2017). The gradual process of providing support to aging parents begins in middle-age for many adults. Increased caregiver demands often results in a decrease in the quality of relationships with parents and higher caregiver burden (Kim et al., 2017). In addition job demands, combined with caregiver demands, result in greater stress (Dich, Lange, Head, & Rod, 2015). However, the caregiver role may be perceived as positive if excessive time is not required.

During the midlife period, interaction with siblings usually revolves around care for aging parents. Sibling connections may bring them closer together or revisit unresolved issues. Other relationships in midlife that may cause stress are children and friends. These relationships can be rewarding or cause depression based on the expectations of adult children or grandchildren. Friendships during this period are fewer, but closer. Friends are an important component of the social network of middle-age adults (Connidis, 2015; Igarashi, Hooker, Coehlo, & Manoogian, 2013).

Older Adults

Although some sources of stress may abate in older adulthood, other stressors, particularly those resulting from loss, are more prevalent. Older adults are particularly vulnerable to negative life events such as the death of a spouse, death of close family members and friends, personal injury or illness, changes in financial status, caregiving responsibilities, and retirement. Diminished sensory acuity, decreased dexterity and strength, and loss of flexibility may cause frustration and limitations in performing activities of daily living. Cumulative stress along with depression can compromise immune function, leaving older adults more vulnerable to chronic diseases mentioned earlier (McEwen, 2017b).

In older adults, years of daily hassles and cumulative major life events increase morbidity and mortality, particularly when coping strategies have been ineffective. Systemic effects on the cardiovascular, gastrointestinal, neurological, endocrine, and immune systems are increasingly apparent. Ethnic and gender-specific coping strategies are especially helpful for older adults to manage their daily stressors more effectively and efficiently (Lee & Mason, 2014). Evidence shows that the ability to manage stressors improves with age. Compared to younger age groups, older adults are more likely to be flexible, willing to compromise, and adjust their expectations. They also report a willingness to express their feelings, potentially contributing to a healthier and more satisfying life (American Psychological Association, 2017a).

STRESS IN THE WORKPLACE

A major source of stress is created by the workplace. Workplace stress is considered physical and psychological responses to undue pressures and demands at work that are health damaging. Workplace stress occurs when job requirements do not match the needs or capabilities of the worker. Low-to-moderate levels of stress in the workplace generate positive performance; however, moderate-to-high stress levels cause deterioration in performance and further escalate already existing stress and tension. Workplace stress leads to disability, absenteeism, and decreased productivity, all of which are very costly to the worker and to business and industry. Common sources of work stress include worker characteristics as well as working conditions and include the following:

- Lack of preparation for the job
- Unrealistic job demands
- Conflicting or lack of clarity about job expectations
- Lack of opportunity for growth
- Lack of support or help from coworkers
- Unpleasant or dangerous job conditions
- Lack of family-friendly policies
- Low decision latitude and poor communication (National Institute for Occupational Safety and Health, 2014).

Organizational changes improve working conditions and reduce the costly effects of chronic stress on workers. Changes that prevent or reduce job stress include clearly defining roles and responsibilities, providing workers opportunities to participate in decisions that affect their jobs, improving communication, and providing opportunities for workers to have social interactions with coworkers. In addition, instituting policies that provide flextime, job sharing, or childcare benefits can ease stressors for parents who must work outside the home and care for young children.

In addition to workplace changes, stress management programs should also be offered. Stress management training teaches workers to identify their sources of stress and learn skills to reduce the stress. However, stress management training should not be implemented without first attending to workplace changes needed to eliminate environmental stressors (Bhui, Dinos, Galant-Miecznikowska, de Jongh, & Stansfeld, 2016).

Support at home can buffer work-related stressors, or the existence of stressors at home together with work stressors may have a cumulative effect. More employers offer worksite stress management programs that include family members. Organizational changes and interventions that focus on individual workers and their families result in greater positive outcomes than interventions that just focus on one entity. The best outcomes for reduction of stress in the workplace occur when a comprehensive framework guides the selected interventions (American Psychological Association, 2017b).

STRESS GENERATED BY TECHNOLOGIES

Before the widespread popularity of wireless devices and personal computers, other technologies were stressors to individuals, families, and the workplace. For example, industrial machinery is disruptive. The presence of clocks and watches causes stressful reminders of schedules and productivity expectations. With the addition of social media and wireless devices, the total effect of technology on the lives of many Americans borders on overload.

In a Pew Research Center Survey, women who frequently used Twitter, e-mail, and photo sharing reported less stress than women and men nonusers of these technologies. There was no difference in reported stress between men users and men nonusers. Women experienced higher levels of stress when they became aware of distressing events in the lives of their families and friends through social media. This type of psychological stress is referred to as "the cost of caring" (Hampton, Raine, Lu, Shin, & Purcell, 2015a). However, the social benefits of digital technologies may reduce the negative effects of the "cost of caring" (Hampton, Raine, Lu, Shin, & Purcell, 2015b).

Another stress associated with electronic devices is the excessive desire of users to constantly check e-mails, texts, and social media sites. Four out of five U.S. adults report checking their accounts frequently or are "constant checkers." Higher stress is reported in constant checkers compared to persons who do not use the technology as frequently. Constant checkers report stress from information received on social media and report feeling more disconnected from family (American Psychological Association, 2017c). Digital devices are important in the daily lives of most adults; however, individuals need to be made aware of the effects of being constantly connected on physical and psychological health.

The significant influence of technology on children requires parents/guardians to limit children's screen time. Parents express feelings of being disengaged from their family even when they are in the same room because of technology. Parents also report stress about the potential influence of social media on the child's mental and physical health (American Psychological Association, 2017c). One strategy to address technology overload is to periodically "unplug" or take a "digital detox." This is particularly important for "constant checkers" and children. Two-thirds of "constant checkers" agree with the idea of a "digital detox"; however, less than one-third report actually doing so. Parents need to make every effort to manage their personal use of technology to role model a healthy relationship with technology for their children (American Psychological Association, 2017c).

STRESS GENERATED BY MIGRATION

Many immigrants face overwhelming experiences when they move to a new country. Experiences in the home country, such as pre-migration exposure to violence, loss, and trauma are stressors that increase risk for mental health problems in immigrant populations. Stress management approaches may depend on their compatible cultural views and beliefs. For example, different cultures may or may not support the use of medications to treat stress-related illnesses. Individuals from Arabic-speaking countries generally support cognitive behavioral therapy because it is consistent with their basic values and beliefs. Concern for stigmatization of mental health illness may hinder Asian Americans from seeking mental health services. The complicated network of resettling problems affects access to all health care services, especially mental health services. However, many immigrants are resourceful and have an optimistic view of their future in the United States, and these characteristics will impact their mental health outcomes (Garcini et al., 2016). Postmigration settlement in areas that provide community social activities, emotional support, and assistance in managing stressful situations promote social engagement and well-being. Nurses must take into consideration the stressors of relocation prominent in all immigrant populations and implement strategies to facilitate their integration into the new culture. Table 8-1 lists some of the major stressors that immigrants confront in the United States, and Table 8-2 describes barriers that prevent immigrants from using mental health services.

Hispanic migrants from Mexico and Central and South America are the largest immigrant group in the United States, making up over half of the foreign born population (Alarcon et al., 2016). Undocumented immigrants in this country are mainly Mexican, including children who migrated with their parents. Undocumented Mexican immigrants face additional stressors and challenges, including psychological, physical, verbal, and sexual abuse, discrimination, isolation, fear of deportation, living in unsafe neighborhoods, and poverty (Garcini et al., 2017). These chronic stressors lead to depression and anxiety disorders, as well as drug and alcohol abuse. Poverty and unemployment play a major role in poor mental and physical health in both documented and undocumented Mexicans, stressing the need to address health inequities in this groups as well as facilitating access to mental health

---

TABLE 8-1   Major Stressors Confronting Immigrants in the United States

Economic insecurity: cost of living, low-paying jobs

Discrimination in housing, school, and workplace

Language differences: lack of language-friendly printed materials

Limited integration into mainstream culture: maintaining own cultural norms

Differing parenting styles: differences in how children are disciplined

Fear of deportation in both documented and undocumented immigrants

TABLE 8–2 Primary Barriers to Seeking Mental Health Services

Stigma of seeking mental health services

Little understanding of mental health services system

Competing cultural practices

Lack of information about health services

Language barriers

Cost of services

---

services (Garcini et al., 2017). Chapter 12 provides information on promoting health equity and health literacy, two major strategies for decreasing stressors in diverse populations.

APPROACHES TO STRESS MANAGEMENT

Nurses understand the importance of the relationship between stress and health and illness as a basis for assessment and stress reduction. They are in key positions to identify individuals and families who are not coping effectively. Observation, active listening, and supportive decision-making enable nurses to help clients identify stressors and select strategies to manage the primary stressors in their client's lives. Assessment findings direct the nurse to structure appropriate interventions and/or make referrals to assist clients in managing stressors *before* health-damaging effects occur.

Strategies to Minimize the Frequency of Stress-Inducing Situations

Individuals continuously adapt to externally imposed change. Nurses can assist clients in minimizing the stress that often accompanies adaptation to these changes by teaching them to (1) change their environment, (2) avoid excessive change, and (3) manage time.

CHANGE THE ENVIRONMENT. In general, changing the environment to decrease the incidence of stressors is the "first line of defense." Widely held values and beliefs shape the environment in any society. Although changing the environment is the most proactive approach to minimize the frequency of stress-inducing situations, it may be the most difficult strategy to implement. For example, a job change may be required to modify the environment. When changing the environment is *not* possible, individual and family coping resources must come into play to reinterpret stress as a challenge and increase resilience. Additional factors that decrease stress include:

- Warm, cohesive, and supportive family members
- Cultural events and customs that promote identity
- Supportive relationships with others outside the family
- Involvement in churches and neighborhood organizations

All of the above factors emphasize the role of supportive relationships for decreasing stress.

AVOID EXCESSIVE CHANGE. During periods of significant life changes, avoidance of additional unnecessary changes is essential. For example, postponement of geographic relocation or pregnancy may be required if a family is experiencing the illness of a family member. Tension created by multiple changes is synergistic. Deliberately postponing changes that result in stress helps clients constructively manage unavoidable change, and postponement prevents the need for multiple adjustments at one point in time.

During periods of moderate or high stress, any lifestyle changes that are initiated should be voluntary and should *challenge*, rather than *threaten*, the client. Increasing positive sources of stress that promote growth can offset the harmful effects of negative stress. For example, learning a new activity or sport may provide a distraction to counterbalance potentially negative stress.

PRACTICE TIME MANAGEMENT.   The time management approach to stress reduction focuses on reorganizing one's time to accomplish the most important goals *within the time available*. Lack of time is a frequently reported reason for not participating in health-promoting activities, so time management skills will help reduce this barrier.

Time management begins with identifying how time is spent and prioritizing goals. When clients identify time wasted on activities unrelated to personal goals, they can restructure how they spend their time. A frequent source of stress is over commitment to others or unrealistic expectations of oneself. Time overload can be avoided by learning to say "no" to demands of others that are unrealistic or of low personal or family priority. *Time overload* results in frustration and loss of satisfaction when work is accomplished, as one's best efforts are seldom applied when under strain and pressure. A task may appear overwhelming; however, accomplishment becomes manageable if the task is broken down into components, and a portion of the task is completed. Breaking down the task allows mastery and a feeling of competence.

Individuals can avoid feelings of overload by delegating responsibilities to others or enlisting their assistance. Making use of friends' and family's willingness to assist provides freedom from the expectation of having to be "all things to all people." Another important aspect of time management is to reduce the perception of time pressure and urgency. Perceptions of time urgency are often needlessly self-imposed. The client should differentiate between time urgencies that are valid and ones that are not. Time urgencies can be avoided by minimizing procrastination, as leaving tasks until the last minute results in needless pressure and stress. Learning to manage distractions, such as e-mails, text messages, and phone calls is another effective time management strategy. When attention is paid to every distraction, time is taken away from the current activity and then additional time is required to refocus on the original activity. Addition time management strategies include learning to prioritize, building in rewards when goals or activities are accomplished, and balancing leisure family time with work.

Strategies to Increase Resistance to Stress

Both physical and psychological conditioning increase resistance to stress. Physical conditioning for stress resistance promotes *healthy behaviors*, such as regular physical activity and good nutrition. Psychological conditioning builds *healthy mental states*, such as positive self-esteem, self-efficacy, assertiveness, and adequate coping resources.

PROMOTE HEALTHY BEHAVIORS.   Regular physical activity and healthy eating behaviors are important during stressful events (see Chapters 6 and 7 for a detailed discussion on exercise and nutrition, respectively). In general, people who exercise regularly report feelings of well-being. However, extreme fatigue, anxiety, and decreased vigor can occur with overtraining. It is well documented that exercise improves a person's mental and physical state and increases one's ability to combat stress.

A healthy, balanced diet contributes to good health and is especially important during periods of stress. Caffeine, alcohol, overeating, and tobacco should be avoided during stressful periods. Overeating may provide immediate satisfaction, but it is only temporary. Chronic stress may also depress the appetite, resulting in weight loss over time. Poor nutrition, regardless of the underlying cause, reduces one's ability to manage stress and maintain good health.

ENHANCE SELF-ESTEEM.   Self-esteem is the value attributed to self or how one feels about oneself. A person's concept of his or her desirable and undesirable attributes, strengths and weaknesses, achievements, and success contributes to his or her self-esteem. Self-esteem develops over time.

One approach to enhancing self-esteem is positive verbalization. In this technique, clients identify positive aspects of themselves or personal characteristics they value daily. They should also ask significant others to comment on their positive attributes. Each characteristic, one per day, is recorded on paper or a wireless device and read several times a day. This technique helps clients spend more time thinking about their positive attributes, and decreases the amount of time spent in self-devaluation. Self-awareness of positive characteristics and their presence in conscious thought encourages behavior that produces positive self-esteem.

ENHANCE SELF-EFFICACY.   Mastery experiences create a self-belief that one has the competence to perform effectively and overcome obstacles. Counseling clients to undertake tasks or new behaviors that are challenging and result in successful outcomes enhances self-efficacy. Self-efficacy or beliefs about personal competency influence motivation, affect, thought, and action. Chapter 2 describes strategies to increase self-efficacy.

Persons with high levels of self-efficacy mentally rehearse successes rather than failures, set high goals, make a firm commitment to attain them, and perceive more control over personal threats. Persons with high self-efficacy also tend to be more assertive in acquiring the support they need to optimize their chances of success (Folkman, 2013).

LEARN ASSERTIVENESS SKILLS.   Substituting positive, assertive behaviors for negative, passive ones enhances one's resistance to stress. *Assertiveness* is the appropriate expression of oneself and one's thoughts and feelings. Assertiveness is more constructive and effective than aggression in managing problems. Assertiveness enables individuals to share their perceptions and feelings with others in a way that facilitates rather than inhibits personal or group productivity. The following strategies enhance assertiveness:

- Make a deliberate effort to greet others by name
- Maintain eye contact during conversations
- Comment on the positive characteristics of others
- Initiate conversation
- Express opinions constructively
- Express feelings
- Disagree with others when holding opposing viewpoints
- Take initiative to engage in a new behavior or learn a new activity

Although it is possible for clients to become more assertive with simple techniques, *very* passive and reserved clients might benefit from more comprehensive assertiveness training. The nurse may need to assist clients in locating a personal counselor or coach.

SET REALISTIC GOALS.   Realistic or attainable goals enable the client to establish an achievable plan to manage stressors. Long-term goals set the direction for stress management, and short-term goals outline the steps to achieve the goal. Short-term goals enable one to experience immediate success and stay on course. Setting goals that are attainable within a reasonable period leads to success, which reinforces the client's desire to continue to set additional stress-management goals. Another useful tenet is to focus on only one goal at a time.

Stress-management goals need a realistic action or implementation plan as they are more likely to be achieved. An action plan might include the where, when, and how of what one will do to achieve the goal. Developing an action plan also enables the client to visualize what is realistic to achieve the goal. For example, a short-term goal might be to take a walk when one feels stressed by a family conflict. The action plan would include how the family member will exit the conflict to walk, where the client will walk, and the length of time to walk. Specific action plans facilitate achievement of goals.

BUILD COPING RESOURCES.   Psychological stress occurs when there is an *imbalance* between appraised demands and appraised coping capabilities. Nurses should teach clients to direct more attention to the *resource* side of the equation or their coping capabilities and resources. General coping resources that enhance stress resistance include the following:

- *Self-disclosure:* Predisposition to share feelings, troubles, thoughts, and opinions with others.
- *Self-directedness:* Degree to which clients respect their own judgement in decision-making.
- *Confidence:* Ability to gain mastery over the environment and control emotions to reach personal goals.
- *Acceptance:* Degree to which clients accept their shortcomings and imperfections and maintain a tolerant attitude toward others.
- *Social support:* Availability and use of a network of caring family and friends.
- *Financial freedom:* Availability of financial resources to maintain one's lifestyle.
- *Physical health:* Overall health; absence of chronic diseases and disabilities.
- *Stress monitoring:* Awareness of situations that may precipitate stress.
- *Stress control:* Ability to lower arousal through relaxation and meditation.
- *Structuring:* Ability to organize and manage personal resources, for example, time and family responsibilities.
- *Problem solving:* Ability to resolve personal problems.

After assessing the extent to which coping resources are present, the client can maximize existing strengths and develop additional resistance resources.

COMPLEMENTARY THERAPIES TO MANAGE STRESS

More than two-thirds of the world's population uses complementary and integrative health (CIH) practices, and approximately one-third of Americans report the use of CIH therapy at some point in their lives. *Complementary therapies* are non-mainstream medical and health care practices and products used together with conventional medicine to manage stress, stress-related illnesses, and other health conditions. *Alternative therapies* are non-mainstream practices that are used in place of convention medicine. *Integrative health care* brings together complementary and conventional practices in a coordinated way for health benefits in many situations (National Center for Complementary and Integrative Health, 2016). The use of the CIH therapy in America is more prevalent among well-educated, higher-income women with chronic and degenerative conditions, and older adults. Among those who use CIH, less than one-third acknowledge they discuss CIH use with their health care providers. In spite of the growth of integrative medicine and health care, traditional or conventional medicine continues to expand, marginalizing both preventive medicine and holistic approaches that are central to integrative medicine (Ali & Katz, 2015). However, conventional health care providers who integrate complementary medicine into their practice report fewer hospital stays and less prescription drug usage in their patients (Kooreman & Baars, 2012).

Complementary therapies used to manage stress and stress-related problems include:

1. Self-regulation techniques, for example, mindfulness
2. Relaxation techniques, for example, progressive relaxation, imagery, self-hypnosis, biofeedback, and deep breathing exercises
3. Meditation techniques, for example, yoga and tai chi
4. Acupuncture
5. Herbal products and dietary supplements

Mindfulness-based stress reduction (MBSR), **relaxation through guided imagery**, and **yoga** are three evidence-based complementary therapies discussed in this chapter.

Mindfulness-Based Stress Reduction

Mindfulness is a mental state that focuses attention and awareness of experiences in the present moment with an attitude of acceptance and openness. Mindfulness focuses attention on awareness of one's body, actions, feelings, and surroundings and deliberately centers on experiences in the present (Kabat-Zinn, 2011). Mindfulness interventions are grounded in exercises that teach individuals to turn inward and focus on moment-to-moment experiences (Creswell, 2017). Mindfulness interventions have proliferated and include mindfulness-based stress reduction, mindfulness-based cognitive therapy (MBCT), and mindfulness-based relapse prevention (MBRP).

Mindfulness-based stress reduction was developed by John Kabat-Zinn almost 40 years ago for people with psychological stress and chronic health problems. Although MBSR is based on ancient Buddhist teachings, it is a secular approach to stress reduction. The duration of the program is usually six to eight weeks, with daily two- or two-and-a-half-hour sessions, conducted by a trained instructor. Daily home practice and a one-day mindfulness retreat, usually in week 6, are also included. The daily sessions focus on mindfulness exercises, yoga exercises, and discussions about using mindfulness to reduce stress (Kabat-Zinn, 2011). Participants are taught how to practice mindfulness during activities such as sitting in a chair and walking, and during daily activities, such as daily chores.

One way to experience and practice MBSR is to experience *mindfulness* while walking. Be aware of the inner chatter of the mind, note it, and return to the present. Listen for the sound of your foot touching the ground, and feel the sensation while just being aware of what you are doing. Being mindful is active yet passive, and practiced anytime or anywhere by simply focusing on what is happening in the present moment.

Systematic reviews of research conducted to understand the role of mindfulness interventions on psychological and biological outcomes have been conducted. The evidence generated by studies looking at psychological outcomes is mixed, as some studies have shown improvement, whereas others have not (Alsubaie et al., 2017; Creswell, 2017). A review of mindfulness-based training to reduce stress in workers did show that these interventions reduced stress (Eby et al., 2017). Reviews of the effects of mindfulness and mind–body interventions on biological outcomes show promising results, including evidence of reduction in inflammatory markers (Bower & Irwin, 2016), and functional and structural brain changes after eight weeks of training similar to traditional long-term meditation (Gotink, Meijboom, Vernooij, Smits, & Myriam-Hunink, 2016).

Almost all of the research conducted to understand the effects of mindfulness-based interventions suffers from multiple weaknesses, including inconsistencies in training programs, small nonrandomized samples, no comparison or control groups, non-blinded participants, and inconsistent or poor-quality outcome measures. The mixed results mentioned above may be due to these limitations. In spite of the weakness, there is enough evidence for mindfulness-based interventions to be used to reduce stress for multiple psychological and physical problems. Very few adverse outcomes have been reported, and it is considered low risk for children and adolescents.

Relaxation through Imagery

Guided imagery is a stress-reducing intervention in which the interrelationship of the body and mind influences physiological responses. This cognitive process uses visual, auditory, olfactory, touch, or other senses to mentally visualize pictures or experiences that bring about positive responses. Recalling the warmth of the sun, the feeling of warm sand, the sensations of a gentle breeze, or the sounds of ocean waves may result in actual changes in muscle tension. For some clients, visualizing specific colors, shapes, or patterns is effective. As concrete images become more vivid, an individual's ability to use less concrete imagery will increase.

Guided imagery has been used to reduce stress pain in patients with cancer, patients undergoing minor surgical procedures, insomnia, and pregnancy. The relaxation technique is inexpensive to implement, as no special equipment is needed and no negative outcomes have been reported. In addition, a single intervention is usually needed to teach the technique. Nurses and other professionals should undergo training before performing guided imagery. An online guided imagery training course for health professionals has been successfully tested (Rao & Kemper, 2017).

Research has shown varying outcomes. Pain reduction is well documented in patients with cancer (Burhenn, Olausson, Villegas, & Kravits, 2014), and self-reported stress reduction has been reported in pregnant adolescents (Flynn, Jones, & Ausderau, 2016). Much of the research has the same weaknesses as research on mindfulness interventions.

Yoga and Tai Chi

Yoga is a traditional, spiritual discipline that combines movement, relaxation, and mindfulness to improve the quality of life. The origin of yoga is rooted in India and has long been an integral part of Indian culture and spiritual life. Hatha yoga is commonly practiced in the Western world, which incorporates postures, breathing, and meditation. Yoga is important in different ways. Some people practice yoga for physical fitness. For others, it is a way to develop a state of mind open to reflection and self-discovery.

Yoga interventions have been implemented to reduce stress and improve acute and chronic health problems. The practice of yoga plays an important role in stress reduction, depression management, pain relief, cognitive function, and balance (Cramer, Anheyer, Lauche, & Dobos, 2017; Field, 2016; Streeter et al., 2017). Research has shown that mindfulness-based interventions, including yoga, are associated with reduced risk of inflammatory disease (Buric, Farias, Jong, Mee, & Brazil, 2017). The limited number of studies warrants additional research. However, the research provides positive evidence for use of these therapies to reduce stress.

Tai chi is a physical activity that originated in an ancient Chinese tradition. It consists of a series of slow, gentle flowing movements performed in a slow focused manner and accompanied by deep breathing. Tai chi, a type of meditative movement, involves strengthening, balance, concentration, relaxation, and breathing control (Chen, Hunt, Campbell, Peill, & Reid, 2016). It is considered a low-intensity exercise that differs from traditional forms of exercise, as it is not designed to burn calories or raise heart rate. Figure 8–3 describes yoga, meditation, exercises, and stretching poses.

Research reviews indicate that tai chi is effective in prevention of falls in the elderly (Hu et al., 2016). The slow, low-intensity movements are suited for older adults

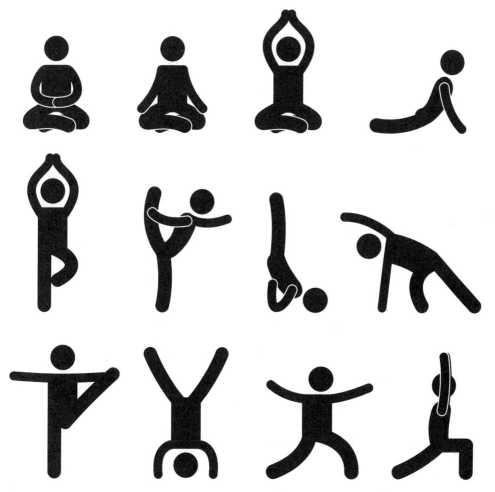

FIGURE 8–3   Yoga, Meditation, Exercises, and Stretches

to improve balance and strength. The effects of tai chi on inflammatory markers in women at risk for cardiovascular disease showed a decrease in inflammatory markers, providing evidence of its potential to reduce cardiovascular risk. Positive results have also been reported in physical performance in patients with cancer, osteoarthritis, pulmonary disease, and heart failure (Chen et al., 2016).

Nurses have many opportunities to implement stress reduction interventions in their practice. Some complementary therapies only require brief instructions by an experienced practitioner. Yoga and tai chi require more instruction and frequent practice to gain skill sufficient to teach others. If the nurse or health care professional does not have the expertise, consultation or referral to professionals with the necessary training is an opportunity to develop collaborative interdisciplinary relationships and referral networks.

CONVENTIONAL APPROACHES TO MANAGE STRESS

The use of prescription and over-the-counter medications to treat stress and stress-related disorders continues to increase. Medications may offer an appropriate short-term option, when an acute, serious stress-related disorder needs immediate relief. However, long-term use often results in adverse side effects and the potential for psychological and/or physiological dependency. Stress management strategies and interventions described in this chapter are realistic alternatives to reduce stress. Medications may be useful temporarily in conjunction with other strategies, but medication therapy alone is *not* likely to be successful in the long term.

Role of Primary Care in Managing Stress

The only mental health care many clients are likely to receive is in primary care settings. Primary care physicians are beginning to assume a greater role in mental health care. However, primary care providers vary in their skills in screening and treating patients with mental health issues, and concerns continue to be raised about the quality of mental health care in these settings (Olfson, 2016). The *Healthy People 2020* mental health goals included two objectives: (1) to seek to reduce the proportion of persons who experience a major depressive episode, and (2) to increase depression screening by primary care providers. Midcourse (2015) results indicate that depressive episodes have decreased over the 2010 baseline in adults, but they have increased in adolescents ages 13 to 17 years (Healthy People 2020, 2017). In addition, overall suicide rates have increased over 2010 baseline rates at midcourse. Although mental health screening by primary care providers has increased, the percentage remains quite small; however, the percentage of primary care facilities that provide mental health treatment has increased to 75.7%. Advanced nurse practitioners are playing a larger role in primary care and need to take responsibility for promoting and conducting early screening and interventions for stress-related problems and depression.

ROLE OF E-THERAPIES IN STRESS MANAGEMENT

The combination of increased demand and increased cost of treating mental health disorders and stress-related conditions, in the face of a shortage of providers, creates an *urgency* to explore innovative methods to provide services. The Internet and wireless devices offer a potential solution to address this critical issue. E-therapies may reduce treatment costs, stigma, travel expenses, and the workload of mental health professionals. The American Psychiatric Association supports online therapy if it meets the same standard as face-to-face treatment (American Psychiatric Association, 2017; Bennion, Hardy, Moore, & Millings, 2017). Computer and Web-based stress reduction interventions can offer anonymity, 24-hour availability, and access for hard-to-reach populations. E-therapies also have the potential to prevent escalation of stress and mental health problems by enabling participants to be reached earlier.

Web-based stress management interventions differ in many ways, including content, length of intervention, guided and unguided formats, and flexible or fixed sessions. Web-based interventions have been used for workplace stress management with some success in managing stress and improving well-being (Ryan, Bergin, Chalder, & Wells, 2017). The interventions are usually individual-focused and identified on a website. Internet and smartphone applications (apps) for mindfulness interventions have proliferated. Although most apps do not offer access to a trained professional, they have been shown to be effective in decreasing perceived stress in nonclinical populations (Jayawardene, Lohrmann, Erbe, & Torabi, 2017). Stress-based interventions are effective in reducing stress-related mental health issues, more so if they have an online coach, are medium in length, and the intervention is based on theory (Heber et al., 2017).

Smartphones are the most popular devices to connect to the Internet and offer the greatest access to mobile interventions (Mani, Kavanagh, Hides, & Stoyanov, 2015). An evaluation of 560 mindfulness-based iPhone apps found that only 23 met the study criteria, and of those only 5 apps provided all the program-based components of mindfulness training. The efficacy of the apps in developing mindfulness could not be determined due to limited data. E-therapy Web and smartphone apps are growing rapidly with little oversight, standardization, or evaluation of effectiveness. Research must address these issues so that these online treatments are safe and effective for managing stress and other mental health conditions.

CONSIDERATIONS FOR PRACTICE IN STRESS MANAGEMENT

Individuals who experience the same stressors often respond differently. Stress-related illnesses are very common and require appropriate interventions or referrals to help clients manage stress before they result in severe mental health problems. Developmentally specific interventions are necessary because children, adolescents, young adults, and older adults use different coping strategies. Awareness of these differences enables the nurse to intervene at the appropriate time and with the appropriate strategy to achieve stress reduction. Nurses need to become familiar with computer and Web-based stress management apps that can be implemented with their clients. In addition, they need to know how to evaluate the quality of apps before recommending them to clients. Although the stress management interventions discussed in this chapter are within the nurse's scope of practice, it may be necessary to gain additional expertise by working with experienced providers, enrolling in courses or seminars, and practicing the newly acquired skills. Research continues to expand to understand the most effective interventions and modes of delivery as well as the underlying mechanisms of nontraditional therapies, mandating that practitioners stay current on the latest evidence-based practices.

OPPORTUNITIES FOR RESEARCH ON STRESS MANAGEMENT

Major advances in understanding the mechanisms of stress and stress-reducing treatments offer new possibilities for more effective management of stress. Further research is needed to overcome the weaknesses of research on these mechanisms. Internet and smartphone apps for stress management are abundant; however, the quality varies and most have not been tested for efficacy, using rigorous research, offering a challenging avenue of research.

Although minority groups suffer from mental health issues, little research has been conducted with these populations. Research should focus on testing interventions that decrease environmental and family stressors. Much of the research needed in stress management requires the collaboration of multiple disciplines. As researchers and practitioners, nurses play a key role as members of these teams.

Summary

This chapter presents multiple evidence-based approaches to assist individuals and families to manage stress. The client and the nurse should make collaborative decisions about the most appropriate interventions to use, taking into account the client's mental and physical health status. Sources of stress and responses to stress need to be assessed, as the information enables the nurse to develop a tailored stress management plan. The role of E-therapies is becoming more important in stress management, although the quality of apps remains an issue. Nurses need to be aware of their level of expertise with stress-reducing interventions and refer clients to other health care providers when appropriate.

Learning Activities

1. Identify three stress management strategies for young and middle adults, and develop a plan to implement the strategies in one of the groups.
2. Select one Web-based app to manage stress and evaluate its quality. Describe your evaluation criteria.
3. Practice mindful walking and describe your feelings, experiences, and sensations.
4. Outline a plan to implement guided imagery with an adolescent who will undergo a dental procedure. Address how you will evaluate its effectiveness.

References

Alarcon, R. D., Parekh, A., Wainberg, M. L., Duarte, C., Araya, R., & Oquendo, M. (2016). *Hispanic immigrants in the USA: social and mental health perspectives. Lancet Psychiatry*, 3(9), 860–870. doi:10.1016/S2215-0366(16)30101-8

Ali, A., & Katz, D. (2015). Disease prevention and health promotion: How integrative medicine fits. *American Journal of Preventive Medicine*, 49(5 Suppl 3), S230–S240. doi:10.1016/j.amepre.2015.07.019

Alsubaie, M., Abbott, R., Dunn, B., Dickens, C., Keil, T., Henley, W., & Kuyken, W. (2017). Mechanism of action of mindfulness-based cognitive therapy (MBCT) and mindfulness-based stress reduction (MBSR) in people with physical and/or psychological conditions: A systematic review. *Clinical Psychology Review, 55*, 74–91. doi:10.1016/j.cpr.2017.04.008

American Psychiatric Association. (2017). *New research: Cognitive behavioral therapy delivered online effective for treating depression.* Press release. Retrieved from https://www.psychiatry.org/newsroom/news-releases/new-research-cognitive-behavioral-therapy-delivered-online-effective-for-treating-depression

American Psychological Association. (2017a). *Report on stress in America: Coping with change: Part 1.* Washington, DC: Author. Retrieved from www.apa.org

American Psychological Association. (2017b). *Coping with stress at work.* Washington, DC: Author. Retrieved from www.apa.org

American Psychological Association. (2017c). *Report on stress in America: Coping with change: Part 2.* Washington, DC: Author. Retrieved from www.apa.org

Bennion, M., Hardy, G., Moore, R., & Millings, A. (2017). E-therapies in England for stress, anxiety or depression: What is being used in the NHS? A survey of mental health services. *BMJ Open, 7*, e014844. doi:10.1136/bmjopen-2016-014844

Bhui, K., Dinos, S., Galant-Miecznikowska, M., de Jongh, B., & Stansfeld, S. (2016). Perceptions of work stress causes and effective interventions in employees working in public, private and non-governmental organizations: A qualitative study. *BJPsych Bulletin, 40*(6), 318–325. doi:10.1192/pb.bp.115.050823

Bot, I., & Kuiper, J. (2017). Stressed brain, stressed heart? *Lancet, 389*, 770–771. doi: 10.1016/S0140-6736(17)30044-2

Bower, J., & Irwin, M. (2016). Mind–body therapies and control of inflammatory biology: A descriptive review. *Brain, Behavior, and Immunity, 51*, 1–11. doi:10.1016/j.bbi.2015.06.012

Boustani, M., Frazier, S., Becker, K., Bechor, M., Dini-zulu, S., Hedemann, E.... Pasalich, D. (2015). Common elements of adolescent prevention programs: Minimizing burden while maximizing reach. *Administration and Policy in Mental Health Services Research,, 42*(2), 209-219. doi:10.1007/s10488-014.0541-9

Burhenn, P., Olausson, J., Villegas, G., & Kravits, K. (2014). Guided imagery for pain control. *Clinical Journal of Oncology Nursing, 18*(5), 501–503. doi:10.1188/14.CJON.501-503

Buric, I., Farias, M., Jong. J., Mee, C., & Brazil, I. (2017). What is the molecular signature of mind–body interventions? A systematic review of gene expression changes induced by mediation and related practices. *Frontiers in Immunology, 8*, 670. doi:10.3389/fimmu.2017.00670

Chen, Y., Hunt, M., Campbell, K., Peill, K., & Reid, W. (2016). The effect of Tai Chi on four chronic conditions—cancer, osteoarthritis, heart failure, and chronic obstructive pulmonary disease: A systematic review and meta-analysis. *British Journal of Sports Medicine, 50*, 397–407. doi:10.1136/bjsports-2014-094388

Chisholm, D., Sweeny, K., Sheehan, P., Rasmussen, B., Smit, F., Cuijpers, P., & Saxena, S. (2016). Scaling-up treatment of depression and anxiety: A global return on investment analysis. *Lancet Psychiatry, 3*(5), 415–424. doi:10.1016/s2215-0366(16)30024-4

Connidis, I. (2015). Exploring ambivalence in family ties: Progress and prospects. *Journal of Marriage and Family, 77*(1), 77–95. doi:10.1111/jomf

Cramer, H., Anheyer, D., Lauche, R., & Dobos, G. (2017). A systematic review of yoga for major depressive order. *Journal of Affective Disorder, 213*, 70–77.

Creswell, J. D. (2017). Mindfulness interventions. *Annual Review of Psychology, 68*, 491–516. doi:10.1146/annurev-psych-042716-051139

Dich, N., Lange, T., Head, J., & Rod, N. (2015). Work stress, caregiving and allostatic load: Prospective results from the Whitehall II cohort study. *Psychosomatic Medicine, 77*(5), 539–547. doi:10.1097/PSY.000000000000191

Eby, L., Allen, T., Conley, K., Williamson, R., Henderson, T., & Mancini, V. (2017). Mindfulness-based training interventions for employees: A qualitative review of the literature. *Human Resource Management Review.* doi:10.1016/j.hrmr.2017.03.004

Field, T. (2016). Yoga research review. *Complementary Therapies in Clinical Practice, 24*, 145–161. doi:10.1016/j.ctcp.2016.06.005

Fink, G. (2016). Eighty years of stress. *Nature, 539*, 175–176.

Flynn, T., Jones, B., & Ausderau, K. (2016). Guided imagery and stress in pregnant adolescents. *American Journal of Occupational Therapy, 70*(5), 7005220020. doi:10.5014/ajot.2016.019315

Folkman, S. (2013). Stress: Appraisal and coping. In M. Gellman & J. Turner (Eds.), *Encyclopedia of behavioral medicine.* New York: Springer.

Garcini, L., Galvan, T., Malcarne, V., Pena, J., Fagundes, C., & Klonoff, E. (2017). Mental disorders among undocumented Mexican immigrants in high-risk neighborhoods: Prevalence, comorbidity, and vulnerabilities. *Journal of Consulting and Clinical Psychology, 85*(10), 927–936. doi:10.1037/ccp0000237

Garcini, L., Murray, K., Zhou, A., Klonoff, E., Myers, M., & Elder, J. (2016). Mental health of undocumented immigrant adults in the United States: A systematic review of methodology and findings. *Journal of Immigrant & Refugee Studies, 14*(1), 1–25. doi:10.1080/15562948.2014.998849

Gerber, M., Endes, K., Herrmann, C., Colledge, F., Brand, S., Donath, L., . . . Zahner, L. (2017). Fitness, stress, and body composition in primary schoolchildren. *Medicine & Science in Sports & Exercise, 49*(3), 581–587. doi:10.1249/MSS.0000000000001123

Gotink, R., Meijboom, R., Vernooij, M., Smits, M., & Myriam-Hunink, M. (2016). 8-week mindfulness based stress reduction induces brain changes similar to traditional long-term meditation practice—A systemic review. *Brain and Cognition, 108,* 32–41. doi:10.1016/j.bandc.2016.07.001

Hampton, K., Raine, L., Lu, W., Shin, I., & Purcell, K. (2015a). *Social media and the cost of caring.* Washington, DC: Pew Research Center. Retrieved from http://www.pewinternet.org/2015/01/15/social-media-and-stress/

Hampton, K., Raine, L., Lu, W., Shin, I., & Purcell, K. (2015b). *Psychological stress and social media use.* Washington, DC: Pew Research Center. Retrieved from http://www.pewinternet.org/2015/01/15/psychological-stress-and-social-media-use-2/

Healthy People 2020. (2017). *Midcourse course review of 2020 goals.* Retrieved June 25, 2017, from HealthyPeople.gov website.

Heber, E., Ebert, D. D., Lehr, D., Cuijpers, P., Berking, M., Nobis, S., & Riper, H. (2017). The benefit of Web- and computer-based interventions for stress: A systematic review and meta-analysis. *Journal of Medical Internet Research, 19*(2), e32. doi:10.2196/jmir.5774

Hu, Y., Chung, Y., Yu, H., Chen, Y., Tsai, C., & Hu, G. (2016). Effect of Tai Chi exercise on fall prevention in older adults: Systematic review and meta-analysis of randomized controlled trials. *International Journal of Gerontology, 10*(3), 131–136. doi:10.1016/j.ijge.2016.06.002

Igarashi, H., Hooker, K., Coehlo, D., & Manoogian, M. (2013). "My nest is full": Intergenerational relationships at midlife. *Journal of Aging Studies, 27*(2), 102–112. doi:10.1016/j.jaging.2012.12.004

Jayawardene, W., Lohrmann, D., Erbe, R., & Torabi, M. (2017). Effects of preventive online mindfulness interventions on stress and mindfulness: A meta-analysis of randomized controlled trials. *Preventive Medicine Reports, 5,* 150–159. doi:10.1016/j.pmedr.2016.11.013

Jones, A., Cochran, S., Leibowitz, A., Wells, K., Kominski, G., & Mays, V. (2015). Usual primary care provider characteristics of a patient-centered medical home and mental health service use. *Journal of General Internal Medicine, 30*(12), 1828–1836. doi:10.1007/s11606-015-3417-0

Kim, K., Bangerter, L., Liu, Y., Polenick, C., Zarit, S., & Fingerman, K. (2017). Middle-aged offspring's support to aging parents with emerging disability. *The Gerontologist, 57*(3), 441–450. doi:10.1093/geront/gnv686

Kabat-Zinn, J. (2011). Some reflections on the origins of MBSR, skillful means, and the trouble with maps. *Contemporary Buddhism, 12*(1), 281–306. doi:10.1080/14639947.2011.564844

Kim, D., Kubzansky, L., Baccarelli, A., Sparrow, D., Spiro, A., & Tarantini, L., . . . Schwartz, J. (2016). Psychological factors and DNA methylation of genes related to immune/inflammatory system markers: The VA normative aging study. *BMJ Open, 6,* e009790. doi:10.1136/bmjopen-2015-009790

Kooreman, P., & Baars, E. (2012). Patients whose GP knows complementary medicine tend to have lower costs and live longer. *European Journal of Health Economics, 13*(6), 769–776. doi:10.1007/s10198-011-0330-2

Lazarus, R. S. (1999). *Stress and emotion: A new synthesis.* New York, NY: Springer.

Lazarus, R. S., & Folkman, S. (1984). *Stress, Appraisal, and Coping,* New York, NY: Springer.

Lee, H., & Mason, D. (2014). Cultural and gender differences in coping strategies between Caucasian American and Korean American older people. *Journal of Cross-Cultural Gerontology, 29*(4), 429–446. doi:10.1007/s10823-014-9241-x

Mani, M., Kavanagh, D., Hides, L., & Stoyanov, S. (2015). Review and evaluation of mindfulness-based iPhone apps. *JMIR mHealth and uHealth, 3*(3), e82. doi:10.2196/mhealth.4328

McEwen, B. (2017a). Neurobiological and systemic effects of chronic stress. *Chronic Stress, 1,* 1–11. doi:10.1177/2470547017692328

McEwen, B. (2017b). Allostasis and the epigenetics of brain and body health over the life course. *JAMA Psychiatry, 74*(6), 551–552. doi:10.1001/jamapsychiatry.2017.0270

National Center for Complementary and Integrative Health. (2016). *Complementary, alternative, or integrative health: What's in a name?* Retrieved on June 26, 2017 from https://nccih.nih.gov/health/integrative-health

National Institute for Occupational Safety and Health (NIOSH). (2014). *Stress at work.* DHHS (NIOSH) Publication 99-11, prepared by NIOSH Working Group, updated June 6, 2014.

Olfson, M. (2016). The rise of primary physicians in the provision of US mental health care. *Journal of Health Politics, Policy and Law, 41*(4), 559–583. doi:10.1215/03616878-3620821

Olfson, M., Blanco, C., Wang, S., Laje, G., & Correll, C. (2014). National trends in the mental health care of children, adolescents, and adults by office-based physicians. *JAMA Psychiatry, 71*(1), 81–90. doi:10.1001/jamapsychiatry.2013.3074

Rao, N., & Kemper, K. (2017). The feasibility and effectiveness of online guided imagery training for health professionals. *Journal of Evidence-Based Complementary & Alternative Medicine, 22*(1), 54–58. doi:10.1177/2156587216631903

Ryan, C., Bergin, M., Chalder, T., & Wells, J. (2017). Web-based interventions for the management of stress in the workplace: Focus, form, and efficacy. *Journal of Occupational Health, 59*(3), 215–236. doi:10.1539/joh.16-0227-RA

Ryan-Wenger, N., Wilson (Sharrer), V., & Broussard, A. (2012). Stress, coping, and health in children. In V. H. Rice (Ed.), *Handbook of stress, coping, and health: Implications for nursing research, theory, and practice* (pp. 226–253). Thousand Oaks, CA: Sage Publications.

Selye, H. (1936). A syndrome produced by diverse nocuous agents. *Nature, 138*, 32.

Shapero, B., Black, S., Liu, R., Klugman, J., Bender, R., Abramson, L., & Alloy, J. (2014). Stressful life events and depressive symptoms: The effect of childhood emotional abuse on stress reactivity. *Journal of Clinical Psychology, 70*(3), 209–223. doi:10.1002/jclp.22011

Sharma, S., Powers, A., Bradley, B., & Ressler, K. (2016). Gene X environment determinants of stress- and anxiety-related disorders. *Annual Review of Psychology, 67*, 239–261. doi:10.1146/annurev-psych-122414-033408

Solecki, S., & Fay-Hillier, T. (2015). The toll of too much technology on teens' mental health. *Journal of Pediatric Nursing, 30*(6), 933–936. doi:10.1016/j.pedn.2015.08.001

Stepler, R. (2017). *Led by baby boomers, divorce rates climb for America's 50+ population*. Washington, DC: PEW Research Center. Retrieved from http://www.pewresearch.org/fact-tank/2017/03/09/led-by-baby-boomers-divorce-rates-climb-for-americas-50-population/

Steptoe, A., & Kivimaki, M. (2013). Stress and cardiovascular disease: An update on current knowledge. *Annual Review of Public Health, 34*, 337–354. doi:10.1146/annurev-publhealth-031912-114452

Streeter, C., Gerbarg, P., Whitfield, T., Owen, L., Johnston, J., Silveri, M., . . . & Jensen, J. (2017). Treatment of major depressive disorder with Iyengar yoga and coherent breathing: A randomized controlled dosing study. *The Journal of Alternative and Complementary Medicine, 23*(3), 201–207. doi:10.1089/acm.2016.0140

Stults-Kolehmainen, M., & Sinha, R. (2014). The effects of stress on physical activity and exercise. *Sports Medicine, 44*(1), 81–121. doi:10.1007/s40279-013-0090-5

Tawakol, A., Ishai, A., Takx, R., Figueroa, A., Ali, A., Kaiser, Y., … Pitman, R. (2017). Relation between resting amygdalar activity and cardiovascular events: A longitudinal and cohort study. *Lancet, 389*(10071), 834–845. doi:10.1016/S0140-6736(16)31713-7

Tottenham, N., & Galvan, A. (2016). Stress and the adolescent brain: Amygdala-prefrontal circuitry and ventral striatum and developmental targets. *Neuroscience & Biobehavioral Reviews. 70*, 217–227. doi:10.1016/neubiorev.2016.07.030

World Health Organization. Calouste Gulbenkian Foundation. (2017). *Improving access to and appropriate use of medicines for mental disorders*. Geneva, Switzerland: Author.

CHAPTER 9

Social Support
and Health

OBJECTIVES

This chapter will enable the reader to:

1. Differentiate between social networks, social integration, and social support.
2. Describe characteristics of social networks that assess the availability of support.
3. Explain the major types of social support.
4. Critique the role of social media in social support.
5. Describe the role of social networks and social support in health promotion.
6. Implement strategies to enhance social support systems.

Understanding the social relationships of individuals is critically important in health promotion. Individuals receive support to engage in healthy behaviors from families, friends, neighbors, and coworkers. Social support is considered a reciprocal process and interactive resource that provides comfort, assistance, encouragement, and information. The amount and types of social support needed fluctuate across the life span and across situations. Social support decreases the occurrence of stressors, buffers the impact of stress, and decreases physiological reactivity to stress.

Much of our understanding of the relationship between social support and health has come from multiple disciplines. An understanding of how social support affects mental and physical health is essential to promote mental, social, and physical well-being. Relationships among social support, health behaviors, and health outcomes are addressed in this chapter. In addition, the nurse's role in assisting clients to assess, modify, and develop effective social support systems to meet their needs is described.

SOCIAL NETWORKS

Although the terms *social networks*, *social integration*, and *social support* are used interchangeably and are overlapping, they are not the same (Gottlieb & Bergen, 2010). *Social networks* refer to the web of social relationships or social ties that surround an individual and the characteristics of those ties. *Social integration* is the degree of involvement or participation in the social network, and *social support* is considered the qualitative, or perceived, functional component. A social network is made up of persons an individual or family knows and interacts with. These interactions may occur frequently or infrequently and may include varying numbers of individuals.

Social integration is the extent to which individuals participate in their social environment at different levels (Gottlieb & Bergen, 2010). The converse of social integration is social isolation or the lack of contact with family, friends, and others in the social network.

Social support refers to resources within the network that are sensed as being available and helpful (perceived support) or are actually provided (received support). The social support system for any given individual or family is usually much smaller than the social network or number of contacts.

Characteristics of *social networks* have been described in various ways. These characteristics or network properties usually include *size* or the actual number of people in a network, *density* or the extent to which network members know each other, *composition* or *type* of members, such as family, relatives, friends, religious organizations, work, etc., and *frequency of contact* with network members. The commonly cited characteristics of social networks are described in Table 9–1.

The density and contacts with others in one's social networks are considered one's social ties. The most commonly studied network characteristics are network size, composition, and frequency of interactions with network members.

Social network is not a static concept, as its structure changes across the life span. The nature of an individual's social relationships can be depicted using Antonucci's hierarchical mapping technique that has progressively enlarging concentric circles around an inner circle (Antonucci, Ajrouch, & Birditt, 2014). *Social networks*, or convoys of social support, are considered a lifetime set of relationships that continue to

TABLE 9–1   Characteristics of Social Networks

Characteristic	Measure
Size	Actual number of persons in network
Density	Extent to which individuals are connected or know each other
Contact	Amount of interaction with network members in a specified time period
Composition	Specific relationship to network member, such as family member, friend, etc.
Duration	Length of time individual has known network members
Reciprocity	Degree of exchange in relationship with network members
Strength	Extent to which network ties are voluntary or obligatory

Source: Adapted from Uchino (1972).

develop and change over the life span. Circles represent the degree of closeness of family members and friends to the individual. The inner circle consists of closest, intimate relationships, such as family and longtime friends who individuals cannot imagine not being in their lives. Individuals in the next circle may be close relatives, friends, and neighbors. The third circle reflects contacts that are somewhat close, such as coworkers or people in one's class or church-affiliated group. In the most outer circle are people who provide services, such as health professionals, including one's physicians and nurses. Throughout the life span, the outer circles are more likely to change, whereas the inner circle tends to be more stable. Inner circle members are difficult to replace, and when they are no longer available, there may be a sense of grief and loss. The hierarchical mapping of social networks is one strategy to assess a client's social network. Figure 9–1 provides an example of how an individual's social network can be assessed using hierarchical mapping.

Social networks determine the availability and adequacy of social support, which are linked to health outcomes. The size of the network is thought to be an important component in social support. However, the types of persons in the network who provide the support, not the network size, have been associated with satisfaction. For example, voluntary social network ties, such as friends and religious affiliation membership, may be more important for well-being than obligatory social network ties such as family, because one usually chooses network ties that are rewarding. Social networks also promote social participation, providing opportunities for companionship and promoting a sense of belonging. This connectedness helps shape activities and behaviors that individuals engage in, including health behaviors.

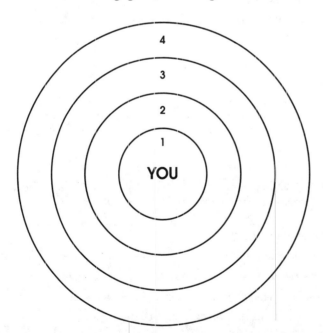

Circle 1: List all persons who you are so close to that you cannot imagine living without them.

Circle 2: List all persons who are important to you and are close to, but not as much as Circle 1.

Circle 3: List all persons you have not listed that are important enough to include in your network.

Circle 4: List all professionals who you can turn to for help if needed, such as physicians, nurses etc.

FIGURE 9–1 Hierarchical Mapping to Assess Social Relationships

Source: Adapted from Antonucci, T. C. (1986). Hierarchical mapping technique. *Generations,* (Summer), 10–12.

SOCIAL INTEGRATION

Social integration, the extent of close family, friends, and community ties, has two components: a behavioral component, or the extent of actively engaging in multiple social activities and relationships; and a cognitive component, the extent of a sense of community and identification with one's social roles. Socially integrated individuals have been reported to live longer than those who are less integrated into their networks. This is thought to be due to less social isolation and a sense of meaning in life. Social isolation, on the other hand, has been associated with an increase in morbidity and mortality (De Jong Gierveld, van Tilburg, & Dykstra, 2016).

SOCIAL SUPPORT

The resources provided by social relationships are considered social support. Social support can be defined as a network of interpersonal relationships that provide psychological and material resources intended to benefit an individual's ability to cope. Social support may be perceived (emotional support) or tangible (supportive acts). Social support is usually described as four broad categories: *emotional, instrumental, informational,* and *appraisal* support. *Emotional* support refers to the demonstration of caring, empathy, love, and trust. *Instrumental* support includes tangible or actual support or actions, including providing money or assistance with services. *Informational* support refers to advice provided, as well as information or suggestions. Last, *appraisal* support refers to the provision of affirmation or constructive feedback. The type of support that is beneficial at any given time may differ, depending on the nature of the situation. For example, emotional support may help in a crisis, whereas informational support may be more useful in assisting individuals to understand how to learn specific tasks, such as the preparation of nutritious meals. Appraisal or affirmation support may encourage individuals to continue to engage in a new health behavior. Table 9–2 describes the major types of support with examples of each.

Social support must be viewed within the context of social relationships. The context includes cultural characteristics that shape receiving and giving support. Cultural boundaries define the major subgroups of American society, such as African Americans, Asian Americans, Hispanics–Latinos, and Native Americans. Within these cultural boundaries, social support operates uniquely within each social context. For example, religious support plays a unique role for African Americans in promotion of health behaviors (Holt, Roth, Huang, Park, & Clark, 2017).

TABLE 9–2 Types and Examples of Social Support

Type	Examples
Emotional	Listening sympathetically, reassuring
Instrumental/tangible	Providing assistance with chores or child care
Informational	Making helpful suggestions, offering advice
Appraisal/affirmation	Giving feedback, assisting in decision-making

Hispanic–Latino Americans and Asian Americans are similar in that the core of their social support system is the family, which includes both close and distant kin. Many Korean and Chinese Americans recognize gender hierarchies (patrilineage) and show respect for older adults (Chung, 2017). Some may use shame and harmony in giving and receiving support. Many Native Americans live in relational networks that foster mutual assistance and support. For many, the extended family and the tribe are the primary support systems (Verbos & Humphries, 2014).

Family social structures reinforce an individual's sense of belonging; however, high-density networks can also exert conformity pressures and social obligations that may promote and even normalize health-damaging behaviors. Although many similarities in social support exist among the various American cultures, the influence of the sociohistorical context differs greatly across populations. Culturally sensitive approaches are needed to understand the role of social support in diverse populations.

Other types of social support systems relevant to health have been described: *natural support* systems (families), *peer support* systems, *religious support* systems, *professional support* systems, and organized *self-help support* groups not directed by health professionals. In most instances, the family remains the primary support group.

Although health professionals have access to information and resources that might not otherwise be available, they are seldom the first source of support for an individual. Initially, family and close friends or peers are sought for advice and support. Health professionals may become the support system only when other sources of support are unavailable, interrupted, or exhausted. Health professionals usually are unable to provide support over long periods of time. In addition, these relationships are not characterized by reciprocity, as they usually involve a power differential and offer limited empathetic understanding due to lack of intimacy. Health professionals can offer short-term emotional and appraisal support as well as informational support in health behavior change.

All support systems of an individual or family are synergistic. In combination, they represent the social resources available to facilitate healthy lifestyles. Various individuals or groups are dominant at different points, depending on the stage of development and the stressors or challenges at hand. For example, in preadolescence and early adolescence, parents are the greatest source of support. The support shifts to a greater reliance on peers for lifestyle choices during middle adolescence with a decreased perception of parental support. Friends remain dominant in young adulthood. Family and friends are important sources of support for the elderly.

Family as the Primary Source of Support

The family is the primary context for learning to give and receive social support. Family cohesion, expressiveness, and lack of conflict are reflected in the supportive behaviors that family members provide to one another. Low family support and poor child–parent interactions influence the life course trajectories of young people. Family stressors, such as unemployment, poverty, changes in family structure (as a death or divorce), crime, and substance use, can decrease family cohesion and increase conflict.

Family social support exerts complex effects on the physical and mental health of its members. The classic Alameda County, California, study provided initial information about the association of social networks, social integration, social support, and mortality, and this association has been substantiated in later research (Berkman & Syme, 1979; Tanskanen & Anttila, 2016). Social isolation in men and women is associated with higher mortality. Depressive symptoms are associated with an adverse family environment that offers low levels of social support. Men who remain socially isolated after losing their partners are at higher risk of developing symptoms of chronic depression, whereas having supportive relationships has been associated with a decreased risk. Having a supportive marital partner or socially supportive relationships helps reduce psychological distress.

Social support has positive effects throughout the life span. According to the well-known convoy model (Ajrouch, Fuller, Akiyama, & Antonucci, 2017), two aspects of social support networks—a greater proportion of kin and the presence of family members—significantly reduce distress. The interplay between family stressors, such as poor relationships and conflict, and family support is depicted in Figure 9–2. Within families, both positive and negative interactions occur. Negative family interactions can be viewed as stressors and are associated with worse well-being, while positive, helpful family interactions constitute support and are associated with positive well-being. Positive, emotional bonds within the family strengthen the family's effective functioning.

Social support is unequally distributed and varies by socioeconomic status. Neighborhood stressors, such as abandoned buildings, litter and graffiti, physical decay, and absence of green space, have been associated with poorer mental health. Neighborhood poverty has consistently been associated with poor mental and physical health status and higher mortality (Marcus, Echeverria, Holland, Abraido-Lanza, & Passannante, 2016). Persons living in disadvantaged neighborhoods may lack supportive relationships, as neighborhood poverty prevents the formation of supportive social networks due to distrust, fear, and self-imposed social isolation. However, if supportive social relationships exist, they may buffer the effects of neighborhood stressors and provide critical resources for day-to-day survival. Women living in poverty are especially vulnerable

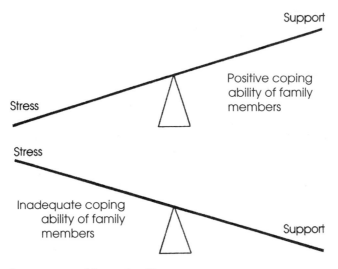

FIGURE 9–2 Family as a source of Support or Stress

and less nurturing due to economic hardship and other stressors (Duncan, Magnuson, & Votruba-Drzal, 2016). Many economically disadvantaged working women rely on minor children for emotional and child support, which may result in worse well-being for the children and poor outcomes for the mother. Burdening the children decreases their well-being, which becomes an additional stressor for the mother. Persons with low socioeconomic status need assistance to find alternate resources to provide social support, such as local organizations or nonprofit institutions. Special attention to social support resources for persons with lower socioeconomic status is critical (Archibald, Stewart, Vo, Diallo, Shabazz, Owens, & Randall, 2017).

Peers as a Source of Support

Informal support from one's peers has consistently been shown to have powerful stress-buffering and health-promoting effects, which are often greater than formal support services. Support from peers is important when there is a breakdown in an individual's usual support network. Peers are nonprofessionals who share similarities, such as age and gender, and possess specific concrete knowledge from personal experiences. Peers have been called community health workers, *promotoras*, health coaches, and lay health advisors. Peer support can be provided through face-to-face or telephone-based sessions, self-help groups, e-mail, and smartphones. Peer support primarily occurs through the provision of emotional, informational, or appraisal support. The more similar the peer is to the individual, the more likely the support will lead to understanding, empathy, and mutual help. Peer support may positively or negatively affect health behaviors. For example, peer support from friends during adolescence has been found to influence consumption of fast-foods, physical activity, and alcohol use initiation.

Peer support groups consist of people who function informally to meet the needs of others. Many of these individuals have encountered an experience that has influenced their own lives and resulted in successful adjustment and growth. Because of personal insight and experiential knowledge, their advice is sought primarily to resolve a problem with which they are familiar.

Peer support leaders must be skilled in communication, active listening, and problem solving. In addition, peers need empathy with the person's difficulties and must be willing to take a supportive role. Peer support commonly includes befriending, mediation/conflict resolution, mentoring, and counseling. Peer support groups have been developed in schools and colleges to decrease aggressive acts and social isolation, as well as to teach skills and promote health. Peer support groups have been implemented in hard to reach, diverse populations with success. Strategies that promote success include being nonjudgmental, showing respect, offering flexibility to meet the needs of the group, involving participants, and working with communities to recruit participants (Sokol & Fisher, 2016).

Community Organizations as Sources of Support

Characteristics of a community and its organizations have a direct bearing on the health of individuals and families. The social interactions of residents contribute positively or negatively to health. Stable communities tend to promote close-knit ties among residents that lessen the effects of crises on community members. Stable communities are characterized by value similarity, mutual assistance, shared trust, and concern for members.

Organized religious support systems, such as churches, temples, mosques, or other faith-based meeting places, may provide support for individuals, as people who attend share similar value systems, a common set of beliefs about the purpose of life, and a similar set of guidelines for living. Even highly mobile individuals may find a support system in the local church, synagogue, or mosque. The place of worship takes primary responsibility for support to enhance the spiritual dimension of health.

Faith-based communities can be a source of support for promoting healthy lifestyles (Levin, 2016). Religious organizations represent miniature, dynamic communities that provide social, emotional, and instrumental support, such as child care, meals, transportation, and counseling. In addition, volunteer helpers are readily available. Religious communities often participate in community programs that promote healthy lifestyles and prevent high-risk behaviors. Religious communities and health care professionals have a long history of partnering for health promotion community programs for diverse populations.

Nurses who function as parish or congregational nurses support health promotion within a community setting. Parish nurses integrate concern for the spirituality of the person with holistic care within a faith-based community.

FUNCTIONS OF SOCIAL SUPPORT GROUPS

The primary functions of social support groups are to augment personal strengths of group members and promote achievement of life goals. Social support groups contribute to health as follows:

1. Create an environment that supports health-promoting behaviors
2. Decrease the likelihood of threatening or stressful life events
3. Provide positive feedback or confirmation for an individual's actions
4. Buffer the negative effects of stressful life events

Support groups function to share common social concerns, provide intimacy, prevent isolation, respect competencies, offer dependable assistance in crises, serve as referral agents, and provide feedback and aid.

Social support groups offer insight about the unique role of social support in reducing stress. They provide a strong sense of community, nonjudgmental acceptance, and invaluable information, which empowers individuals to gain control over their lives. The type of group leader (professional or peer) does not matter, as long as the group provides a supportive environment, a sense of belonging, and meets an individual's perceived needs.

Self-Help Groups

Organized support groups that are not directed by health professionals include voluntary service groups and self-help groups. These groups do not have an expert leader, which distinguishes them from support groups that are led by a trained facilitator. Self-help groups do not attempt to change the behavior of members or promote lifestyle change. They share a common problem or concern and address issues defined by group members. Self-help groups reach individuals who may not be able to afford professional services.

Self-help groups have been called "mutual help groups" to reflect the fact that group members give and receive advice, encouragement, support, and firsthand knowledge. One therapeutic factor, in addition to mutual support, is the group's ability to normalize a stigmatizing condition and to take away the embarrassment of having an undesirable behavior. This is a necessary step for making cognitive, emotional, and behavioral changes.

Examples of self-help groups include Narcotics Anonymous, Alcoholics Anonymous, Mended Hearts, The Compassionate Friends, and physical fitness clubs. Necessary components to form a group include a critical mass of interested persons, a form of publicity or recruitment to attract members, and a central goal or activity that gives the group purpose and sustains the investment of its members.

The question has been raised as to why individuals use self-help groups rather than other resources, such as professional services. Two possible reasons are offered:

1. Self-help groups fulfill a need for services not being offered
2. Self-help groups form because of disappointment with traditional medical models and lack of meaningful resources within the community

Self-help groups enable group members to expand their social networks as well as receive support. Self-help groups empower individuals by increasing self-worth. Some consider the term *self-help* misleading because members are not involved just to help themselves. Instead, they help each other, so the term *mutual-aid group* has been suggested, which implies that each person is both a helper and a receiver of help. However, self-help group members prefer the term *self-help*.

The success of self-help groups in assisting individuals cope with different life experiences attests to their continuing viability as a health resource. Self-help groups are particularly effective for individuals who do not receive support from other relationships.

Social Media as a Source of Support

Social media, including social networking sites and virtual social worlds, provide a new platform for clients to explore and obtain information, interact and share experiences with others, and receive support from groups with similar interests and needs. Users of social media sites can upload messages and videos and link their pages with others, expanding their social network. Social media enable individuals to form groups to communicate with others about common health issues or interests. These technologies are accessible on the Internet. They are inexpensive, have a broad reach, and are easy to use, making them appealing to persons of all ages. Social media provide a vehicle for the provision and maintenance of social support (Levac & O'Sullivan, 2016). Examples of social media technologies include microblogs such as Twitter, video sites such as YouTube, and social networking sites such as Facebook (Househ, Borycki, & Kushniruk, 2014).

Social networking sites (SNSs) are an example of social media that enable users to access support. These Internet-based applications enable individuals to create and communicate information with others 24 hours a day. These sites provide health information, support for a specific issue, or help to engage in healthy behaviors, such as losing weight or becoming physically active. Facebook and Twitter are two currently popular SNS tools. These online communities enable individuals to interact and share information.

In online social support communities, groups of individuals interact with a purpose. Online communities overcome geographic distance and access to information.

They are accessible for those with limited time or persons who do not have access to or desire face-to-face groups. Individuals are motivated to join these groups to obtain informational as well as emotional support. Online communities also offer educational information and discussion forums. Technologies for online communities include online message boards, forums, asynchronous or synchronous communication, video-conferencing, and virtual world environments.

Individuals who prefer online support groups over offline groups may have limited access to traditional social support networks, are dissatisfied with the lack of support from their personal social networks or health care professionals, have a stigmatizing health issue, such as obesity, and perceive that they are similar to members of online support communities (Wright, 2016). Active participation in online support communities has been associated with positive outcomes and less social isolation. This is thought to be due to the development of a sense of community within the group and feelings of connectedness.

Communication in online communities is most helpful if it

- Does not threaten the individual's self esteem
- Is sensitive to the individual's feelings
- Clearly supports the individual's intentions
- Uses explicit language in presenting messages

Online support groups enable members to be selective in presenting information about themselves and allows for greater openness in sharing feelings. The downsides of online support groups include the following:

- Membership changes frequently
- Instrumental support is not provided
- Inaccurate or outdated information may be presented
- Problematic behavior may be promoted
- Sharing personal information poses a potential risk
- Potential exists for deception or manipulation

The Centers for Disease Control and Prevention (CDC) has developed useful guidelines and best practices for using social media and virtual worlds to communicate science-based health promotion and prevention information (see the CDC website). In addition, guidelines for designing, implementing, and evaluating online social support groups are available in the literature (Effing & Spil, 2016).

Internet technology has been shown to be acceptable across ethnically diverse groups. However, socioeconomic status continues to be a limiting factor. A "digital divide" continues to exist, as minorities, the elderly, and rural residents have greater barriers to accessing new technology due to limited literacy and education, and lack of economic resources. The major predictors of social media use are a home computer and Internet access, both of which require resources to acquire (Lin et al., 2015). In addition, limited literacy and education increase one's discomfort with the technology and a belief that it is too complicated to learn. However, when minorities learn to access social media, they become empowered, as they are able to obtain health information and support (Nguyen, Mosadeghi, & Almario, 2017). Women and young people are more likely to use social media, and older people are the least likely group to use new communication technologies. Online communities could play a powerful role in meeting the informational and support needs of the elderly. Online support groups among the elderly have the potential to overcome many barriers, including mobility limitations, lack of transportation, and finances. Facebook has great appeal to young adults. Although fewer persons over age 65 access Facebook, research has shown that online social networking sites, such as Facebook, can improve cognitive executive function. This is thought to be associated with the cognitive demands of online social networking and social engagement (Myhre, Mehl, & Glisky, 2016). As older adults become more active participants, multiple sites have been developed to discuss topics such as health, difficult life transitions, and caregiver issues.

Privacy concerns remain a challenge for social networking sites. Inappropriate access to, misuse of, and illegal disclosure of personal information are potential issues if electronic data are not protected from unauthorized users. Individuals should share only the minimum amount of data to accomplish their purpose and learn how to protect personally identifiable information.

Social media play an important role in enabling individuals across the life span to access informational and emotional social support. The rapid growth of the Internet has occurred without concurrent attention to policy, ethical, and legal issues. As nurses and other health care providers adopt these technologies, they need to implement protocols that address security concerns and implement strategies to evaluate the usefulness of the protocols and the usefulness of the technologies in promoting healthy behaviors.

ASSESSING SOCIAL SUPPORT SYSTEMS

All health care providers need to be aware of available sources of social support for clients and their families. Approaches for assessing social support networks of clients are described in Chapter 4. These approaches provide insight into existing support resources. Culture, stage of life-span development, social context (school, home, work), and role context (parent, student, professional) should be considered. Multiple measures are available to assess social networks, social integration, perceived and received social support, loneliness, and social isolation. Successful health promotion depends on support from friends and/or families, so an assessment of an individual's support systems is essential.

SOCIAL SUPPORT AND HEALTH

The importance of social support to mental and physical health is now well established. Lower levels of support are consistently linked to higher rates of morbidity and mortality. Although the actual mechanisms linking social support to health are less well understood, several processes have been proposed (Mason, 2016). First, social support may be directly linked to health by promoting healthy or unhealthy behaviors, supplying information, or making available tangible resources, such as child care or opportunities to participate in health promotion activities at work. Social support may foster a sense of meaning in life or be associated with more positive affective states, such as enhanced sense of self-worth and increased sense of control.

Social support may also contribute to health by buffering the effects of stress on an individual. Social support decreases the negative effects of stressful experiences on one's mental and physical health. Stress promotes negative coping patterns and activates physiological systems that place a person at risk for developing illnesses. Social support is thought to buffer the negative effects of the stress response by promoting less-threatening interpretations of adverse events and effective coping strategies. Even when faced with extremely stressful events, having individuals available who provide support can reduce the intensity of stress.

Social support and social integration have been associated with a reduction in biomarkers of inflammation, a major predictor of chronic diseases, including cardiovascular disease and type 2 diabetes (Yang et al., 2016). Studies consistently link low levels of social support and social isolation with high levels of inflammatory markers in persons of all ages. Longitudinal evidence also substantiates the relationship between supportive family and friends and decreased inflammation. These results have been reproduced in animal models (Kanitz, Hameister, Tuchscherer, Tuchscherer, & Puppe, 2016). In addition, supportive relationships have been associated with longer telomere length (Lincoln, Lloyd, & Nguyen, 2017). The telomere is considered to be a cellular indicator of aging, as it has been found to shorten over the life span. These findings suggest that social support is associated with the aging process and reinforce the positive effects of supportive relationships on health. Nurses are in unique positions to intervene to provide short-term support and to assist clients in identifying and developing supportive relationships.

Social Support and Health Behavior

Social network and support systems influence health behavior. Significant others function as lay referral systems for individuals who are considering seeking professionals for health promotion, illness prevention, or care. Concurrence by the lay referral system often determines the extent to which advice from health professionals is actually followed.

Social support from spouses or partners is associated with health behaviors. Spouses or partners may or may not encourage and support the new health behavior by showing their approval or disapproval. They may also have some control over aspects of the proposed change, such as food shopping and preparation; or they may participate in the behavior change, such as walking together. High levels of warmth, encouragement, and assistance characterize spousal and partner support. A non-supportive family network can interfere with successful implementation of health habits by limiting the individual's time and energy available for health behavior, introducing stressors that compromise healthy behaviors, or sabotaging planned health behaviors.

Social support and social integration have consistently been associated with positive health behaviors and reduced risky behaviors. Greater family involvement and positive family relationships and community-based support have been found to be helpful in promoting physical activity. Social support and interactions with friends promote healthy behaviors through the development of social norms. For example, exercising with a friend or playing team sports makes exercise more enjoyable. Social norms may also prevent the initiation of unhealthy behaviors, such as smoking and alcohol consumption.

Adoption and maintenance of health behaviors over time is difficult unless the behavior is supported by family members and friends. All health care providers need to help clients understand the importance of naturally occurring support and connect them with informal support systems if natural ones are not available.

TABLE 9–3 Definitions of Autonomy Support

Specialty	Definition
Health promotion	Acknowledging other's perspective, offering choices, minimizing pressure and control
Education	Providing explanatory rationales, using non-controlling language, showing patience for self-paced learning
	Providing choice within limits, acknowledging other's feelings and perspectives, providing opportunities for initiative taking, providing non-controlling feedback, avoiding controlling behaviors
Communication	Understanding and validating the other person's frame of reference, respecting other's experiences, promoting choice through clarification of goals, emphasizing ownership and personal responsibility

Autonomy Support and Health Behaviors

Autonomy support, a concept in self-determination theory (SDT), refers to understanding and validating another's perspectives and feelings. Autonomy supportive persons offer support by respecting an individual's experiences, promoting choices, using non-controlling language, displaying patience, acknowledging negative feelings, minimizing pressure and control, and providing relevant information. Table 9–3 offers definitions of autonomy support used by various clinical specialties, including health promotion, education, and communication. Effective components of autonomy support are similar to emotional and informational support, such as using non-controlling language, acknowledging perspectives and feelings, providing rationale, and nurturing motivational resources. Autonomous supportive actions support individuals and families in implementing and maintaining health behaviors.

ENHANCING SOCIAL NETWORK AND SUPPORT SYSTEMS

Support-enhancing strategies have three goals:

1. Strengthen existing supportive relationships
2. Establish new interpersonal ties
3. Prevent disruption of social relationships from evolving into mental or physical illness

When developing strategies to increase social support, it is important to consider the type of social support that will be targeted. Will it be emotional or informational support or an increase in social contacts? The kind of support, who will provide the support, and contextual issues all play a role. For example, strategies to increase perceived support should focus on helping persons recruit supportive others into their social network by teaching them relationship-building skills. Conditions that warrant recruitment of additional supportive network members include the following:

- The existing network is conflictual
- The existing network reinforces unhealthy behaviors
- The existing network is unable or unwilling to offer support

Social support is complex and includes characteristics of the person who needs or desires support (perceiver), characteristics of the person who gives the support (supporter), characteristics of the situation, and the interaction of these factors. All of these facets need to be considered when designing strategies and groups to improve social support.

Facilitating Social Interactions

Interpersonal skills are central in developing supportive relationships. Social skills training teaches individuals how to develop supportive interpersonal relationships, as they learn to express positive and negative feelings honestly and communicate effectively. Training can be conducted with individuals or groups who have similar skill needs. Social skills training is based on the belief that socially competent responses can be learned. Initially, training is directed toward assessing and modifying perceptions of appropriate behavior in social situations. In addition, persons are taught to re-evaluate their thoughts about themselves more positively. Attempts are made to improve social interaction patterns using social cognitive theory concepts (modeling, role playing, performance feedback), coaching, and homework assignments. Skills taught include learning to do the following:

- Initiate conversations
- Give and receive emotional and instrumental support
- Handle periods of silence
- Recognize nonverbal communication
- Become a good listener
- Handle criticism and conflict.

Individuals learn to identify positive and negative ways of communicating; how to use clear and accurate messages; how to differentiate between assertive, aggressive, and passive behaviors; and how to say no when necessary. More effective interpersonal communication skills enable individuals to increase social ties and foster supportive relationships.

Enhancing Coping

Limited social networks and support may result in serious psychological and physical problems during major negative life events. Support groups for widows, children of separated or divorced parents, and parents who have lost a child, for example, can assist persons to learn to cope effectively with these stressful life events. Effective coping skills help individuals understand emotional reactions, reduce feelings of alienation, and move ahead into the future.

Problem-solving coping strategies are aimed at reducing stressful situations. These coping strategies enable one to identify the stressful situation, perceive it to be controllable, identify and implement a potential solution, and evaluate the outcome. Effective coping skills enable individuals to see a stressful event as a challenge or opportunity rather than a threat and to believe that a solution is possible. Effective coping enhances social support, as it functions as a resource to positively respond to stressful life events.

Preventing Social Isolation and Loneliness

Social isolation is a state in which individuals have little or no contact with family members, friends, or neighbors, and limited social participation. Loneliness is an individual's subjective feeling of social isolation due to dissatisfaction with the frequency and quality of social contacts (De Jong Gierveld et al., 2016). Both social isolation and loneliness place individuals at increased risk for chronic illnesses. Preventing loneliness or social isolation is a more desirable approach than treatment of loneliness and isolation after they have occurred. Two approaches to prevention include:

1. Identifying high-risk groups
2. Implementing strategies to develop social support ties and supportive relationships

Young, unmarried, unemployed, low-income, minority persons and the elderly are particularly vulnerable to limited support and loneliness. Programs to decrease social isolation and loneliness must be congruent with the individual's wishes. Strategies should increase social interactions and reduce isolating behaviors. Programs may include transportation to social events or groups, respite programs for caretaker relief, religious support, and community support such as neighborhood watch groups for elders and families. Telephone and Internet online support are additional resources to decrease isolation, including online social support groups.

Educational approaches to prevent loss of social support and subsequent loneliness include classroom experiences for schoolchildren to help them gain skills in making friends, working cooperatively with others, and learning to resolve differences or conflict constructively. A body of evidence over the past 30 years has substantiated that poor social functioning in children often leads to serious personal adjustment problems in later life.

Social disconnectedness and perceived isolation in older adults have consistently been associated with increased morbidity and mortality. Older adults have reduced social networks and social contacts due to death of family and friends. They must build new social relationships among people they have not previously known and create new social support systems in the face of decreasing economic resources or mobility issues. Many older persons need to learn skills to promote successful relationships, as well as skills to resolve interpersonal conflicts with people they already know. Programs to decrease loneliness in older women have focused on improving their relational competence and developing friendships (Martina, Stevens, & Westerhof, 2016). Practice of new skills is essential and includes listening well, setting boundaries, expressing appreciation, and managing conflict. Assisted living facilities may be beneficial for some elders to help them stay connected, as these facilities have ready-made social networks. In addition, community programs and neighborhood activities can be designed to help persons build relationships or to reach out to others who may need emotional or instrumental support. As mentioned earlier, the digital divide exists in the elderly, so strategies are needed to facilitate the availability of computers and classes to learn Internet skills for this group.

Other general suggestions for enhancing social support for all ages include the following:

- Set mutual goals with family members or friends to achieve common needs for support
- Learn to constructively resolve conflict between support network members
- Offer assistance to individuals within one's social network to show concern and promote trust

- Seek counseling, if needed, to resolve marital and/or family conflict
- Engage nurses and other health professionals as community support resources
- Increase ties with online or face-to-face social groups

Clients should be encouraged to articulate specific goals to enhance personal support networks. By focusing on one or two realistic changes, clients can build effective social support systems.

CONSIDERATIONS FOR PRACTICE IN SOCIAL SUPPORT

The connection between social relationships and health across the life span emphasizes the critical role of assessing a client's social network and social support system, and implementing strategies, if necessary, to enhance these systems. Appraisal of social networks and support systems should be part of an initial assessment. Culturally sensitive information about support systems should be obtained to assess the adequacy of support. If the social network needs to be increased and social support is limited, strategies can be implemented to teach clients skills to access and develop supportive relationships. Nurses should also assist clients in exploring new sources of support, including families, friends, neighbors, self-help, Internet and telephone support groups, and community organizations. Strategies to decrease social isolation and loneliness in the elderly should be implemented to enable them to develop new social relationships. The role of the Internet in accessing information and support offers many opportunities for individuals of all ages. Accessing these resources increases the potential for success in health promotion and lifestyle change. All health care professionals need to be familiar with online resources that have been evaluated for quality, ease of use, and accuracy.

OPPORTUNITIES FOR RESEARCH IN SOCIAL SUPPORT

The positive relationship between social networks, social support, and health has consistently been documented. However, questions still need to be investigated to understand the mechanisms of social support on health outcomes. In addition, the effectiveness of social media in providing support has not been well evaluated.

1. The long-term effectiveness of social media in sustaining health behaviors needs evaluation.
2. The types of social relationships (family, friends) and support (emotional, informational) that are most effective in promoting health behaviors should be explored.
3. Social ties and relationships that decrease chronic neuroendocrine responses to stress warrant further investigation.
4. The most effective strategies to decrease social isolation in the elderly need to be identified and tested.
5. The short- and long-term effectiveness of strategies to promote positive social supportive behaviors in children need to be tested.

Nurses play a major role in social support research and can provide leadership to investigate these issues.

Summary

Social support plays an important role in health behaviors and health outcomes across the life span. The extent to which stressful events threaten health and health-promoting behaviors may well depend on the support available from primary (family) or extended (friends, community, and professional) social networks. Social support groups can help clients cope with everyday hassles and major, stressful life experiences. The design and evaluation of strategies and interventions to increase social support need to include online social media resources.

Learning Activities

1. Perform a social network review with a young adult and an elderly client, using the hierarchical model presented in Figure 9–1.
2. Detail three strategies to increase your client's social support, based on the assessment you performed in Learning Activity 1. Take current sources as well as potential sources of support into consideration.
3. Develop four strategies to increase family support for an adult who has expressed a desire to lose weight.
4. Design a plan to prevent social isolation in elderly living alone in an apartment complex for seniors, using both face-to-face and online strategies.

References

Ajrouch, K. J., Fuller, H. R., Akiyama, H., & Antonucci, T. C. (2017). Convoys of social relations in cross-national context. *The Gerontologist*, 1–12. doi:10.1093/geront/gnw204

Antonucci, T. C., Ajrouch, K. J., & Birditt, K. S. (2014). The convoy model: Explaining social relations from a multidisciplinary perspective. *The Gerontologist*, 54(1), 82–92. doi:10.1093/geront/gnt118

Archibald, M., Stewart, J. Vo, L., Diallo, D., Shabazz, W., Owens, R., & Randall, L. (2017). The role of social support for women living in poverty. In *Poverty in the United States*, 113–132. Springer.

Berkman, L., & Syme, S. L. (1979). Social networks, host resistance, and mortality: A nine-year follow-up study of Alameda County residents. *American Journal of Epidemiology*, 109(2), 186–204. doi:10.1093/oxfordjournals.aje.a112674

Chung, A. (2017). Behind the myth of the matriarch and the flagbearer: How Korean and Chinese American sons and daughters negotiate gender, family, and emotions. *Sociological Forum*, 32(1), 38–49. doi:10.1111/socf.12316

De Jong Gierveld, J. J., van Tilburg, T. G., & Dykstra, P. A. (2016). Loneliness and social isolation. In A. Vangelisti & D. Perlman (Eds.), *The Cambridge handbook of social relationships* (pp. 1–30). New York, NY: Cambridge University Press.

Duncan, G., Magnuson, K., & Votruba-Drzal, E. (2016). Moving beyond correlations in assessing the consequences of poverty. *Annual Review of Psychology*, 68:413–434. doi:10.1146/annurev-psych-010416-044224

Effing, R., & Spil, T. (2016). The social strategy cone: Towards a framework for evaluating social media strategies. *International Journal of Information Management*, 36(1), 1–8. doi:10.1016/j.ijinfomgt.2015.07.009

Gottlieb, B. H., & Bergen, A. E. (2010). Social support concepts and measures. *Journal of Psychosomatic Research*, 69(5), 511–520. doi:10.1016/j.jpsychores.2009.10.001

Holt, C. L., Roth, D. L., Huang, J., Park, C., & Clark, E. M. (2017). Longitudinal effects of religious involvement on religious coping and health behaviors in a national sample of African Americans. *Social Science & Medicine*, 187, 11–19. doi:10.1016/j.socscimed.2017.06.014

Househ, M., Borycki, E., & Kushniruk, A. (2014). Empowering patients through social media: The benefits and challenges. *Health Informatics Journal*, 20(1), 50–58. doi:10.1177/1460458213476969

Kanitz, E., Hameister, T., Tuchscherer, A., Tuchscherer, M., & Puppe, B. (2016). Social support modulates stress-related gene expression in various brain regions of piglets. *Frontiers in Behavioral Neuroscience, 10*, 227. doi:10.3389/fnbeh.2016.00227

Levac, J. J., & O'Sullivan, T. (2016). Social media and its use in health promotion. *Interdisciplinary Journal of Health Sciences, 1*(1), 47–53.

Levin, J. (2016). Partnership between the faith-based and medical sectors: Implications for preventive medicine and public health. *Preventive Medicine Reports, 4*, 344–350. doi:10.1016/j.pmedr.2016.07.009

Lin, C. A., Atkin, D. J., Cappotto, C., Davis, C., Dean, J., Eisenbaum, J., . . . Vidican, S. (2015). Ethnicity, digital divides and uses of the Internet for health information. *Computers in Human Behavior, 51*, 216–223. doi:10.1016/j.chb.2015.04.054

Lincoln, K. D., Lloyd, D. A., & Nguyen, A. W. (2017). Social relationships and salivary telomere length among middle-aged and older African American and White adults. *Journals of Gerontology: Social Sciences*, 1–9. doi:10.1093/geronb/gbx049

Marcus, A. F., Echeverria, S. E., Holland, B. K., Abraido-Lanza, A. F., & Passannante, M. R. (2016). The joint contribution of neighborhood poverty and social integration to mortality risk in the United States. *Annals of Epidemiology, 26*(4), 261–266. doi:10.1016/j.annepidem.2016.02.006

Martina, C. M., Stevens, N. L., & Westerhof, G. J. (2016). Change and stability in loneliness and friendship after an intervention for older women. *Ageing & Society*, 1–20. doi:10.1017/S0144686X16001008

Mason, H. O. (2016). Multiple measures of family and social support as predictors of psychological well-being: An additive approach. *Journal of Educational and Developmental Psychology, 6*(2), 97–112. doi:10.5539/jedp.v6n2p97

Myhre, J. W., Mehl, M. R., & Glisky, E. L. (2016). Cognitive benefits of online social networking for healthy older adults. *Journals of Gerontology: Psychological Sciences, 72*(5), 752–760. doi:10.1093/geronb/gbw025

Nguyen, A., Mosadeghi, S., & Almario, C. V. (2017). Persistent digital divide in access to and use of the Internet as a resource for health information: Results from a California population-based study. *International Journal of Medical Informatics, 103*, 49–54. doi:10.1016/j.ijmedinf.2017.04.008

Sokol, R., & Fisher, E. (2016). Peer support for the hardly reached: A systematic review. *American Journal of Public Health, 106*(7), e1–e9. doi:10.2105/AJPH.2016.303180

Tanskanen, J., & Anttila, T. (2016). A prospective study of social isolation, loneliness, and mortality in Finland. *American Journal of Public Health, 106*(11), 2042–2048. doi:10.2105/AJPH.2016.303431

Uchino, B. N. (1972). *Social support & physical health* (p. 12), New Haven, CN: Yale University Press.

Verbos, A. & Humphries, M. (2014). A Native American relational ethic: An indigenous perspective on teaching human responsibility. *Journal of Business Ethics, 123*:1–9. doi:10.1007/s10551-013-1790-3

Wright, K. B. (2016). Communication in health-related online social support groups/communities: A review of research on predictors of participation, applications of social support theory, and health outcomes. *Review of Communication Research, 4*, 65–87. doi:10.12840/issn.2255-4165.2016.04.01.010

Yang, Y. C., Boen, C., Gerken, K., Li, T., Schorpp, K., & Harris, K. M. (2016). Social relationships and physiological determinants of longevity across the human life span. *Proceedings of the National Academy of Sciences, 113*(3), 578–583.

PART 4

Evaluating the Effectiveness of Health Promotion

CHAPTER 10

Evaluating Health Promotion Programs

OBJECTIVES

This chapter will enable the reader to:

1. Describe the purpose of evaluation for health promotion.
2. Compare three approaches to evaluation and provide examples of each.
3. Discuss types of outcomes to consider when evaluating health promotion programs.
4. Describe the steps in program evaluation.
5. Discuss criteria to evaluate the quality of mobile applications for health behavior change.

Credible evidence to guide health promotion programs is established by evaluating program outcomes. Evaluation is necessary to assess the effectiveness of health promotion programs for clients and communities. Knowledge of the success of health promotion is based on both research and program evaluations. Nurses and other health care professionals are continually being asked about the benefits of health promotion and prevention activities. This question can be answered by carefully examining the cumulative evidence produced by program evaluations.

PURPOSE OF EVALUATION

Evaluation, the process of systematically collecting and analyzing information, is undertaken to assess the value of a health promotion program or intervention. Program evaluations are considered decision oriented, whereas research evaluations generate scientific knowledge. Health promotion evaluations serve many purposes: to determine if program objectives were achieved, to identify strengths and weaknesses of the program, to increase stakeholder and community support, to provide accountability to funding agencies, to contribute to the scientific knowledge base of health promotion, and to inform policy decisions (McKenzie, Neiger, & Thackeray, 2012).

Evaluations also provide information to guide decisions about resource allocation, as funds can be eliminated if programs are shown to be ineffective. Health promotion evaluations enable the nurse to increase the success of health promotion activities, to make choices between health promotion activities, and to assess if a new intervention with documented efficacy will translate to practice.

Questions that may be answered by a comprehensive evaluation include the following:

- Is the health promotion intervention effective in an ideal situation? (efficacy)
- Does the health promotion intervention produce the same benefits when it is translated to a practice setting? (effectiveness)
- How does the health promotion intervention work? (theory)
- What are the intended and unintended effects? (outcomes)
- How long do the effects last? (sustainability)
- What resources are needed to implement the program? (costs, time, personnel)
- Is the program cost effective?
- Are the clients satisfied?
- Who will benefit most from the program?
- How can the program be refined?

Resources, including cost, time, and number of personnel required, pose limitations on evaluations. All stakeholders must be engaged in the evaluation process, including those who have an investment in the program as well as intended users. Credible evidence is critical to make accurate conclusions. In addition, performing an evaluation requires knowledge, skills, and administrative support. If these components are not present, the evaluation may not produce useful information.

APPROACHES TO EVALUATION OF HEALTH PROMOTION PROGRAMS

Evaluation approaches provide a road map for systematically collecting, analyzing, and reporting information. Knowledge of differences in efficacy and effectiveness evaluations, process and outcome evaluations, and quantitative and qualitative evaluation approaches is needed to design an appropriate evaluation plan. Other approaches such as systems analysis, goal-based evaluations, decision-making evaluations, social return on investment (SROI), and empowerment evaluations are not reviewed in this chapter.

Efficacy or Effectiveness Evaluation

Efficacy refers to changes in program outcomes that are achieved under ideal circumstances. The health promotion program is implemented and evaluated under controlled or optimal conditions to demonstrate that the changes observed are due to the program and not due to chance or other factors unrelated to the intervention. *Efficacy* is best demonstrated with research using randomized controlled trials.

The *effectiveness* of a program or intervention is the result it achieves in the real world, with limited resources, in entire populations or specified subgroups of a population. *Effectiveness* addresses the usefulness of a program in practice, as it is implemented and evaluated in a typical practice setting. *Effectiveness* can also be demonstrated in research using randomized control trials as well as less rigidly structured evaluation methods.

Efficacy studies test the usefulness of programs or interventions under ideal, controlled circumstances. Efficacy evaluations are followed by effectiveness evaluations that assess the program in real-life settings for feasibility, costs, and its usefulness and acceptance by diverse groups. If the efficacy of a health promotion program has been scientifically documented, its effectiveness can then be evaluated in practice settings.

Process or Outcome Evaluation

Process evaluation of a health promotion program refers to verifying the content of the program and whether it was delivered as intended, whereas *outcome* evaluations focus on the results or effects of the program. Although the terms *formative, implementation,* and *process evaluations* are used interchangeably, some authors state that formative evaluations focus on programs that are under development, while process evaluations focus on programs that are underway.

Process evaluations concentrate on program implementation, so it provides information to help improve the delivery of the program and better define the needs and preferences of the targeted group. Variations in delivery among sites and clients are identified as well as breakdowns between what was intended and what was actually delivered.

Process evaluations provide insights into factors that hinder or facilitate the implementation of the program to achieve program goals. Did the program fail because of a poorly conceived or designed program, or because of breakdowns in delivery? What contextual factors may have been operating to influence delivery of the program?

Process evaluations also assess whether the intended "dosage" of the program was delivered. Did the client attend all program sessions, or only half of the sessions? Dosage is important to track, as the amount of participation or exposure needs to be strong enough to produce the desired results. Ideally clients should attend all program components. However, in the evaluation process, one may find that attending two-thirds is just as effective in meeting the desired outcomes. Process evaluations are necessary, as they offer valuable insight into the reasons for the success or failure of the program. Table 10–1 describes essential elements that need to be tracked in a process evaluation to assess if the program has been implemented as intended (Aarestrup, Jorgensen, Due, & Kroiner, 2014; Moore et al., 2015).

Outcome evaluations focus on the results or changes brought about by the program, either intended or unintended. Unintended outcomes refer to unforeseen effects of the program. Unintended outcomes, also called side effects, may be positive or negative. For example, an intended outcome of a school-based activity program may be increased physical activity. However, teachers may also observe a decrease in aggressive or combative behavior among students, an unintended positive outcome. The choice of outcomes to measure is determined by the program goals. If the goal is to achieve weight loss, weight should be measured prior to program initiation and at the end of the program. If the program goal is primary prevention of cancer, clients should be followed for years to learn if cancer occurs. *Outcome* evaluations enable one to assess if changes occurred as a result of the program. In other words, was the program successful in promoting the desired change?

Outcomes may include short-term, intermediate, or long-term assessments of change. Short-term outcomes are usually measured immediately after completion of

TABLE 10–1 Process Evaluation Elements to Consider in Assessing Program Implementation

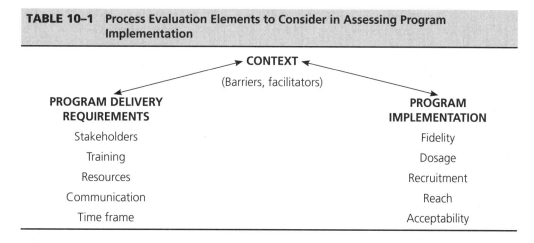

PROGRAM DELIVERY REQUIREMENTS	CONTEXT (Barriers, facilitators)	PROGRAM IMPLEMENTATION
Stakeholders		Fidelity
Training		Dosage
Resources		Recruitment
Communication		Reach
Time frame		Acceptability

the program to assess the program's immediate impact, whereas intermediate outcomes measure broader health and social outcomes. Long-term outcomes measure lasting or sustained effects of health promotion programs.

Quantitative or Qualitative Evaluation

The randomized controlled trial (RCT) is considered the gold standard to evaluate the intended outcomes of a program. Rigorously developed and precisely implemented programs (interventions) are typically evaluated with predetermined measures that can be converted to *numeric* (quantitative) information (data). For example, paper-and-pencil measures may be used to assess changes in attitudes or knowledge, or laboratory measures can be used to assess changes in body fat or blood glucose. This information can then be analyzed to evaluate the program effects. Although quantitative measures are objective and provide evidence of the program effects, this objective information may fail to account for the client's perspective.

Qualitative evaluations represent a different perspective, as clients participating in the program are asked to provide input about the program. Information (data) may be obtained in individual or group interviews (focus groups). The recorded conversations (words) are then organized into themes or categories. This approach provides additional insight into the success or failure of the program. Qualitative evaluations that include multiple stakeholders are called *participatory evaluations* (Braithwaite et al., 2013). Participatory evaluations are essential for integrating the multiple perspectives into the evaluation process.

Qualitative evaluation approaches focus on the perception of the client, providing information about the program that may not be captured with quantitative information. Outcomes that can be identified with qualitative interviews include self-awareness, motivation, social connectedness, and control over daily life. These types of outcomes convey information on factors that may lead to or hinder the desired behavior change.

Complex programs with multiple components present many challenges and often require the use of multiple evaluation methods. *Mixed methods* evaluations incorporate both quantitative and qualitative data. The premise of mixed methods evaluations is that no one method is adequate to evaluate a program, and multiple methods are complementary. When using mixed methods to evaluate a program, issues to consider include how and in what sequence the methods will be implemented, and how the different types of information will be used to describe the program outcomes.

DECIDING OUTCOMES TO MEASURE

Choice of health promotion outcomes to measure is dependent on the desired goals, the purpose and type of program, and the ability to access the information needed to measure the intended results. The challenge is to select outcomes that are comprehensive, comparable, meaningful, and accurate in reflecting the program outcomes. In addition, measurement of the outcomes must be feasible.

Nurse-Sensitive Outcomes

Although quality of care has always been a concern for nursing, quality improvement programs have focused on structure and process. The shift to effectiveness (outcomes) has posed a challenge, as nurses practice in interdisciplinary teams in which health outcomes are influenced by more than one discipline. For example, in many health promotion programs, nurses, nutritionists, psychologists, and exercise physiologists may all be involved in implementing the program. The challenge is to identify and measure outcomes that are influenced by nursing actions.

Nurse-sensitive outcomes are indicators of care considered to be influenced by nursing. Examples of nurse-sensitive categories that reflect health promotion and community outcomes are summarized in Table 10–2. **Biological** outcomes are commonly used in health promotion and may include weight, blood pressure, and laboratory values, such as lipid levels. **Psychosocial** outcomes measure patterns of behavior, communication, and relationships. Measures may include attitude, mood, emotions, coping, and social functioning. **Functional** outcomes include activities, mobility, and self-care outcomes. **Behavioral** outcomes involve the client's actions, such as participation in regular physical activity. Knowledge, the **cognitive** level of understanding, is a common nurse-sensitive outcome because teaching is a major component of nursing practice.

Home functioning outcomes focus on the performance of the client and family in the home environment. Measures of these outcomes may include family support and role function. **Safety** is also a nurse-sensitive outcome, as nurses implement interventions to promote safe home, community, and work environments. For example, the nurse may work with clients in the community to promote a safe neighborhood environment with lighted walking paths.

Symptom control outcomes involve the management of symptoms that may result from changing undesirable behaviors. For example, dietary restrictions to lose weight may produce negative symptoms, such as craving. Strategies will be needed to manage the unpleasant symptoms to promote adoption of the new diet.

Goal attainment outcomes refer to helping clients accomplish their health promotion goals, such as walking daily for 30 minutes or losing 20 pounds. **Client satisfaction** is a global measure of contentment with the services received. Measures of satisfaction or dissatisfaction with health promotion programs provide valuable information needed to make program changes.

The Nursing Outcomes Classification (NOC) is a standardized classification of patient–client outcomes developed to evaluate the effects of nursing interventions (Moorhead, Johnson, Maas, & Swanson, 2012). Seven categories have been identified: physiological health, functional health, psychosocial health, family health, health

TABLE 10–2 Categories of Nursing–Sensitive Outcomes

Category	Examples
Biological	Blood pressure
	Weight
	Laboratory values
Psychosocial	Attitudes
	Emotions
	Moods
	Social functioning
Functional	Activities of daily living
	Mobility
	Self-care
Behavioral	Actions
	Activities
Cognitive	Knowledge
Home functioning	Family support
	Family roles
Safety	Noise-free environment
Symptom control	Smoking withdrawal
Goal attainment	Behavior change
Satisfaction	Program/service contentment
Costs	Cost effectiveness

knowledge and behavior, perceived health, and community health. NOC is one of the standardized languages recognized by the American Nurses Association (ANA). Information about the NOC system is available on its website.

Outcomes that are sensitive to nursing practice are necessary to document the effectiveness of health promotion programs planned and implemented by nurses. To date, most of the efforts to validate nurse-sensitive indicators have occurred in the acute care setting, with less attention to the community. Work is needed to assess the validity of these outcomes with nursing activities in health promotion settings. Validation of nurses' influence on changing behavior provides evidence of nurse's central role in health promotion and prevention.

Individual, Family, and Community Outcomes

Health promotion outcomes can be measured at three levels: (1) individual or client focused, (2) family focused, and (3) community focused.

Individual- or **client-focused outcomes** measure the effects of health promotion programs on individuals. These outcomes can be classified as *biological* or *behavioral*. *Biological* outcomes are objective physiological changes in clients. For example, a nutritional intervention may result in a change in body mass index or a decrease in the client's triglyceride level.

Behavioral outcomes are measures of social, emotional, spiritual, and intellectual wellness. Behavioral outcomes may include psychosocial functioning, positive affect, self-care, knowledge, perceptions, and quality of life. Monitoring behavioral outcomes is important in health promotion programs, as these outcomes may be detectable before longer-term biological effects are observed.

Family-focused outcomes have received less attention due to the challenges in measuring the contributions of family members to health outcomes. The significant role the family plays in the development of both health-promoting and health-damaging behaviors, beginning at a very early age, is well documented. Measurable family-focused outcomes include changes in family eating behaviors, such as a change in the frequency of shared family meals or changes in consumption of high-fat foods; or changes in leisure activity patterns, such as an increase in the number of family activities that include physical activity.

Community-focused outcomes are global measures in health promotion; they focus on the effectiveness of the program at the community level. Community outcomes include community participation, empowerment, and an increase in community resources for health promotion, such as biking paths and wellness centers. Community outcomes are measured at the neighborhood or group level. Broader measures present multiple challenges since multiple factors may be operating in the community to affect the program outcomes, other than the program itself.

Short-Term, Intermediate, and Long-Term Outcomes

Health promotion programs pose challenges for measuring outcomes, as the intended outcomes may not be evident for many years. For this reason, different levels of outcomes, that is, short-term, intermediate, long-term, have been described. An example of a model for health promotion differentiating outcomes is shown in Figure 10–1. The model distinguishes health promotion (short-term) health outcomes (long-term)

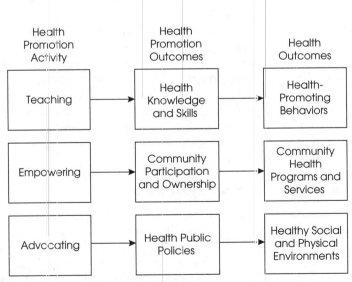

FIGURE 10–1 Outcomes for Health Promotion Activities

TABLE 10–3 Hierarchy of Potential Outcomes in Health Promotion

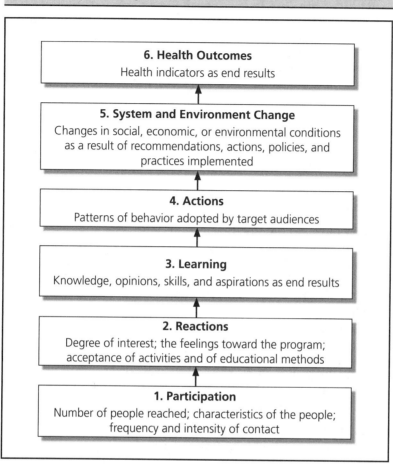

Source: Centers for Disease Control and Prevention (2006).

outcomes, which may not be evident for many months or years. The model reflects outcomes associated with various types of health promotion activities.

The Centers for Disease Control and Prevention (CDC) has published a hierarchy of outcomes that also suggests levels of outcomes to measure, beginning with short-term outcomes, such as number of participants reached (Centers for Disease Control and Prevention, 2006). The hierarchy, which is a mainstay for CDC public health program evaluations, is shown in Table 10–3.

Lack of effectiveness of health promotion programs may be due to measuring outcomes at the wrong time. If information is collected immediately following the program, it may be too soon to capture desired changes in lifestyle behaviors. If the effects are measured many months after the program has ended, other factors may intervene to influence the expected results. Therefore, the timing of measurements should be planned carefully to capture the anticipated effects. Measurement at multiple time points usually is necessary. **Short-term outcomes** are measured immediately following the program to measure the immediate effects. Examples of short-term outcomes include knowledge or a readiness to change. **Intermediate outcomes** are targeted at a longer time point following the intervention when a behavior change is expected to have occurred. Intermediate outcomes are measured soon enough to capture the effects before they may be due to other possible reasons. Intermediate outcomes are useful in reflecting attitude changes or attempts to change, although sustained lifestyle change has not yet occurred. **Long-term outcomes** are the final or end results of health promotion programs. Long-term outcomes include such things as sustained weight loss and improved quality of life. When interpreting the results of long-term change, it is important to account for other potential factors that may have influenced the outcomes.

Economic Outcomes

Effective delivery of health promotion programs requires resources, including people, time, facilities, and equipment and supplies. These economic costs need to be evaluated in relation to program benefits for consumers, health care payers, and policy makers. Results of economic evaluations provide stakeholders information that enables them to make decisions about investing in effective programs that make the best use of limited resources. Economic evaluations are used to quantify and measure the costs and benefits of alternative programs and are not undertaken until program effectiveness is established. These types of evaluations compare the costs of the program with the outcomes gained.

Economic evaluations include *cost-minimization analysis, cost-effectiveness analysis, cost-utility analysis,* and *cost-benefit analysis.* One way to describe the different types of analyses is by the questions they answer.

- A *cost-minimization analysis* answers the question, "What are the monetary costs of the resources needed to implement the program?"
- *Cost-effectiveness analysis* (CEA) answers the question, "What is the most inexpensive way to achieve a given outcome?"
- In *cost-utility analysis*, the question answered is, "What is the cost per quality-adjusted life year?"
- In *cost-benefit analysis*, the question answered is, "What is the net benefit of a given alternative?"

Economic analysis begins with merely reporting the cost of the program implemented. This is followed by cost-benefit analysis, which places a monetary value on a health outcome. Cost-benefit analysis compares the monetary value of resources used in the program with the value of outcomes produced by the program.

Several challenges are inherent in economic evaluations of health promotion programs. First, health promotion programs sometimes include groups that may not be representative of the general population. Second, health promotion programs and economic analyses are designed for different purposes. Economic analysis can also be time consuming. Last, health promotion programs are often complex, while economic evaluations focus on single interventions with clearly defined outcomes.

Broader outcomes of health promotion encompassed in the Ottawa Charter for Health Promotion (see Chapter 1), such as empowerment, or nonhealth outcomes like self-awareness, are not easily captured, raising multiple challenges for economic evaluations.

Ethical issues in economic analysis occur when evaluators attach costs to values such as individual quality of life, with measures such as quality-adjusted life years (QUALYs) or potential life years gained. All types of economic analyses have potential limitations that need careful consideration. However, nurses and other health care professionals need to show that health promotion is cost effective, so they should be considered when planning health promotion evaluations.

Economic evaluations have begun to assume an important role in health care policy decisions. The approach has been standardized with principles and procedures for reporting the results. Regulatory bodies now consider cost-effectiveness part of the approval process for new medications and technologies. However, the analytic techniques are not simple and have many methodological pitfalls, so only individuals with expertise should conduct the analysis.

STEPS IN EVALUATION OF HEALTH PROMOTION PROGRAMS

Evaluations shed light on the process and effectiveness of health promotion programs in real-world settings. One method for evaluating program effectiveness is the Centers for Disease Control and Prevention's Framework for Program Evaluation, which outlines essential steps of program evaluation (see Figure 10–2). The comprehensive

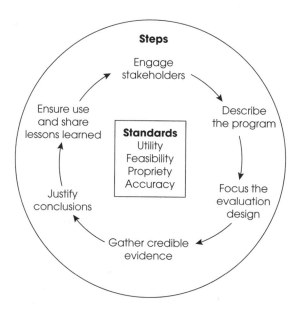

FIGURE 10–2   Centers for Disease Control and Prevention Framework for Program Evaluation (CDC, 1999)

framework has become a template for program evaluation because of its focus on planning, designing, implementing, and using the results and lessons learned (Centers for Disease Control and Prevention, 2000). Each step incorporates both planning and evaluation activities. The steps are briefly described. An in-depth discussion can be found in the CDC program evaluation self-study guide available on the CDC website (U.S. Department of Health and Human Services, 2011).

ENGAGE STAKEHOLDERS. Initially, four groups of stakeholders are identified to participate in the evaluation. They include persons who have an investment in the program, including (1) persons who implemented the program; (2) clients who attended the program; and (3) potential users of the results, such as community agencies; and (4) agencies that provided resources. It is critical to engage stakeholders in the evaluation process as well as to assess their expectations. When they are not involved, the results of the evaluation may not reflect their needs and could be criticized or rejected.

DESCRIBE THE PROGRAM. A clear description of the program includes an overview of the need for the program, the program objectives, program strategies and activities, and expected measurable outcomes. Logic models (conceptual maps) may be used at this stage to visually display the program components and their relationships. A clear description of the program is needed, along with how it will be implemented and how it is expected to work.

FOCUS THE EVALUATION DESIGN. The type of evaluation design will be determined by the resources available and the time constraints of the evaluators. Focusing the evaluation design means deciding in advance what questions will be answered and what data will be collected to answer the questions. Any ethical and confidentiality issues need to be considered during this stage. Both process and outcome evaluations should also be considered.

GATHER CREDIBLE EVIDENCE. Prior to information gathering, the kind of information (qualitative or quantitative) and type of data collection methods (questionnaires or interviews) need to be decided. All data should be obtained as rigorously as possible so that it is perceived as believable and relevant by stakeholders. Sources of information, how it was obtained, and who collected it should be transparent.

JUSTIFY CONCLUSIONS. After all information collected is carefully analyzed, the results need to be interpreted and presented as accurately as possible. The information should enable the evaluators to make recommendations for needed program changes as well as identify which aspects of the program were useful and effective in promoting change.

ENSURE USE AND SHARE LESSONS LEARNED. Dissemination of the evaluation results should include all stakeholders, as well as potential users of the program. In addition, the lessons learned can be used to increase the effectiveness of the program. The information, including lessons learned, should be presented to a wider audience through written reports and publications.

EVALUATING EVIDENCE FOR HEALTH PROMOTION PRACTICE

Credible, scientific evidence for one's health promotion practice is obtained from many sources: a synthesis of relevant research literature; standards of practice; clinical expertise; and client preferences. Evidence is frequently obtained by critically evaluating the research base for a program intervention and then integrating the findings into one's practice to guide health promotion decisions for clients. This process is called *evidence-based practice* or *evidence-based health promotion*. Evidence-based practice focuses on applying interventions that have been shown to be effective, based on predefined criteria (Mackey & Bassendowski, 2017). The concept has evolved from a clinical procedure to a more holistic approach and is relevant for health professionals concerned with the scientific base of health promotion interventions. Evaluation questions include the following:

- Can I trust this information? (validity)
- Will the information make an important difference in my practice? (significance)
- Will I be able to use the information in my practice? (applicability)

Evidence-based practice involves identifying a client problem, conducting a literature search to find the best evidence to address the problem, critically evaluating the evidence, translating the evidence into one's practice, and re-evaluating the outcomes in one's own practice (Melnyk & Newhouse, 2014). The evidence-based process does not replace clinical expertise, as the nurse must evaluate new knowledge in light of its relevance to the target population as well as its costs in terms of resources and time.

Current best evidence can be obtained from the Cochrane Collaboration, an organization committed to improving global health through systematic reviews of the effectiveness of health interventions. The Cochrane Collaboration's website is a valuable resource (see www.cochrane.org).

STRATEGIES FOR PROMOTING EFFECTIVE HEALTH PROMOTION OUTCOMES

Evaluation of results of health promotion has led to understanding program components that facilitate successful behavior change. Although knowledge about long-term maintenance of change—the last step in the change process of health promotion—is limited, several strategies have been identified.

Designing the Program

Theory-based, tested interventions provide a greater understanding of how the program is expected to promote or change behavior. Theories describe the factors (concepts) that facilitate behavior change, suggesting strategies that influence behavior change. For example, Bandura's social cognitive model theorizes that people learn by observing and modeling the behavior of others, thereby increasing their self-efficacy to perform the behavior. This relationship has been substantiated. Research has documented that observing others who role model physical activity behavior helps clients develop self-efficacy to perform physical activity. An understanding of the theoretical basis of a program intervention is critical to choosing strategies that are known to promote behavior change.

Health promotion programs are complex and usually involve multiple components. For example, programs may contain several interacting components, such as weight loss and physical activity. When designing programs, the nurse first assesses whether the intervention is appropriate and feasible for the target population. The program may also need to be changed to be culturally relevant or appropriate to the context. For example, a high-intensity community walking program may not be appropriate for a sample of obese, older adults who live in a high-crime neighborhood. Feasibility questions to ask include the following:

Are facilities or other resources needed accessible in the community?

Will the proposed program reach the intended audience?

Will the program be acceptable to the intended audience?

Will the program be affordable to the intended audience?

Is the program compatible with existing programs in the community?

Programs that are costly or resource intensive will result in poor participation. In addition, community agencies may not be committed or offer the needed support. Programs that are easy to implement and fit with existing programs have a greater chance of being successfully implemented. Evidence of the efficacy of the program should be available. If the efficacy of the intervention has not been tested, the intervention should be rigorously evaluated.

Selecting Outcomes

Program results should be evaluated with realistic, measurable outcomes. The outcome evaluation component needs careful planning so that outcomes reflect the purpose of the program. Self-report measures, using paper-and-pencil questionnaires, are used to measure knowledge, attitudes, and self-report health behaviors. Objective measures are more precise and sensitive to change, and may include actual physical activity recorded with technology such as pedometers or smartphones. Measurement of weight, for example, is a more accurate indicator of dietary change than self-reported eating habits. Community-level outcomes, although less well developed, also may be appropriate to measure, such as the number of new public physical activity facilities and walking paths or the number of restaurants that provide healthy choices. These broader outcomes provide information about how the program has improved the overall community, independent of behavior change of individual members. Outcomes that measure the client's perspective also should be considered. Although interviews may be time consuming, the client's perspective may offer valuable information about the strengths and weaknesses of the program.

When long-term outcomes may not be realistic, an evaluation may include such things as program participation rates or client satisfaction. Although these outcomes do not measure effectiveness, they provide information about the acceptance of the intervention and its implementation. As discussed earlier, process measures are also useful to assess implementation effectiveness. Measurement of the "delivered dose," an assessment of aspects of the program that were implemented, and "received dose," the number of people who participated in the program, is a useful aspect of process evaluation.

Deciding Time Frame

A realistic time frame is necessary to properly conduct the program and evaluate the results. What is realistic depends on the type, comprehensiveness, and complexity of the program and the target population. In an individual-focused intervention targeting a small group, six weeks may be a realistic period to implement and evaluate short-term results. However, five years may be needed to implement and evaluate a complex, community-based program in primary schools. The time frame should be acceptable to the target population or community, as it may backfire if it is rushed or too long.

Sustaining Behavior Change

Most of the progress in health promotion has been in promoting health behavior change; less progress has been seen in identifying strategies that sustain these changes. The current theoretical models of health behavior focus on how people decide to adopt healthy behaviors. Exceptions are Bandura's cognitive theory, which asserts that self-efficacy beliefs are a critical determinant of both the initiation and maintenance of behavior change, and Prochaska and DiClemente's transtheoretical model, which includes a maintenance stage. However, neither model offers detailed guidance about the process of maintenance and how it differs from initiation and adoption of behaviors.

In health promotion programs, factors that have been shown to be associated with sustainability of the behavior change include *duration of the program, continuing contact or booster follow-up sessions, ongoing self-monitoring,* and *family support.* Ongoing self-monitoring has consistently been found to be effective in both eating and physical activity interventions (Bardus, van Beurden, Smith, & Abraham, 2016). Interventions that provide ongoing support, such as telephone calls or text messages, and ongoing self-monitoring and positive reinforcement of change have been shown to be effective in promoting long-term (2 years) weight loss. Continued professional support and contact are also needed for sustained change. Professional support includes helping clients maintain the health benefits achieved through the initial program and building the capacity of the community to continue the program.

Sustainability of health promotion programs in the community is influenced by the *design of the program, implementation factors, facilitators and barriers within the targeted community,* and *factors in the broader community environment.* Potential barriers include *insufficient human and financial resources, lack of buy-in, reliance on volunteers,* and *inability to get the support of powerful persons in the community.*

Factors that promote sustainability include *partnership formation, networking,* and *community capacity building* (Hanson & Salmoni, 2011). Sustainability is facilitated when community capacity building has occurred and program goals have included long-term maintenance. Program sustainability is an ongoing process that is ever changing as new knowledge is gained. Building an infrastructure that integrates resources to support the program, beginning in the planning stage, is critical.

USING MOBILE TECHNOLOGIES IN PROGRAM EVALUATIONS

New technologies, including mobile health applications (apps), Internet-based technologies, and text messaging (short message service), are beginning to play an important role in program evaluations (Materia et al., 2016). These technologies serve as useful data collection devices for both process and outcome evaluations. Specifically, they can be used to implement Web-based surveys that have the advantages of less preparation and administration time, and reminders can be sent through e-mail or text messaging. Other types of stored data may be downloaded, such as daily steps taken or time spent in physical activity.

The usefulness of technology in evaluations depends on the quality of data collected and analyzed. Planning for data collection, storage, and analysis needs to be done early in the evaluation process. The target population must also be taken into account. Although persons under 50 years of age easily adapt to new technologies and new apps, the elderly, rural, minority, and persons with low socioeconomic backgrounds may have more difficulty. In addition, an assessment of the time, skill, and resources available must be known prior to planning to use technology in the evaluation. Last, confidentiality of the data must be a priority.

Evaluating Mobile Health Applications

Health mobile apps continue to evolve. Applications enable health behavior interventions to be implemented to increase physical activity and healthy eating and weight loss; promote tobacco cessation; and decrease alcohol intake. They are inexpensive, offer tailoring, promote self-monitoring behaviors, and have a wide reach. Although evaluation of the efficacy of the apps on behavior change is limited, evidence indicates that they may produce modest, positive short-term outcomes. Using American Heart Association criteria to evaluate mobile interventions and prospective observational studies, short-term improvements were noted in diet, physical activity, body weight, and tobacco use when Internet interventions were used (Afshin et al., 2016). Although multiple reviews of health apps have been conducted, the actual number of studies has been quite small, and almost all research evaluating the technologies to date has not been done using randomized controlled trials with adequate sample sizes, and they suffer from multiple types of bias.

Another limitation is the lack of standard evaluation criteria to assess the efficacy and effectiveness of apps for behavior change. Health care professionals need to know which apps and strategies are successful for changing behaviors before recommending them to clients. One model currently available to evaluate mobile health apps is the Mobile Application Rating Scale (MARS; Stoyanov et al., 2015). The MARS is a simple, reliable rating scale that assesses four categories of quality: *engagement*, *functionality*, *aesthetics*, and *information quality*. The scale is still considered a research tool, as it has not been validated with multiple types of health apps (Bardus et al., 2016).

Evaluation of the types of behavior change strategies or techniques used by apps should also be done. The criteria and examples of measures for the criterion are described in Table 10–4. Even if a formal evaluation is not possible, the nurse should review the criteria to the extent possible before recommending an app to clients.

CONSIDERATIONS FOR PRACTICE IN EVALUATING HEALTH PROMOTION PROGRAMS

Nurses perform informal assessments daily to evaluate their practice. However, knowledge and skills are also needed to perform systematic evaluations of programs that promote behavior change. Evaluation provides useful information to be able to

TABLE 10–4 Criteria to Assess Quality of Mobile Health Applications with Examples

Criteria	Examples of Evaluation Measures
Engagement	Entertainment
	Interest
	Interactivity
Functionality	Ease of use
	Navigation
Aesthetics	Graphics
	Visual appeal
Information	Accuracy of app description
	Quality and quantity of information
	Credibility
Change techniques	Goal setting
	Tailoring
	Feedback
	Self-monitoring
	Social networking

Sources: Adapted from Stoyanov et al. (2015); Bardus et al. (2016).

recommend and/or implement relevant, feasible, and effective programs for individuals and communities. The CDC's evaluation model is realistic to implement in practice settings. Involvement of multiple stakeholders increases the likelihood of successful evaluations.

Nurses in community settings are in pivotal positions to evaluate new delivery models of health promotion. New technologies can augment individual counseling and follow-up and facilitate ongoing contact, social support, and real-time expertise to answer questions with individuals across the life span, including the elderly. Web-based health promotion programs have shown positive effects on behavior change and can also be a component of self-help programs. Program delivery using Web-based technologies has a wide reach for delivery. Mobile technologies have special relevance for youth and individuals living in rural areas. However, programs that incorporate mobile technologies should be tailored to the populations, with attention to age, health literacy, and socioeconomic background.

Evaluation continues when the program has ended, as maintenance continues to be a major problem in health behavior change. Evidence supports the need for ongoing support and reinforcement to sustain change. Follow-up of clients who have been successful in implementing new health-promoting behaviors is needed to provide support and to promote continued self-monitoring to sustain the changes. Nurses are in a good position to identify the most effective strategies for maintenance of healthy behaviors through observations and discussions with clients and their families.

OPPORTUNITIES FOR RESEARCH IN EVALUATING HEALTH PROMOTION

Evaluation of health promotion programs offers many avenues for research. First, it is evident that current theories of health promotion should be expanded and tested, as most theories have not focused on sustaining behavior change. In addition, the use of theories and models to guide and evaluate mobile technology interventions has been limited, offering a new avenue for research and evaluation.

Accurate and sensitive measures of behavior change are needed to evaluate behavioral outcomes in health apps. Although data are collected with most of the apps, the reliability and validity of the information obtained is unknown. Outcome measures of health behaviors also need to be standardized across technologies to enable researchers and practitioners to compare findings.

Research to evaluate the efficacy and effectiveness of mobile apps on both short-term and long-term behavior change needs to be tested with rigorous clinical trials using adequate sample sizes across the life span. In addition, the relevance and effectiveness of mobile apps for diverse and low-economic-status populations is lacking and is an important area for investigation.

Summary

Evaluation of health promotion programs documents which components are most effective to promote behavior change as well as what does not work. Evaluation facilitates the development of a knowledge base on which to make decisions about programs. The evaluation process is complex, time consuming, and requires advanced knowledge. However, learning to evaluate programs provides valuable information to promote successful health behavior change.

Learning Activities

1. Select a health promotion intervention of interest, such as promoting physical activity in the elderly, and evaluate the literature to establish the most effective strategies to use in a program for the group.
2. Develop an evaluation plan for a health promotion program to teach primary school children healthy nutrition behaviors.
   a. What would you consider in designing the program?
   b. What factors will you need to consider when assessing the feasibility of the program for your population?
   c. Develop a process evaluation plan, describing how you will evaluate the dosage of the intervention.
   d. Describe your outcome evaluation plan. Which outcomes will be appropriate to measure, and how will you measure them? Consider both short-term and intermediate outcomes.
   e. Describe the time frame you will use to implement and evaluate the results of the program and the rationale for choosing it.
3. Choose a mobile app designed for physical activity or weight reduction and evaluate its potential usefulness for adolescents, ages 14–16 years, using the criteria provided in Table 10–4. What additional health promotion strategies might be used for weight loss in this group?

References

Aarestrup, A. K., Jorgensen, T. S., Due, P., & Kroiner, R. (2014). A six-step protocol to systematic process evaluation of multicomponent cluster-randomized health promoting interventions illustrated by the Boost study. *Evaluation and Program Planning, 46,* 58–71. doi:10.1016/j.evalprogplan.2014.05.004

Afshin, A., Babalola, D., Mclean, M., Yu, Z., Ma, W., Chen, C., . . . Mozaffarian, D. (2016). Information technology and lifestyle: A systematic evaluation of internet and mobile interventions for improving diet, physical activity, obesity, tobacco, and alcohol use. *Journal of the American Heart Association, 5*(9), e003058. doi:10.1161/JAHA.115.003058

Bardus, M., van Beurden, S. B., Smith, J. R., & Abraham, C. (2016). A review and content analysis of engagement, functionality, aesthetics, information quality, and change techniques in the most popular commercial apps for weight management. *International Journal of Behavioral Nutrition and Physical Activity, 13,* 35. doi:10.1186/s12966-016-0359-9

Braithwaite, R. L., McKenzie, R. D., Pruitt, V., Holden, K. B., Aaron, K., & Hollimon, C. (2013). Community-based participatory evaluation: The Healthy Start approach. *Health Promotion Practice, 14*(2), 213–219. doi:10.1177/1524839912443241

Centers for Disease Control and Prevention. (1999). *Framework for program evaluation in public health.* Morbidity and Mortality Weekly Report, 48 (No. RR–11).

Centers for Disease Control and Prevention. (2000). *Overview of the framework for program evaluation.* Retrieved May 22, 2017, from http://www.cdc.gov/eval/framework/index.htm

Centers for Disease Control and Prevention. (2006). *Introduction to program planning for public health programs: Evaluating appropriate antibiotic use programs.* Atlanta, GA: Author.

Hanson, H. M., & Salmoni, A. W. (2011). Stakeholders' perceptions of programme sustainability: Findings from a community-based fall prevention programme. *Public Health, 125*(8), 525–532. doi:10.1016/j.puhe.2011.03.003

Mackey, A., & Bassendowski, S. (2017). The history of evidence-based practice in nursing education and practice. *Journal of Professional Nursing, 33*(1), 51–55. doi:10.1016/j.profnurs.2016.05.009

Materia, F. T., Miller, E. A., Runion, M. C., Chesnut, R. P., Irvin, J. B., Richardson, C. B., & Perkins, D. F. (2016). Let's get technical: Enhancing program evaluation through the use and integration of Internet and mobile technologies. *Evaluation and Program Planning, 56,* 31–42. doi:10.1016/j.evalprogplan.2016.03.004

McKenzie, J. F., Neiger, B. L., & Thackeray, R. (2012). *Planning, implementing, and evaluating health promotion programs* (6th ed.). San Francisco, CA: Pearson/Benjamin Cummings.

Melnyk, B., & Newhouse, R. (2014). Evidence-based practice versus evidence-informed practice: A debate that could stall forward momentum in improving healthcare quality, safety, patient outcomes, and costs. *Worldviews on Evidence-Based Nursing, 11*(6), 347–349. doi:10.1111/wvn.12070

Moore, G. F., Audrey, S., Barker, M., Bond, L., Bonell, C., Hardeman, W., . . . Baird, J. (2015). Process evaluation of complex interventions: Medical Research Council guidance. *British Medical Journal, 350,* h1258. doi:10.1136/bmj/h1258

Moorhead, S., Johnson, M., Maas, M. L., & Swanson, E. (2012). *Nursing outcomes classification (NOC)* (5th ed.). St. Louis, MO: Elsevier Mosby.

Stoyanov, S. R., Hides, L., Kavanagh, D. J., Zelenko, O., Tjondronegoro, D., & Mani, M. (2015). Mobile app rating scale: A new tool for assessing the quality of health mobile apps. *JMIR mHealth and uHealth, 3*(1), e27. doi:10.2196/mhealth.3422

U.S. Department of Health and Human Services, Centers for Disease Control and Prevention, Office of the Director, Office of Strategy and Innovation. (2011). *Introduction to program evaluation for public health programs: A self-study guide.* Atlanta, GA: Centers for Disease Control and Prevention.

Approaches for Promoting a Healthy Society

CHAPTER 11

Empowering for Self-Care to Promote Health

OBJECTIVES

This chapter will enable the reader to:

1. Differentiate between self-care and self-management.
2. Discuss experiential educational approaches to empower individuals for self-care.
3. Apply strategies to promote self-care empowerment across the life course.
4. Describe strategies to overcome barriers to self-care empowerment.
5. Critique the role of the Internet and social media in self-care empowerment to promote health.

Professional nurses play a major role in empowering clients for self-care to promote health throughout the life span. Activation of individuals to take a participatory role in their health is based on the assumptions that they have the desire, ability, and resources to do the following:

1. Be actively involved in solving their health problems
2. Make rational, informed decisions about their health and health care
3. Gain the knowledge, competencies, and skills needed to foster health
4. Strive for greater mastery over environmental conditions that influence health
5. Promote public policy to build healthy communities

Self-care is considered a basic form of primary care. Self-care includes health-promoting activities, such as eating a healthy diet, being physically active, getting adequate rest, and avoiding harmful substances and environments, as well as other behaviors to enhance well-being. *Family self-care* focuses on supporting the self-care of family members, and *community self-care* focuses on self-care groups to create enabling environments. Common characteristics of self-care include the following:

- It is situation and culture specific.
- It is influenced by one's social and physical environments.
- It involves the capacity to make choices and act.
- It is influenced by knowledge, skills, values, motivation, and self-efficacy.
- It focuses on aspects of health under an individual's control.
- It occurs independently of health care professionals.

OREM'S THEORY OF SELF-CARE

Dorothy Orem, a pioneer in nursing theory development, began publishing about the concept of self-care in 1959. She went on to develop the theory of self-care, also known as the self-care deficit theory, which continues to be tested and expanded. The theory is reviewed briefly, as it has relevance for self-care in health promotion.

In Orem's self-care model, three types of conditions or needs that require self-care are described: (1) *universal*, (2) *developmental*, and (3) *health deviation* (Orem, 1995, 2001; Orem & Taylor, 2011). *Universal* self-care needs are required by everyone to maintain life processes and include sufficient air, water, food, elimination, a balance between activity and rest, a balance between isolation and social interaction, protection from hazards, and protection of human functioning and development. *Developmental* self-care needs are also required by all and are concerned with maintaining conditions that support development across the life span, or prevent the deleterious effects of environments on human development. *Universal* and *developmental* self-care needs are considered *essential enduring requisites*, as they are necessary throughout the life span. *Health deviation* self-care needs are *situation-specific requisites*, as they occur in illness or injury and adversely affect health and well-being.

Three concepts are central to the model: *self-care*, *self-care agency*, and *self-care requisites* (*basic conditioning factors*) (Orem, 2001). Orem's definition of self-care is similar to the one provided in the introduction. *Self-care agency* refers to the complex abilities needed to perform self-care, such as one's knowledge and skills. *Self-care agency* includes internal capabilities such as memory, self-concept, and self-awareness; and capabilities specific to self-care actions, such as motivation and decision-making. *Basic conditioning factors* are those that influence an individual's self-care and self-care agency, such as age, developmental state, life experiences, sociocultural background, resources, and current health state. Self-care activities are learned in everyday life. To promote health, nurses should focus on basic conditioning factors, as many of these are amenable to change. In Orem's model, individuals perform self-care to meet needs and demands consistent with their age, maturation, experiences, resources, and sociocultural background.

Three systems of care are described by Orem within professional practice: a *compensatory* system, a *partially compensatory* system, and an *educative-developmental* system. In the *compensatory system*, total care is provided for the client. This can be considered self-management support or dependent care and is most common in acute-care settings, such as hospitals during acute illness episodes. The *partially compensatory system* of care is implemented when there can be shared responsibility for care (shared care). Care during rehabilitation from illness is partially compensatory. In contrast, in the *educative-developmental system* the client has primary responsibility for personal health, with the nurse functioning as a consultant or collaborative partner. The educative-developmental system is compatible with self-care in health promotion.

Orem's model of self-care has been criticized because it is based on the assumption that individuals are able to exert control over their environments in the pursuit of health. However, many individuals and families do not have control over their physical and social environments, two components that influence health and health behaviors. Therefore, it is important to evaluate the client's context, as it may not be possible to change many external factors without community or policy changes that provide resources and improve access to health-promoting environments.

SELF-CARE OR SELF-MANAGEMENT

Self-care is more comprehensive than performing activities of daily living. Self-care for health promotion can be defined as deliberate activities initiated or performed by an individual, family, or community to achieve, maintain, or promote maximum health (Orem, 2001; Webber, Guo, & Mann, 2013). According to the World Health Organization (WHO) definition, self-care activities are undertaken to maintain and promote health, prevent disease, and cope with illness or disability with or without health care professional support (World Health Organization, 2009). Self-care approaches represent empowerment and autonomy. Active involvement in self-care is widely acknowledged as an important strategy to achieve one's health goals. The government initiative, *Healthy People 2020*, emphasizes the importance of prevention and health promotion. Self-care is the basis for implementing health promotion and prevention strategies.

Self-care and *self-management* are used interchangeably. However, many consider the concepts distinctly different. *Self-management* is an individual's ability to detect and manage symptoms, treatments, physical and psychosocial consequences, and lifestyle changes associated with living with a chronic illness. In self-management, an individual participates in activities to manage the illness, such as adjusting medication, eating special diets, or taking direct action such as making a doctor's appointment. Clients and families assume responsibilities that previously were carried out by health professionals.

Self-care refers to individual responsibility to promote one's health and well-being, whereas self-management *focuses* on managing an illness. Self-management may be considered *shared care*, as health care professionals and clients work together to manage health conditions. In *dependent care*, individuals completely rely on health professionals with little opportunity for self-care. Self-care to promote health across the life span continues to gain significance as consumers become empowered and decrease their dependence on traditional medical care.

Although differences in the two concepts have been well established, the terms continue to be used interchangeably. Some authors include both health promotion activities and illness management activities in self-care (Jaarsma, Riegel, & Stromberg, 2017). In this chapter, self-care refers to activities undertaken to promote health. However, self-care health promotion activities are performed by healthy and chronically ill individuals.

Client Activation and Self-Care

Consumer activation refers to an individual's capability and willingness to manage his or her health and health care (Hibbard, 2017). Specifically, it refers to an individual's knowledge, skills, and confidence to manage one's health and health care. Individuals are ready to engage in self-care activities to promote health when they have the necessary knowledge, skills, and self-efficacy.

Activation is commonly measured with the Patient Activation Measure (PAM), a scale that assesses self-reported knowledge, skills, and confidence necessary to be an activated consumer in both health promotion and health care decision-making (Hibbard, 2017; Kenney, 2017). The authors of the scale have validated four stages in the activation process.

Stage 1: Clients believe that taking an active role in their health is important.

Stage 2: Clients have the confidence and knowledge to take action to manage or promote their health.

Stage 3: Clients take action to promote their health.

Stage 4: Clients maintain the new behaviors and have confidence that they can continue the behaviors under stressful situations.

Clients who score high on activation measures are more likely to engage in self-care and self-management behaviors. Supportive social environments are precursors to activation, as individuals in supportive, less stressful environments report higher levels of activation, are engaged in more health-promoting behaviors, and report better health outcomes including health behaviors (Greene, Hibbard, Sacks, Overton, & Parrotta, 2015). Research is beginning to explore how educational strategies can be tailored to each stage of activation, similar to tailoring strategies using Prochaska's stages of change.

Self-Efficacy and Self-Care

The concept of *self-efficacy* is related to activation, but it is not the same. Self-efficacy, as described in Chapter 2, is one's beliefs or confidence about one's ability to successfully perform a behavior or task. Self-efficacy focuses on beliefs; activation includes an individual's beliefs as well as his or her willingness to carry out the behavior or task (Shellman, 2014). Self-efficacy and activation are preconditions to empowerment for self-care. Persons with low self-efficacy and/or low activation need additional role modeling, sustained practice with success, and positive feedback to gain the confidence needed to perform health behaviors. The four concepts, self-care, self-management, activation, and self-efficacy, are summarized in Table 11–1.

TABLE 11–1   Definitions of Concepts Associated with Self-Care to Promote Healthy Behaviors

Self-Care	Self-Management
Deliberate activities initiated or performed by an individual, family, or community to achieve, maintain, or promote maximum health	An individual's ability to detect and manage symptoms, treatments, physical and psychosocial consequences, and lifestyle changes associated with living with a chronic illness
Consumer Activation	**Self-Efficacy**
An individual's knowledge, skills, confidence, and willingness to manage his or her health and health care	An individual's beliefs or confidence about his or her ability to successfully perform a behavior or task

THE PROCESS OF EMPOWERING FOR SELF-CARE

The goal of empowerment is to enable people to control and make changes in their personal lives as well as their environments to promote and maintain a healthy life. Empowerment for self-care refers to a complex social process of recognizing, promoting, and enabling individuals, families, and communities to meet personal needs, solve problems, and access resources necessary to control and enhance their health and well-being (Bridges, Loukanova, & Carrera, 2017). Empowerment is embedded in health promotion, as both are based on the assumption that individuals have the capacity to bring about changes in their personal behaviors as well as their communities. Characteristics of the empowering process to promote self-care include the following:

- A helping process
- A partnership in which both individuals and health professionals are valued
- Client decision-making
- Freedom to make choices
- Willingness to accept responsibility

Empowered persons actively participate in self-care, are well informed about the need to engage in healthy behaviors, are actively involved in health-related decisions, and are committed to their health (Palumbo, 2017). In the nurse–client relationship, knowledge, values, and power are shared. Empowerment emphasizes rights and abilities of individuals and communities, rather than deficits and needs.

Health education to empower individuals for self-care is multidimensional and complex. The client brings a unique personality and learning style, established social interaction patterns, cultural norms and values, environmental influences, and a level of readiness to adopt self-care behaviors. The nurse brings innate personality characteristics, values, attitudes, and social circumstances that affect the nature of the interaction.

In empowered relationships, health professionals are not in control; they are facilitators. Client choice, mutual decision-making, nonjudgmental responses, and experiential learning are components of empowerment-based educational strategies. Self-care results when clients determine their own goals and the strategies to reach these goals. The essential elements of self-care empowerment are shown in Figure 11–1. When clients are empowered for self-care, they have developed self-awareness and seek information needed to promote a healthy lifestyle. Empowered individuals also have the knowledge and skills to perform self-care activities. In addition, they actively participate in decisions concerning their health and are self-directed to make healthy lifestyle changes.

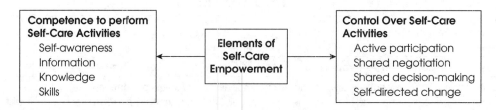

FIGURE 11–1 Essential Elements of Self-Care Empowerment

Education to Empower Clients

Health education is the critical link for empowering individuals and families for self-care. Empowerment education moves away from didactic lectures to focus on knowledge and skills that enable clients to perform healthy behaviors in daily life. An experiential, client-centered approach is considered central to empowerment education (Shellman, 2014).

Experiential learning approaches are based on the philosophy that individuals need to interact with the world to understand it. Active learning experiences are followed by focused reflection on the learning experience. Experiential learning strategies include *sharing and discussing information, practicing new skills,* and *self-reflection.* Role modeling of skills, such as negotiating or information seeking, enables clients to see how to successfully perform the behaviors, which they then practice. Immediate feedback is provided to increase understanding and skill mastery. The nurse collaborates with the client to share information about issues raised by the client and teaches the client how to track progress toward health promotion goals. Clients are taught to self-monitor their progress and make appropriate changes based on the information they gather. Last, they are taught focused self-reflection where they mentally review the knowledge and skills they have gained.

In experiential learning, clients develop knowledge and behavioral skills that can be applied in interactions with families and health care providers. Nurses partner with clients and families to understand their needs and desires for health promotion. In the education process, the nurse partners with clients to enable them to be able to perform the following:

- Identify personal health goals
- Choose realistic strategies to meet goals
- Problem solve barriers to achieving goals
- Track progress toward goals
- Reflect on learning experiences undertaken to meet goals

The self-care education empowerment process is depicted in Figure 11–2. Self-care empowerment education brings the professional expertise of nurses and other health care professionals together with the knowledge and goals of the client. Mutual information sharing enables the client to clarify goals and identify realistic strategies to meet goals, including gaining the knowledge and skills necessary to perform health behaviors or make lifestyle changes. The following elements are essential to the empowerment process:

- Be sensitive to and respect the client's culture
- Enable the client to express concerns
- Promote a participatory partnership
- Provide information to facilitate client decision-making
- Support choice
- Identify structural barriers and facilitators
- Promote skill building

Barriers to learning and implementing self-care behaviors are identified by the client and directly addressed. Failure to identify and decrease barriers can result in frustration and lack of progress toward self-care goals. For example, barriers to weight reduction

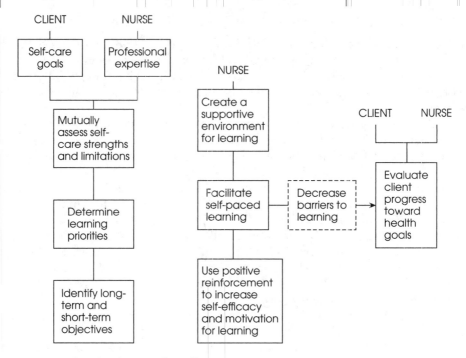

FIGURE 11–2   Educational Process for Self-Care Empowerment

might include time and financial constraints, family or friend saboteurs, and the client's attitudes and beliefs. Lack of attention to these barriers results in a sense of failure, low self-efficacy, and low self-esteem.

SELF-CARE EMPOWERMENT STRATEGIES

Specific strategies can be implemented to empower clients for self-care. These strategies are based on health promotion and experiential learning.

Mutually Share Information to Assess Strengths and Limitations

The client often comes to the encounter with certain self-care goals in mind. Competencies related to these goals can be assessed through informal discussion where information about the client's goals is shared. Clients are asked to describe their personal knowledge, abilities, and experiences that might facilitate or hinder goal attainment. Informal discussions are recommended. Observation of actual behavior can also provide useful insights, if this is possible. Apathy, lack of interest, and inattention should alert the nurse to a lack of motivation or low activation. Reasons for lack of interest should be explored so that strategies can be designed to increase motivation and activation for self-care.

The empowerment process enables clients to take control and make decisions about what they want to know and what is important to them to meet their goals. Sometimes their priority may not be the area of greatest threat to personal health. For example, a client may smoke but be more interested in starting to exercise than to quit smoking.

Although the nurse may believe that smoking constitutes a more serious threat than does a sedentary lifestyle, it is important that the client's choice be honored. If an exercise program is implemented, the client may develop a heightened awareness of the negative impact of smoking on lung capacity and physical endurance. At a later point, the client may exhibit readiness to discuss approaches to smoking cessation based on symptoms during exercise. The nurse is a supportive partner in the process; however, the client plays a crucial role in making choices and developing goals to promote their health.

Identify Strategies to Meet Goals

Once goals have been determined, the nurse and client work together to identify appropriate strategies to meet them. The process begins with mutual identification of both short- and long-term objectives. Long-term objectives guide large segments of learning. Short-term objectives identify the specific content or activities that must be progressively mastered to meet long-term objectives. Short-term objectives are the small steps taken to meet the long-term goal. The objectives should be realistic, not so easy to result in boredom, and not so difficult to cause discouragement. An example of a Goal and Objectives Tracking Form is presented in Table 11–2. The form enables the client to track each objective as it is attained and maintain awareness of the desired health outcomes. The form, either digital or paper, is kept by the client and serves as a self-monitoring device to track progress toward meeting the goal.

Facilitate Self-Paced Learning

The pace at which the client meets each short-term objective will vary, and expectations of both the client and the health professional should be adjusted accordingly. Adding a time frame to the short-term objectives is often a motivator to facilitate goal obtainment. However, the important factor is not how rapidly knowledge or skill is attained but the extent of mastery.

The nurse must be realistic and accept both good and bad days in clients of all ages. Sometimes the nurse and client will be elated with the results, sometimes discouraged. When efforts are less rewarding than anticipated, the pace of learning as well as

TABLE 11–2 Goal and Objectives Tracking Form	
Health Goal: Increased Physical Activity	
Long-Term Objective: To walk for 30 minutes five times a week	
Short-Term Learning Objectives	**Objectives Met**
Demonstrate how to check pulse by counting beats for 10 seconds and multiplying by 6.	
Read activity tracker to check recorded steps after walking.	
State heart rate to achieve during walking.	
Demonstrate two warm-up exercises to use before walking.	
Demonstrate two cool-down exercises to use after walking.	
Plan a weekly schedule for walking.	
Map three different routes to take when walking.	

the short-term objectives should be reviewed carefully and renegotiated. Focusing on resources rather than deficits and praising small steps are important to maintain motivation. Expanding the time frame for learning may also facilitate success. This is especially true for young children and adolescents, who have less experience in the learning process than adults.

Use Autonomy Support to Increase Motivation for Learning

Persons are more likely to be internally motivated to implement new behaviors when they feel supported, and feelings of being pressured by others are minimized. In empowerment education for self-care, the client, nurse, and family play important roles in supporting the client's autonomy. The nurse should be attuned to small steps in client progress and use positive support such as frequent praise and compliments to enhance feelings of success and self-efficacy. Frequent contact is important to provide feedback and recommend new strategies or options to meet goals. Specific information about the proposed change needs to be discussed without pressure. Skills should be practiced to gain mastery, and immediate feedback provided to correct any performance errors. When feedback is intermingled with autonomy support, it is helpful and nonthreatening. After learning has occurred, intermittent support strengthens the behavior making it more resistant to extinction. Autonomy support is congruent with experiential learning as it promotes self-determination. Autonomy supportive strategies are described in Table 11–3.

Family support without pressure or criticism is critical to successful behavior change. Family members are sources of support for one another in developing health behaviors. For example, achievement of a specific goal may be rewarded by the family spending time together in a favorite activity. By providing mutual support, a sense of healthy interdependence rather than crippling dependence is created within the family.

Actual performance of new behaviors that lead to success is a powerful strategy to strengthen self-efficacy, as successfully performing the new behaviors promotes self-confidence to continue the behavior. Other strategies to promote self-efficacy

---

TABLE 11–3   Strategies to Support Autonomy in Self-Care Empowerment Education

- Use neutral language, avoiding terms like "should" or "must."
- Provide multiple choices instead of only one way.
- Promote a sense of ownership of the change.
- Acknowledge the client's feelings and perspective.
- Focus on strengths, not weaknesses.
- Handle lack of progress or relapses with positive and constructive feedback.
- Remain neutral; avoid telling clients what they should do. Help them see what they are doing.
- Avoid criticism and judgment.
- Avoid controlling and pressuring language.

Source: Adapted from Deci and Ryan (2012).

(e.g., modeling, observational learning, and verbal persuasion) can be used during the educational sessions.

Clients should be taught to practice self-reward or self-support. Self-reward of one's own efforts and achievements is important because support and reinforcement for self-care are not always available from others. Rewards can be tailored to personal preferences. Use of foods or unhealthy behaviors as rewards should be discouraged. Instead, such things as an outing with family or friends or a small purchase of a favorite item can be rewarding. Clients should learn to use self-praise and self-compliments. Learning to use internal self-reward in an appropriate manner enables the client to be less dependent on others or tangible objects to facilitate the learning process.

Create a Supportive Environment for Learning

The environment for self-care education is important for successful educational efforts. Tables, chairs, and sofas should be placed in a conversational setting. Pictures and textured materials should be used to create a supportive and nonthreatening climate. Visual aids such as flip charts or bulletin boards should be at a comfortable height to see while seated in a chair. If very young children are present during the sessions, an area with toys and books should be provided for their use. This will minimize distraction of the parents. If children are old enough to be included in the sessions, they should be actively involved. Often use of bright colors and interesting figures or designs on flip charts will amuse children and maintain their interest. Children can play an important role in reinforcing learning or in reminding parents and other family members to engage in the recommended behaviors.

To the extent possible, materials available in the home should be used in teaching. If a client will be preparing low-salt foods, food labels on cans or packages should be reviewed. If the client is learning relaxation techniques, videos for practice should be available for the client following the sessions. Well-illustrated materials should be available in hard copy or Web/mobile applications (apps) for the client to use at home to provide reinforcement of knowledge and skills practiced during sessions. Pictures are especially important for clients with low health literacy.

The minimum time span needed for most health instruction is 15 to 30 minutes. Either individual or small-group teaching methods may be used. Groups should be kept small (four to six individuals) to facilitate interaction and attention to the specific needs of group members. A combination of group and individual instruction often is helpful. A combined approach meets the needs of clients of diverse backgrounds.

Track and Evaluate Progress Toward Goals

Evaluation is a collaborative process by which the nurse and client judge the extent to which short- and long-term objectives and goals have been met. Evaluation involves direct or indirect assessment of behavior change. Although the target behaviors may be observed during limited nurse–client encounters, it must be kept in mind that this may not reflect actual behaviors. Self-report behavior change also is limited, as clients may not be completely honest, or they may ascribe a "halo effect" to themselves, seeing their performance as more frequent or more intensive than it actually is.

Tracking or monitoring one's progress in meeting self-care goals is a successful behavior change strategy and evaluation tool (Harkin et al., 2016). Self-monitoring enables clients to become aware of their behaviors. Information about the behavior may be recorded either digitally (smartphone apps) or in paper journals. In addition, the information can be used to assess progress toward meeting goals.

The success of self-monitoring is determined by its accuracy. In addition, the regularity of monitoring and the timing of monitoring to the actual behavior performed are important. Individuals who self-track frequently (5 days versus 2 days), comprehensively, and consistently are more likely to be successful in changing behaviors (Peterson et al., 2014). Health literacy also plays a role in tracking progress toward goals. Clients must have the language skills to understand the behavior to be monitored and to record the information. Persons with low health literacy skills often record information inaccurately or have difficulty understanding how to record the target behavior (Porter et al., 2016).

Multiple methods can be used to evaluate progress toward goals. These might include client checklists, client digital or paper journal records, laboratory results, verbal reports, and direct observation. The primary purpose of evaluation is to provide an accurate picture of the progress that has been made in attaining health promotion goals, so multiple methods may be necessary.

BARRIERS TO SELF-CARE EMPOWERMENT

Clients who are empowered to perform health-promoting self-care activities are equipped with the information, knowledge, and skills to do so. They are partners with health care professionals, participating in shared decision-making and communicating their preferences and needs. Clients who have control over their health are able to use their acquired skills to promote healthy families and communities. However, many barriers hinder an individual's ability to participate in self-care behaviors. Multiple factors, including health literacy, culture, knowledge and skills, social support, confidence, prior experiences, access to resources, and cognitive abilities, may serve as barriers (Jaarsma et al., 2017; Kambhampati, Ashvetiya, Stone, Blumenthal, & Martin, 2016).

Health care professionals also serve as barriers to self-care empowerment when they continue to practice within a traditional approach, believing that they know what is best. Clients are empowered when health care professionals acknowledge their role and partner with them and their families to offer the information and tools desired to participate in healthy behaviors.

Each client's *desire for change* must be assessed as a potential barrier. Some individuals do not want to be responsible for their own self-care but instead wish to function in a highly dependent role. Their desire for self-care competence may have been frustrated by *prior health care experiences*, which may have made them feel dependent and helpless. It is critical to assess the extent to which clients desire to assume responsibility for their own health when they are given the opportunity to gain the knowledge and skills to do so.

Culture, gender, and *age* may also serve as barriers. In some cultures, it is inappropriate to question authority. Also, in some cultures women are unable to participate in a collaborative health care relationship. Older generations may view questioning authority figures as disrespectful. The nurse will need to identify cultural norms and plan self-care education within the client's frame of reference. Although these norms may limit the empowerment process, the process can be introduced through shared decision-making and a supportive, nonthreatening environment.

Clients' *conceptualization of health* also will play a role in the type of content to share in self-care health promotion education. When health is defined as maintaining stability or avoiding overt illness, prevention behaviors such as immunization, self-examination for signs of cancer, and periodic multiphasic screening may be the priority. When health is defined as self-actualization or well-being, emphasis is placed on health-promoting behaviors, such as physical activity, relaxation techniques, and healthy eating.

Barriers to learning present major challenges for self-care empowerment. For this reason, if the client is not making progress, personal and environmental factors should be explored. In addition, family barriers should be assessed and reduced or eliminated to the extent possible.

Strategies to manage obstacles to healthy behavior should be an integral part of the health education plan. In this way, problems are addressed systematically, and progress in decreasing barriers can be periodically assessed. The client may be unaware of what is inhibiting progress or reluctant to share information. A climate of trust facilitates effective communication and enables the client to discuss perceived and real obstacles to learning and performance.

Health Literacy as a Barrier to Self-Care

Health literacy is defined as an individual's ability to obtain, understand, and use information to make appropriate decisions for self-care. Health literacy is an empowerment strategy as it enables individuals and families to learn the knowledge and skills to take responsibility for their health. Health literacy skills enable clients and families to participate fully in health promotion activities and practice self-care behaviors to promote wellness (Schulz & Nakamoto, 2013).

Limited health literacy is a barrier to empowerment and self-care. Inadequate levels of health literacy are associated with less knowledge and skills, unhealthy behaviors, and less access to and use of screening and preventive health services (Castro-Sanchez, Chang, Vila-Candel, Escobedo, & Holmes, 2016).

Reading and comprehension levels should be assessed prior to beginning health education sessions to promote self-care. Health literacy screening questions can be asked using available measures in the literature (see Chapter 12). Health information should be written in a language and at a level the client and family members can understand. Strategies to promote understanding of information include the following:

- Simple, oral communication using lay terms
- Plain, culturally appropriate language materials
- Pictorial illustrations and models
- Audiovisual aids
- Group educational sessions
- Tailored individual sessions

Health policy makers and health professionals must be sensitive to the extent to which problems of literacy and poverty present barriers to becoming empowered for self-care. Health education programs that are literacy appropriate must be economically feasible for individuals and families living in poverty. This requires coordination of public, private, and volunteer services to provide literacy-appropriate self-care education and realistic options for people of all age groups who are trying to engage in healthy behaviors.

SELF-CARE TO PROMOTE HEALTH THROUGHOUT THE LIFE SPAN

Self-Care for Children and Adolescents

Children represent the potential for a healthy society. However, they face multiple challenges, as the assumption that school-aged children are healthy is no longer valid. The prevalence of obesity in industrialized societies continues to increase, and childhood obesity is a global epidemic with far-reaching public health consequences (Kumar & Kelly, 2017). Childhood is a critical period for the adoption of healthy behaviors and lifestyles. Behaviors are developed and learned based on developmental level, social and physical environments, and family and personal experiences. Thus, health promotion efforts need to begin before unhealthy behavior patterns are established, as these early-learned behaviors will likely continue into adulthood.

During childhood, social and cognitive skills for autonomous decision-making and health behaviors are developed. Health behaviors can be linked to family structure and support, family functioning and stress, level of parental authority, and socioeconomic variables (Sangawi, Adams, & Reissland, 2015). A supportive family shapes the child's behavior through the use of rewards for healthy behavior choices. Family role modeling of self-care behaviors facilitates the development of healthy behaviors such as physical activity. Socioeconomic status also plays a significant role in health behaviors, as increased socioeconomic status enables the family to provide resources, such as a home in a safe neighborhood, a more affluent school system, healthy food choices, and access to community programs.

Parents exert influence over their child's health-promoting behaviors by serving as role models. For example, in families where one or two parents smoke, the risk of the child becoming a future smoker is increased. Programs that target parents as well as children can reduce high-risk behaviors such as tobacco use, sedentary habits, and unhealthy food choices. Parents can become positive role models by being actively involved in school-based programs with their children whenever possible to promote physical activity and healthy eating. Although it may be difficult to involve parents due to work and other commitments, flexible options for their inclusion should be available as the success of these programs warrants the effort.

The family also influences eating patterns. Dietary patterns, such as eating breakfast, are established in childhood and adolescence. Eating breakfast regularly has been shown to have multiple positive effects for children and adolescents, including being less likely to be overweight (Vic et al., 2016). However, breakfast is the most frequently skipped meal in young people. Parental breakfast eating and living in a two-parent family have been shown to be associated with adolescent breakfast consumption (McCullough, Robson, & Stark, 2016). Adolescents in nontraditional families (single parent, step-parent, and no parent) are more likely to display unhealthy eating behaviors such as skipping breakfast and lunch, eating fewer vegetables, and eating more fast-foods than adolescents in traditional (two-parent) households. Strategies to decrease these unhealthy behaviors, which will include schools and the community, need to be implemented. Parents can also role model positive behaviors when eating out, such as ordering healthy choices at fast-food restaurants.

Strategies to reduce time in sedentary activities should be implemented in the home as well as in the school setting. For example, computer and television use or screen time can be limited daily. Instead, family outdoor activities should be planned and fostered. Physical activities can be planned for recess times, and physical activity time can be extended in schools. At both family and community levels, physical activity programs should involve participation by peers as well as family members. Walking instead of riding should be rewarded and parents should be encouraged to take regular walks with their children. Communities can map safe walking areas if school tracks are not available in the neighborhood. The walking school bus program for elementary children to promote walking to school is an example of a strategy to promote physical activity in children (Smith et al., 2015). Other walking interventions have been successful in promoting physical activity in children, especially those conducted in schools (Carlin, Murphy, & Gallagher, 2016).

Children and youth who have dropped out of school or are homeless need special attention to develop self-care behaviors for health promotion. Homeless youth do not have family ties and depend on peers for support. Education sessions may have to take place in parks, food kitchens, or homeless shelters. Children of one-parent families and youth of two working parents also may require special attention, as unsupervised time has been associated with high-risk behaviors such as alcohol, tobacco, and marijuana use (Atherton, Schofield, Sitka, Conger, & Robins, 2016). Special sensitivity to the lack of resources for daily living, lack of parental influence and supervision, and low levels of motivation because of life conditions is critical to promote healthy lifestyles (Keys et al., 2015).

Adolescence is a critical period of physical, cognitive, emotional, and social development in a dynamic and uncertain period between childhood and adulthood. Developmentally, it is a time characterized by change and transitions. Cognitively, adolescents begin to think more abstractly. However, they lack the ability to apply their cognitive skills to solving problems in stressful situations. The mismatch between biological and social maturity has implications for behavioral choices under stress such as being pressured by peers to drink alcohol or experiment with illegal drugs. Socially, the family remains an important source of support. Parents can provide emotional support and encouragement and promote healthy peer interactions, as peers also serve as a source of support and important role models.

The positive youth development approach has been shown to promote positive adolescent development (Bowers, Geldhof, Johnson, Lerner, & Lerner, 2014). Positive youth development is an umbrella term or framework to describe programs that focus on helping adolescents develop and enhance their strengths and capabilities through active engagement with their peers, families, schools, and communities. The approach prevents adolescents from engaging in risky behaviors. Common components include the following:

- Increasing specific youth competencies
- Focusing on youth assets instead of weaknesses
- Encouraging youth to avoid risky behaviors
- Developing opportunities to promote strengths
- Fostering caring relationships with adults

Youth development programs encompass the "five Cs" developed by Zarrett and Lerner (2008) and include *competence, confidence, connection, character,* and *caring/compassion.*

Competence refers to a positive view of one's actions, including social, academic, cognitive, health, and vocational capability. *Confidence* is an internal sense of positive self-worth and self-efficacy and *character* refers to respect for societal norms, a sense of right and wrong, and respect for standards of correct behavior. *Connection* focuses on positive bonds with people, including family, peers, schools, and the community. Last, *caring/compassion* is a sense of empathy and sympathy for others (Lerner, Lerner, Bowers, & Geldhof, 2015).

When empowering for self-care, adolescents need to actively participate in all aspects of the educational empowerment process. Engagement in the process promotes adoption of healthy behaviors. Hart's "ladder of participation" is helpful to understand the levels of the adolescent's participation or engagement, so that changes can be made if they are not being involved as partners in the process (Hart, 1992). Hart's model has been adapted for adolescents by the United Nations International Children's Emergency Fund (UNICEF) to promote youth engagement (French, Bhattacharya, & Olenik, 2014). The ladder is shown in Figure 11–3. The stages of participation begin with the bottom rung of the ladder representing manipulation of adolescents to the top rung representing adults and adolescents sharing decision-making. Increased participation motivates adolescents to commit to positive self-care behaviors, as they are provided opportunities to become stakeholders in their personal health. They become empowered as family members and other adults begin to recognize their ability to make positive decisions that affect their health.

EMERGING ADULTHOOD.   The period of 18 to 25 years, emerging adulthood, is considered a period of time between adolescence and adulthood. Contextual factors that shape the health of young adults in the transition to adult roles and responsibilities include the weakening of the family support safety net. Young adults pursue multiple pathways,

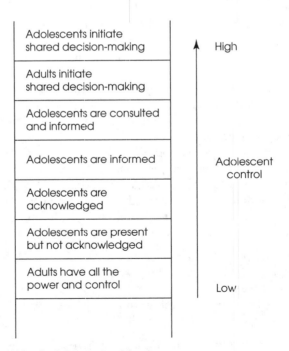

FIGURE 11–3   The Ladder of Adolescent Participation

Sources: Adapted from French et al. (2014) and Arnstein (1969).

such as college, military service, employment, parenthood, and marriage. Each path has its unique set of role expectations and potential barriers to health. Many health problems peak during this period, including homicide, motor vehicle injuries, substance abuse, and sexually transmitted infections. University students frequently engage in unhealthy behaviors, including poor diet, little physical activity, alcohol consumption, and smoking. Although parental involvement diminishes during the transition to adulthood, evidence indicates that parental, community, and institutional support is needed to address the health behaviors of this group. Connectedness to family is protective against developing health-compromising behaviors. Being connected to family and friends promotes positive well-being, which has been associated with fewer risk behaviors and better perceived health during young adulthood (Jimenez-Iglesias, Moreno, Ramos, & Rivera, 2015). The importance of parental factors reinforces the need for a parental component in adolescent health promotion programs. Although these programs may vary in the amount of parental involvement, evidence continues to show that strengthening parent–adolescent relationships promotes healthy adolescent self-care behaviors.

During emerging adulthood, youth may choose to focus on health or engage in risky behaviors such as alcohol consumption and illicit drugs (Schwartz, 2016). Although diet and physical patterns may have been established in childhood, influences from close friends, newly formed social networks, and exposure to new lifestyles may exert pressure to change established behaviors. Physical activity and overall diet quality decrease in college students living away from home. Health promotion efforts need to be focused on strategies to change campus food environments and promote physical activity for college students. Students who do not attend college are more susceptible to engaging in high-risk behaviors. Mechanisms to reach noncollege students to reduce risks include community programs to promote health. Since peers have a greater influence than parents during this period, programs involving peers, including online support groups and apps, can also be used to promote health. The life course of young adults can be redirected during this period as their personal identity is developing, so strategies to promote positive behaviors are paramount.

Self-Care for Young and Middle-Aged Adults

Young and middle-aged adulthood is the time in the life cycle when many young people are intensely involved in careers and child rearing. The momentum of everyday life and demands of dependent others may leave little time to focus on health in the absence of an illness crisis. Strengthening support within the family for self-care is particularly important at this time. Young adults need to learn to accept responsibility for modeling and teaching children competent self-care by increasing their family self-care knowledge and skills and learning how and when to access health care resources for the family. Adult learners bring many assets to self-care education, including life experiences, self-direction, problem- or interest-centered (as opposed to subject-centered) learning needs, and interest in immediate rather than delayed application. Self-care education for adults should include approaches shown in Table 11–4.

Adults who are aware of their own needs for self-care may be more effective in reducing stress inherent in multiple roles. Systematically incorporating health promotion activities into daily routines at work or with family members can both enhance health in a busy lifestyle and model healthy lifestyles to family members. For example, physical activities in place of watching television can be planned prior to dinner or, if feasible, children can walk to school rather than be driven. Adequate attention to

TABLE 11–4   Teaching Approaches to Promote Adult Self-Care

1. Provide time to express feelings.
2. Express a supportive attitude.
3. Reinforce client's self-esteem.
4. Provide or teach how to access health information.
5. Teach self-care skills that can be applied immediately.
6. Present alternative views on health issues.
7. Provide timely feedback and reinforcement.
8. Offer flexible learning pathways.

self-care during the young and middle-age years lays the groundwork for a healthy and productive retirement and old age.

Activities of everyday life shape and influence the health of family members. Family practices either promote or hinder the development of good health habits and well-being in children. Life transitions and traditional caregiving roles by women may result in lack of attention to their own self-care needs. Nurses should offer health promotion strategies that take into consideration family roles and demands, employment status, educational levels, cultural traditions, and available resources.

Self-Care for Older Adults

Active or healthy aging is described as the process of developing and maintaining optimal functioning to enable well-being in older age (World Health Organization, 2015). Domains of optimal functioning include

- Being mobile
- Building and maintaining relationships
- Meeting one's basic needs
- Continuing to learn, grow, and make decisions
- Continuing to contribute

The above domains are integrated into the four components of healthy aging, which are shown in Figure 11–4 (Healthy Aging Subgroup, 2002; Rowe & Kahn, 1997). The four components are: promoting health and preventing disease and injury, optimizing mental cognitive and physical functioning, engaging with life, and managing any chronic conditions.

Promoting health and preventing disease and injury in elderly persons are strategies to compress morbidity in later years. The term "compression of morbidity" is based on the hypothesis that healthy living and healthy living conditions result in a reduction in time spent in disability at the end of life (Fries, 2012; Geyer, 2016). Research has substantiated this relationship. In the Chicago Heart Association Detection Project in Industry, individuals with fewer cardiovascular risk factors in early middle age lived longer, healthier lives than those with less favorable cardiovascular risk factors (Allen et al., 2017). In the Cardiovascular Health Study, community-dwelling elderly who had normal body mass indexes (BMIs), better quality diets, and walked greater distances had fewer or no years of disability before death than those who were either obese or underweight,

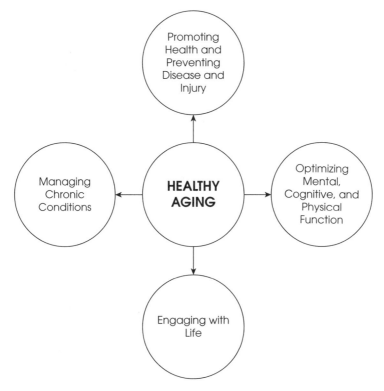

FIGURE 11–4 Components of Healthy Aging

Source: Adapted from Healthy Aging Subgroup (2002).

had unhealthy diets, and spent less time walking (Jacob et al., 2016). These findings document the value of diet and physical activity in older age to prevent or reduce disability in later life. They also reinforce the importance of establishing programs to promote healthy diets and a physically active lifestyle and maintaining a healthy weight early in life.

Physical activity is considered the most important determinant of healthy aging. Physical activity can enhance the self-esteem of older adults and, in some cases, decrease depression and anxiety. Sedentary activities, such as television viewing or computer time, should be limited. Frequency of activity has been shown to be protective, so strategies that promote regular walking and other active leisure-time physical activities should be facilitated. Neighborhood environments that support walking need to be facilitated, including short walking paths with benches, safe pedestrian areas, and parks.

Physical inactivity may be due to lack of opportunities to participate in activities as well as lack of encouragement. Homebound community-dwelling elderly should be encouraged to go outdoors on a regular basis to maintain functional capacity. Loneliness and depression are common psychological barriers to participating in activities in the elderly. Health barriers may include vision and hearing difficulties. Regular participation in activities, such as walking, cycling, and strength and balance training, has the potential to reduce the burden of chronic diseases and disability and improve quality of life in this group. Community-based interventions in senior centers are ideal places to promote physical activity and healthy eating behaviors. Physical activity programs that include chair exercises or chair yoga and promotion of walking improve physical function.

Self-care for older adults focuses on *maximizing independence, engagement, and life satisfaction*. The ability for self-care is high for many older adults, and most function well. Personal autonomy, or the ability to make self-directed choices, is important in older adults. The older person should be a partner in the self-care educational process rather than a passive recipient. Information should promote informed decision-making and independence. Self-care education must also take into account any physical, sensory, mobility, and psychosocial changes. Coping styles do not change significantly with age. Thus, persons who develop positive coping skills early in life are able to meet social demands in later years, find meaning in life, and direct energy to appropriate self-care activities. Older individuals who have been characterized as information seekers have more effective health-promoting behaviors. Other patterns linked with health-promoting self-care behaviors include positive perceptions of one's health and aging, education, social integration, involvement in groups and organizations, and being connected with family.

Promotion of self-care activities to maintain and improve functional ability includes strategies for safe mobility and prevention of falls, and activities that promote social engagement. All evidence to date indicates that the elderly can become physically fit. However, it is much easier to remain physically active if physical activity behaviors are developed earlier in life.

Self-care activities in the elderly also include eating a healthy diet and maintaining a normal weight. The health benefits of the Mediterranean diet are well established and should be part of a program to promote healthy nutrition (Michel, Dreux, & Vacheron, 2016). The health protective effects of the diet against chronic diseases have also been established, including cardiovascular disease, diabetes, hypertension, and inflammatory markers. The diet has been the traditional diet in the Mediterranean basin where olive oil is a staple. The diet is represented by a pyramid, in which plant-based foods (fruits, vegetables, and whole grains) are at the base to indicate a greater consumption of these foods (Bach-Faig et al., 2011). The basic elements of the Mediterranean diet that promote health and reduce disease risk are shown in Table 11–5. These recommendations should be included in self-care education for adults and older adults.

Adopting a Mediterranean diet should not be difficult as it can be adapted to different cultural patterns. The major challenge is overcoming long-term consumption of a

---

TABLE 11–5   Healthy Eating Recommendations for Older Adults

- Consume vegetables, fruits, and whole-grain cereals in two to three meals daily
- Use dairy products in the form of low-fat yogurt and cheeses or other fermented dairy products
- Include extra-virgin olive oil as the major source of dietary lipids
- Eat olives, nuts, and seeds for snacks
- Eat fish, white meat, and eggs twice a week
- Limit amounts of red and processed meats to less than twice a week
- Drink red wine in moderation (one glass for women, two glasses for men)
- Drink at least six glasses (8 ounces each) of water every day

Source: Bach-Faig et al. (2011).

Western diet that includes large amounts of red meats, processed foods, refined flour, sugary beverages, and sweets. The beneficial effects should be stressed as well as strategies for gradually adapting to the dietary changes. The pyramid can serve as a guide for teaching clients.

SELF-CARE IN OLDER WOMEN. Self-care to promote health in older women needs special attention because of different experiences of aging. Women live longer than men, although the mortality rates for both non-Hispanic and white midlife women increased between 1999 and 2013 (Case & Deaton, 2015). Women are more likely to live their later years alone with substantially lower incomes, more vulnerability to poverty, and more chronic health conditions than are men in the same age group. Women are also more likely to have no or inadequate insurance coverage, resulting in barriers to health care.

Unsafe environments and living alone negatively influence the performance of healthy self-care behaviors. Personal, social, and environmental barriers that prevent elderly women from being able to participate in healthy behaviors need to be addressed, including fear of leaving their home, lack of transportation, and inadequate financial resources. Socioeconomic conditions influence participation in health behaviors. Low-cost interventions such as walking groups can be implemented in communities. Interventions that take into account the social context in which women live their lives, as well as their perceptions of their health and well-being, must be incorporated into all health promotion activities.

SELF-CARE DURING RETIREMENT. Retirement is a significant life event that presents major financial, social, and emotional challenges for the older population. The challenges are likely to increase, as the length of time an individual will live following retirement continues to grow. Employment is a fundamental role central to an individual's identity, so retirees may feel that they have lost an important role if it is not replaced with new activities. Appropriate self-care in the form of anticipatory planning in the preretirement phase is associated with successful adaptation. Self-care actions that have been shown to facilitate healthy retirement are shown in Table 11–6.

TABLE 11–6   Self-Care Actions to Facilitate a Healthy Retirement

1. Plan ahead to ensure adequate income.
2. Re-examine your social network. Develop friends not associated with work.
3. Decrease time at work in the last years before retirement if possible by taking longer vacations, working shorter days, or working part-time.
4. Develop routines to replace the workday structure. Focus on developing regular physical activities and avoiding sedentary activities for long periods.
5. Rely on other people and groups in addition to spouse or partner to fill leisure time.
6. Develop leisure-time activities before retirement that are realistic in energy and financial cost.
7. Engage in volunteer work in the community.
8. Assess living arrangements, and if relocation is necessary, take time to develop new social networks.

Although retirement is considered a positive life transition, a growing number of retired adults need to continue to work part-time or are delaying retirement for several reasons. Many older adults have had professional careers and desire to continue to contribute. The baby boomer generation is considered less financially secure, and many people have little or no retirement plans. The number of women over age 65 in the workforce is increasing faster than that of men (Lusardi & Mitchell, 2017). For this group, self-care strategies to promote healthy lifestyles need to consider financial resources as well as limited leisure time.

Retirement has been shown to have both positive and negative effects on health (Eibich, 2015). Potential reasons for better health include decreased stress, increased sleep, and more opportunities for physical activities. Retired adults have more time available to pursue healthy behaviors than younger adults. Research has documented that total sedentary time decreases in retirement; however, leisure-time sedentary activities, such as television and reading, increase (Sprod, Ferrar, Olds, & Maher, 2015). Physical activity interventions that target persons who are getting ready to retire may help reverse this trend. Retired adults should be challenged to plan active leisure-time activities and counseled about resources available within the community to facilitate healthy behaviors. Strategies to stay engaged with friends and community should also be presented.

THE ROLE OF *HEALTHY PEOPLE 2020* IN PROMOTING SELF-CARE

Healthy People 2020's 10-year agenda was introduced in 2010 to continue the national objective to improve the health of all Americans (see the HealthyPeople.gov website). Self-care is implicit in one of the four overarching goals, which is to promote quality of life, healthy development, and healthy behaviors across all life stages. In addition, new information was added for early and middle childhood, adolescent health, and older adults. For both early and middle childhood and adolescents, the critical role of being connected to a parent or positive adult caregiver is explicit in the objectives. In addition, health education in schools is articulated as an objective as well as supportive and safe environments. The goal for older adults is to increase health, function, and quality of life, reinforcing the need to implement self-care strategies in this group. Increasing physical activity is also an objective for this group. The midcourse results for all of these objectives have been reported on the Healthy People website. Although several of the progress indicators have improved, health indicators for obesity among children, adolescents, and adults, and average daily intake of total vegetables are unchanged (Office of Disease Prevention and Health Promotion, 2014).

The *Healthy People 2030* framework, which includes its vision, mission, overarching goals, plan of action, and foundational principles, has been completed and forwarded to the Secretary of Health and Human Services in 2017 (these are available on the healthypeople.gov website). *Healthy People 2030* is the fifth edition of Healthy People. The plan contains achievable national health promotion and disease prevention goals that are adopted across the nation. Over the past 50 years, efforts toward achieving the goals have resulted in reducing the major causes of death by reducing risk factors and increasing childhood vaccines.

THE ROLE OF THE INTERNET IN EMPOWERING FOR SELF-CARE

Health care costs and the shortage of qualified health professionals to deliver effective health promotion programs reinforce the importance of empowering individuals and families to take responsibility for their health. Internet and mobile technology offer viable, effective, lower-cost options to deliver health information and self-care interventions to large segments of the population. Internet technology is now an essential part of everyday life. Millions of people are seeking health information and finding self-help groups who want to learn from each other. Internet virtual communities fulfill the need for affiliation, information, and support. The potential of the Internet as a platform for self-empowerment through development of feelings of competence and control is beginning to be realized. Information that traditionally was not available is now accessible on almost any topic. The information can be accessed at any time in almost any geographical location. This has important implications for persons living in rural or inaccessible areas, who are homebound, and who work. However, the quality of health information available is highly variable, indicating that clients need to be taught how to evaluate the information.

The Internet is still inaccessible to many who do not have adequate financial resources or lack computer or health literacy skills. The "digital divide" refers to the gap in computer and Internet access between groups based on income, age, and education. Emerging issues that will have to be addressed by this technology include the possibility of diminished involvement in face-to-face interactions with family members and friends, as well as weakening attachments to one's local environment, but greater access to remote people and places. Privacy and confidentiality of information continue to be challenges as well.

Advantages of online self-help groups have been identified. These groups are convenient to access, and there is increased access of diverse members, including people in rural or remote areas. They provide access to peers with similar interests and issues, and the fear or embarrassment of public speaking is removed. In addition, lasting relationships may be formed. Disadvantages include misunderstanding that may result from text-based relationships; few controls to prevent erroneous information; absence of rules and guidelines; and ethical issues related to identity, deception, privacy, and confidentiality.

Information and education available through digital technology is changing the way the public obtains health information and relates to health professionals. Online health communities, such as WebMD, are transforming the client–health provider relationship to engage clients as partners in their health (Petric, Atanasova, & Kamin, 2017). Digital technologies promote client empowerment and engagement through information sharing and self-monitoring. Youth perceive the Internet as a primary source of information and support, not an adjunct to traditional informational modes. Older persons engage with mobile technologies in a more limited capacity. Evidence also indicates that mHealth interventions can reduce health disparities (Peek, 2017).

Nurses should work to ensure that the information revolution is used to empower individuals and communities and is accessible to those who do not currently benefit because of poverty or their social, environmental, and cultural conditions. In addition, health care professionals must monitor the content and quality of the sites they recommend. Last, formal evaluation of participants' health outcomes and satisfaction with information must be conducted. Formal evaluations will provide evidence of the effectiveness of this application to health promotion.

CONSIDERATIONS FOR PRACTICE IN SELF-CARE

The nurse's role as collaborator, facilitator, resource, and teacher has become more important than ever as clients express the desire to assume more responsibility for their health. Empowering clients for self-care should be considered a priority for all health care professionals. Empowering clients for self-care moves from the traditional paternalistic controlling view of health promotion to a client- and family-centered approach. The new approach takes longer, as clients and their families are partners in all steps of the educational process. However, engaged clients are more likely to change high-risk behaviors and adopt health-promoting ones if they have choices and are provided with the knowledge and skills needed to promote their health and well-being. A life span approach is necessary, as children, as well as older adults, need to participate in decisions that influence their health. Digital technologies offer many possibilities to engage all ages in promoting healthy behaviors.

OPPORTUNITIES FOR RESEARCH IN SELF-CARE

Although self-care has been practiced for centuries, it did not become the focus of research for health professionals until the 1980s. The theoretical work by Orem (2001) was the initial driving force in nursing for empirical work on the various dimensions of self-care and related nursing care systems. Opportunities for research in self-care include the following:

1. Rigorously evaluate mHealth interventions that use smartphones to promote health behaviors (weight loss, physical activity).
2. Develop and test strategies to promote engagement of adults over age 70 with digital technologies to communicate with health care professionals and promote their health.
3. Develop and test mHealth health literacy intervention to increase self-care behaviors in individuals with limited literacy skills.
4. Test culturally appropriate interventions using digital technologies to enhance self-care empowerment among diverse individuals and families, such as first-generation immigrants.
5. Conduct intervention studies to increase self-care health behaviors, such as physical activity, in community-dwelling older persons.

In addition, a synthesis of the literature is needed to evaluate current standards used to judge the usefulness and accuracy of mHealth interventions.

Summary

Health education to empower individuals and families for self-care is complex. However, use of digital technologies, including social media, and active engagement of individuals and their family members in the process can help ensure the adoption of healthy behaviors. Empowerment for self-care emphasizes the competencies of clients for self-direction and self-responsibility in promoting and managing their health. Environmental constraints that impair self-care must be addressed and resolved to optimize client success. Education to empower and support autonomy enables clients to achieve their health goals. As a major resource, the nurse can enhance the client's success in becoming empowered by teaching them the needed knowledge and skills.

Learning Activities

1. Plan a preschool-based program for children to decrease television or other screen time and replace it with physical activities.
2. Develop a program to increase physical activity in community-dwelling, older adults, identifying and addressing potential barriers in this group.
3. Design a program to promote healthy eating for adolescents using the steps in the empowerment education process to implement the program. Describe how you plan to evaluate the program's effectiveness.
4. Choose a commonly used app that promotes physical activity for middle-age women and develop strategies to increase self-monitoring. Interview three women to learn the strengths and limitations of the app for promoting physical activity and self-monitoring.

References

Allen, N. B., Zhao, L., Liu, L., Daviglus, M., Liu, K., Fries, J., . . . Lloyd-Jones, D. (2017). Favorable cardiovascular health, compression of morbidity, and healthcare costs. *Circulation, 135*, 1693–1701. doi:10.1161/CIRCULATIONAHA.116.026252

Arnstein, S. R. (1969). A ladder of participation. *Journal of the American Institute of Planners, 35*(4), 216–224.

Atherton, O. E., Schofield, T. J., Sitka, A., Conger, R. D., & Robins, R. W. (2016). Unsupervised self-care predicts conduct problems: The moderating roles of hostile aggression and gender. *Journal of Adolescence, 48*, 1–40. doi:10.1016/j.adolescence.2016.01.001

Bach-Faig, A., Berry, E. M., Lairon, D., Reguant, J., Trichopoulou, A., Dernini, S., . . . Serra-Majem, L. (2011). Mediterranean diet pyramid today. Science and cultural updates. *Public Health Nutrition, 14*(12A), 2274–2284. doi:10.1017/S1368980011002515

Bowers, E., Geldhof, J., Johnson, S., Lerner, J., & Lerner, R. (2014). Special issue introduction: Thriving across the adolescent years: A view of the issues. *Journal of Youth and Adolescence, 43*(6), 859–868. doi:10.1007/s10964-014-0117-8

Bridges, J. F., Loukanova, S., & Carrera, P. M. (2017). Patient empowerment in health care. In S. R. Quah (Ed.), *International Encyclopedia of Public Health* (2nd ed., Vol. 5, pp. 416–425). New York, NY: Elsevier.

Carlin, A., Murphy, M., & Gallagher, A. (2016). Do interventions to increase walking work? A systematic review of interventions in children and adolescents. *Sports Medicine, 46*, 515–530. doi:10.1007/s40279-015-0432-6

Case, A., & Deaton, A. (2015). Rising morbidity and mortality in midlife among white non-Hispanic Americans in the 21st century. *Proceedings of the National Academy of Sciences of the United States of America, 112*(49), 15078–15083. doi:10.1073/pnas.1518393112

Castro-Sanchez, E., Chang, P., Vila-Candel, R., Escobedo, A., & Holmes, A. (2016). Health literacy and infectious diseases: Why does it matter? *International Journal of Infectious Diseases, 43*, 103–110.

Deci, E. L., & Ryan, R. M. (2012). Motivation, personality, and development within embedded social contexts: An overview of self-determination theory. In R. M. Ryan (Ed.), *The Oxford handbook of human motivation* (pp. 85–110). New York, NY: Oxford University Press.

Eibich, P. (2015). Understanding the effect of retirement on health: Mechanisms and heterogeneity. *Journal of Health Economics, 43*, 1–12. doi:10.1016/j.healeco.2015.05.001

French, M., Bhattacharya, S., & Olenik, C. (2014). *Youth engagement in development: Effective approaches and action-oriented recommendations for the field.* U.S. Agency for International Development (USAID). Retrieved from http://pdf.usaid.gov/pdf_docs/PA00JP6S.pdf

Fries, J. F. (2012). The theory and practice of active aging. *Current Gerontology and Geriatrics Research, 2012.* doi:10.1155/2012/420637

Geyer, S. (2016). Morbidity compression: A promising and well-established concept? *International Journal of Public Health, 61*(7), 727–728. doi:10.1007/s00038-016-0853-5

Greene, J., Hibbard, J. H., Sacks, R., Overton, V., & Parrotta, C. D. (2015). When patient activation levels change, health outcomes and costs change, too. *Health Affairs, 34*(3), 431–443. doi:10.1377/hlthaff.2014.0452

Harkin, B., Webb, T. L., Chang, B. P., Prestwich, A., Conner, M., Kellar, I., . . . Sheeran, P. (2016). Does monitoring goal progress promote goal attainment? A meta-analysis of the experimental evidence. *Psychological Bulletin, 142*(2), 198–229. doi:10.1037/bul0000025

Hart, R. (1992). *Children's participation: From tokenism to citizenship.* Innocent Essays No. 4, New York, NY: UNICEF. Retrieved from http://www.unicef-irc.org/publications/pdf/

Healthy Aging Subgroup. (2002). *Alberta's Healthy Aging and Seniors Wellness Strategic Framework 2002–2012.* Edmonton, Alberta: Health and Wellness. Retrieved from http://www.health.alberta.ca

Hibbard, J. B. (2017). Patient activation and the use of information to support informed health decisions. *Patient Education and Counseling, 100*(1), 5–7. doi:10.1016/j.pec.2016.07.006

Jaarsma, T., Riegel, B., & Stromberg, A. (2017). Reporting on self-care in research studies: Guidance to improve knowledge building. *Journal of Cardiovascular Nursing, 32*(4), 315–316. doi:10.1097/JCN.0000000000000405

Jacob, M. E., Yee, L. M., Diehr, P., Arnold, A., Thielke, S., Chaves, P., . . . Newman, A. (2016). Can a healthy lifestyle compress the disabled period in older adults? *Journal of the American Geriatric Society, 64*(10), 1952–1961. doi:10.1111/jgs.14314

Jimenez-Iglesias, A., Moreno, C., Ramos, P., & Rivera, E. (2015). What family dimensions are important for health-related quality of life in adolescence? *Journal of Youth Studies, 18*(1), 53–67. doi:10.1080/13676261.2014.933191

Kambhampati, S., Ashvetiya, T., Stone, N., Blumenthal, R., & Martin, S. (2016). Shared decision-making and patient empowerment in preventive cardiology. *Current Cardiology Reports, 18*, 49. doi:10.1007/s11886-016-0729-6

Kenney, M. (2017). *2nd Place: Patient activation among diverse populations: A systematic review.* Final research paper. Kevin and Tam Ross Undergraduate Research Prize. Retrieved from http://digitalcommons.chapman.edu/undergraduateresearchprize/18

Keys, K. M., Vo, T., Wall, M., Caetano, R., Suglia, S., Martins, S., . . . Hasin, D. (2015). Racial/ethnic differences in use of alcohol, tobacco, and marijuana: Is there a cross-over from adolescence to adulthood? *Social Science & Medicine, 124*, 132–141. doi:10.1016/j.socscimed.2014.11035

Kumar, S., & Kelly, A. S. (2017). Review of childhood obesity: From epidemiology, etiology, and comorbidities to clinical assessment and treatment. *Mayo Clinic Proceedings, 92*(2), 251–265. doi:10.1016/j.mayocp.2016.09.017

Lerner, R. M., Lerner, J. V., Bowers, E. P., & Geldhof, G. J. (2015). Positive youth development and relational-developmental-systems. In W. F. Overton & P. Molenaar (Eds.), *Handbook of child psychology and developmental science* (Vol. 1, pp. 607–651). Hoboken, NJ: Wiley.

Lusardi, A., & Mitchell, O. (2017). Older women's labor market attachment, retirement planning, and household debt. In C. Goldin & L. Katz (Eds.), *Women working longer: Increased employment of older ages.* Chicago, IL: University of Chicago Press.

McCullough, M. B., Robson, S. M., & Stark, L. J. (2016). A review of the structural characteristics of family meals with children in the United States. *Advances in Nutrition, 7*, 627–640. doi:10.3945/an.115.010439

Michel, J. P., Dreux, C., & Vacheron, A. (2016). Healthy ageing: Evidence that improvement is possible at every age. *European Geriatric Medicine, 7*(4), 298–305.

Office of Disease Prevention and Health Promotion. (2014). *Healthy People 2020 leading health indicators: Progress update.* Retrieved from https://www.healthypeople.gov/2020/leading-health-indicators/Healthy-People-2020-Leading-Health-Indicators%3A-Progress-Update

Orem, D. E. (1995). *Nursing: Concepts of practice* (5th ed.). St Louis, MO: Mosby.

Orem, D. E. (2001). *Nursing: Concepts of practice* (6th ed.). New York, NY: Mosby.

Orem, D. E., & Taylor, S. G. (2011). Reflecting on nursing practice science: The nature, the structure, and the foundation of nursing sciences. *Nursing Science Quarterly, 24*(1), 35–41. doi:10.1177/0894318410389061

Palumbo, R. (2017). Contextualizing patient empowerment. In R. Palumbo (Ed.), *The bright side and the dark side of patient empowerment: Co-creation and co-destruction of value in the healthcare environment* (pp. 1–21). Ham, Switzerland: Springer International Publishing.

Peek, M. (2017). Can mHealth interventions reduce health disparities among vulnerable populations? *Diversity and Equity in Health and Care, 14*(2), 44–45.

Peterson, N. D., Middleton, K. R., Nackers, L. M., Medina, K. E., Milsom, V. A., & Perri, M. G. (2014).

Dietary self-monitoring and long-term success with weight management. *Obesity*, *22*(9), 1961–1967. doi:10.1002/oby.20807

Petric, G., Atanasova, S., & Kamin, T. (2017). Impact of social processes in online health communities on patient empowerment in relationship with the physician: Emergence of functional and dysfunctional empowerment. *Journal of Medical Internet Research*, *19*(3), e74. doi:10.2196/jmir.7002

Porter, K., Chen, Y., Estabrooks, P., Noel, L., Bailey, A., & Zoellner, J. (2016). Using teach-back to understand participant behavioral self-monitoring skills across health literacy level and behavioral condition. *Journal of Nutrition Education and Behavior*, *48*(1), 20–26. doi:10.1016/j.jneb.2015.08.012

Rowe, J. W., & Kahn, R. L. (1997). Successful aging. *The Gerontologist*, *37*(4), 433–440. doi:10.1093/geront/37.4.433

Sangawi, H., Adams, J., & Reissland, N. (2015). The effects of parenting styles on behavioral problems in primary school children: A cross-cultural review. *Asian Social Sciences*, *11*(22), 171–186. doi:10.5539/ass.v11n22p171

Schulz, P. J., & Nakamoto, K. (2013). Health literacy and patient empowerment in health communication: The importance of separating conjoined twins. *Patient Education and Counseling*, *90*(1), 4–11.

Schwartz, S. (2016). Turning point for a turning point: Advancing emerging adulthood theory and research. *Emerging Adulthood*, *4*(5), 307–317. doi:10.1177/2167696815624640

Shellman, A. (2014). Empowerment and experiential education: A state of knowledge paper. *Journal of Experiential Education*, *37*(1), 18–30. doi:10.1177/1053825913518896

Smith, L., Norgate, S., Cherrett, T., Davies, N., Winstanley, C., & Harding, M. (2015). Walking school buses as a form of active transportation for children—A review of the evidence. *Journal of School Health*, *85*(3), 197–210. doi:10.1111/josh.12239

Sprod, J., Ferrar, K., Olds, T., & Maher, C. (2015). Changes in sedentary behaviors across the retirement transition: A systematic review. *Age and Ageing*, *44*(6), 918–925. doi:10.1093/ageing/afv140

Vic, F. N., Velde, S. J., Van Lippevelde, W., Manios, Y., Kovacs, E., Jan, N., . . . Bere, E. (2016). Regular family breakfast was associated with children's overweight and parental education: Results from the ENERGY cross-sectional study. *Preventive Medicine*, *91*, 197–203. doi:10.1016/jypmed.2016.08.013

Webber, D., Guo, Z., & Mann, S. (2013). Self-care in health: We can define it, but should we also measure it? *Self Care*, *4*(5), 101–105.

World Health Organization. (2009). *Self-care in the context of primary care*. Report of the Regional Consultation, Bangkok, Thailand, January 2009. Retrieved on July 8, 2017, from http://apps.who.int/iris/bitstream/10665/ 206352/1/B4301.pdf

World Health Organization. (2015). *World report on ageing and health*. Geneva, Switzerland: WHO Press. Retrieved from http://apps.who.int/iris/bitstream/10665/186463/1/978924069 4811_eng.pdf

Zarrett, N., & Lerner, R. (2008). Ways to promote the positive development of children and youth. *Child Trends*, *11*, 1–5.

CHAPTER 12

Health Promotion in Diverse Populations

OBJECTIVES

This chapter will enable the reader to:

1. Discuss the social determinants of health and their role in health disparities.
2. Differentiate the concepts of health disparities and health equity.
3. Discuss approaches to promote health equity in diverse populations.
4. Implement strategies to promote health literacy.
5. Describe the continuum of interpersonal skills necessary for cultural competence.
6. Apply strategies that facilitate culturally competent communication in diverse populations.
7. Describe approaches to ensure culturally competent health promotion programs.

The United States has become a nation of racial, ethnic, and cultural diversity. This transition to diversity has occurred as a result of the aging, largely Caucasian baby boomers', persons who were born in the several decades after the second world war, exit from the workforce and the massive immigration of diverse racial and ethnic groups over the past decades (Alba & Barbosa, 2016). Diverse racial groups, including Hispanic Americans, Native Americans, African Americans, and Asian Americans, are changing America from a predominately Caucasian majority of European ancestry into a multicultural, heterogeneous nation. Culturally diverse ethnic groups represent multiple languages, religions, values and ideologies, traditions, eating patterns, kinship and neighborhood boundaries, and social interests. Public attitudes toward these differences influence how diverse populations are treated and gain access to educational and economic opportunities and health care.

Culturally diverse ethnic individuals are more likely to be younger persons from disadvantaged groups who have traditionally migrated for job opportunities (Alba &

Barbos, 2016). Even though diverse racial and ethnic groups may be employed, many are at an economic disadvantage due to factors such as limited education and discrimination (Alba & Barbosa, 2016). Immigrant families are more likely to live in high poverty neighborhoods. At all levels of income, Latina families are more likely to live in high poverty neighborhoods than their white counterparts (Abraido-Lanza, Echeverria, & Florez, 2016). Only 12% of white children are likely to live in poverty, compared to 36% of black children and 31% of Hispanic children (Kids Count Data Center, 2015). Children living in poverty are exposed to multiple risks and are more likely to have poor health. Diverse racial and ethnic cultural groups are at greatest risk for poor physical, psychological, and social outcomes. These diverse groups also have fewer resources to improve their conditions.

Racial and ethnic culturally diverse groups fit the description of vulnerable populations. Vulnerable populations include persons who may experience discrimination, stigma, intolerance, and subordination. Vulnerable groups are often politically marginalized, disenfranchised, and frequently denied their human rights. Vulnerable groups also include people living in poverty, non-English-speaking persons, and recent immigrants and refugees; homeless persons, individuals who experience mental illness or disability, gay, lesbian, bisexual, transgender, and queer (LGBTQ), and people who abuse substances are also considered vulnerable populations.

SOCIAL DETERMINANTS OF HEALTH DISPARITIES AND HEALTH INEQUITIES

Social determinants of health are the structural and economic conditions in which people are born, live, work, and age (Commission on Social Determinants of Health, 2008). These social and economic conditions are shaped locally, nationally, and globally by economic distribution, social policies, and politics. In other words, money, power, and resources are responsible for the major disparities and inequities in health. *Health disparities* are avoidable differences in the incidence, prevalence, mortality, and burden of diseases and other adverse health conditions that exist in individuals because of their racial or ethnic group, religion, socioeconomic status, gender identity, geographic area, sexual orientation, mental health, and other characteristics that have been linked to discrimination or exclusion (Healthy People 2020, 2010a). Health disparities are linked with social and/or economic disadvantage.

Health inequities are avoidable differences in health between groups of persons that arise from social and economic conditions; these differences increase their risks for illness and limit access to health and preventive services. *Health inequities* are avoidable, unfair, and can be eliminated. *Health equity*—the absence of inequities in health across populations, genders, and geographic areas—underlies the commitment to eliminate health disparities (Braveman, 2014a). Health equity is social justice in health (Braveman, 2014b).

Structural determinants are the root causes of health inequities (Irwin, Solar, & Vega, 2017). Structural determinants of health generate and reinforce social stratification and class divisions in a society and define an individual's socioeconomic position. Socioeconomic position brings access to power, prestige, and resources and is based on a person's social class, income, education, and occupation. The major structural social determinants include the following:

- Social class
- Income
- Education

- Occupation
- Gender
- Race/ethnicity

Socioeconomic position shapes intermediary health determinants. Intermediary health determinants are individual-level influences that result from social class. Intermediary determinants influence differences in exposure to risks and vulnerability to health-compromising conditions. They are considered "downstream" determinants that affect an individual's health and well-being. Intermediary determinants include material and social circumstances, behavioral factors, biological factors, and the health care system. Examples of these determinants are provided in Table 12–1.

The World Health Organization (WHO) model shown in Figure 12–1 describes the social determinants of health. This model was first drafted at the WHO Commission on Social Determinants of Health meeting in 2005 and the final model was published in 2010 (Solar & Irwin, 2010). The conceptual framework illustrates how the socioeconomic and political context influences a person's socioeconomic position through the distribution of resources. Individuals are placed in social hierarchies based on the structural determinants listed above, which give them power and prestige. The socioeconomic and political context and the structural mechanisms (social class, gender, ethnicity, education, occupation,

TABLE 12–1   Intermediary Social Determinants of Healthy Inequities

Health Determinant	Examples
Material Circumstances	
Neighborhood and physical environment	Housing density, housing quality, traffic density, air pollutants, hazardous wastes, drinking water quality, urban or rural, zoning policies, and proximity to health care and quality food
Working conditions	Physical, chemical, ergonomic, and psychological factors
Buying potential	Financial means to buy healthy foods, warm clothing, and other necessary items
Behavioral and Biological Factors	
Health-damaging behaviors	Tobacco use, illicit drug use, alcohol consumption, dietary habits, physical activity habits, and sexual practices
Biological factors	Age
Psychosocial Factors	
Living circumstances	Poverty, debt, and neighborhood violence
Interpersonal stressors	Coping resources, social support, social isolation, job insecurity, and unemployment
Health System Factors	
Health care	Insurance, access to health care services, access to prevention and screening services, regular physician, and medication affordability

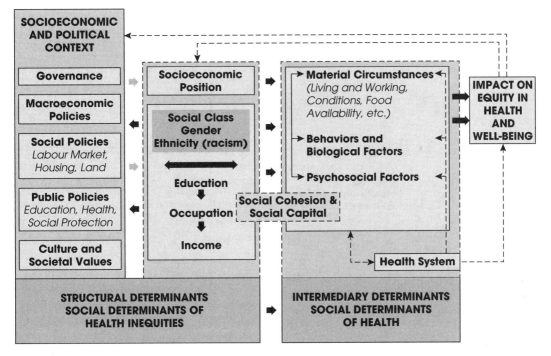

FIGURE 12–1   WHO Framework Describing Structural Determinants of Health

Source: From Solar and Irwin (2010).

income) are the social determinants of an individual's socioeconomic position. These social determinants operate through a set of intermediary determinants to shape a person's health and well-being, including vulnerability to health-compromising conditions. The health system is a social determinant because it has a role in reducing differences in risk exposures and vulnerability, and differences in access and treatment of illness based on a person's socioeconomic position.

In spite of spending more money on medical care than any other nation, the United States ranks near the bottom on key indicators of health, and health disparities persist, based on an individual's racial/ethnic background and socioeconomic characteristics (Bradley, Sipsma, & Taylor, 2017). The U.S. ratio of social service spending to health care spending is the lowest of all developed countries. Countries with low ratios report worse health outcomes. In addition, an examination of funds spent on social services by states indicates that states with a higher ratio of social service to health care spending have better health outcomes, further documenting the need to address the social determinants of health (Bradley et al., 2016).

Healthy People 2020 developed a "Place-based" organizing framework that describes five social determinants of health (Healthy People 2020, 2010a). The five key areas in the model and the critical components of each are shown in Figure 12–2. A "place-based" approach emphasizes conditions (social, economic, and physical) in the environments and settings, including schools, workplace, neighborhoods, and churches, where people live, learn, work, play, worship, and age. One of the five overarching goals of *Healthy People 2020* addresses social determinants, which guided the development of

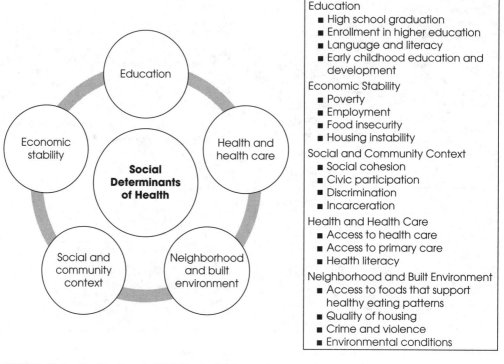

FIGURE 12–2 *Healthy People 2020* Key Social Determinants and Components
Source: From Healthy People 2020 (2010).

objectives to address the key determinants in the model. The Centers for Disease Control and Prevention (CDC) provides a social determinants of health (SDOH) Web portal that offers tools and policy resources to address the SDOH. The CDC resources support the *Healthy People 2020* framework. The foundational principles of the *Healthy People 2030* framework address eliminating health disparities, and achieving health equity.

Socioeconomic Determinants and Health Inequities

Socioeconomic status (SES) is a complex concept with multiple components. It is usually measured as income. However, SES also includes education, occupation, social class, financial resources, and neighborhood socioeconomic conditions. Socioeconomic position is a concept that is also used and includes income, education, and social status. Regardless of which dimensions have been used, SES has been substantiated to be the root of health inequities, measured at the population level (Irwin et al., 2017).

Low economic status is the most consistent predictor of life expectancy, morbidity and mortality, and health status (Hardy, 2017). Although there is great diversity among racial and ethnic populations, overall, racial/ethnic minorities have substantially lower incomes and educational levels than do most White people. Low income and education levels result in economic hardship, such as the inability to meet living expenses, whereas higher incomes and educational levels facilitate access to care, better housing in safer neighborhoods, increased opportunities for healthy food purchases, and access to club memberships and health promotion programs. Neighborhood socioeconomic status has consistently predicted health. In a longitudinal study of persons who stayed in the same community for 10 years, for every $10,000 increment in income, the odds of developing two or more health issues were significantly less (Robinette, Charles, & Gruenwald, 2017). Income is a powerful variable that influences health status.

The effects of low socioeconomic status are long lasting. Low socioeconomic status in childhood has consistently been associated with poorer health in adulthood. In 2009, over 40% of children in the United States lived in low-income families, and were more likely to be African American, Latino, or Native American children with parents who had less than a college education (Chen, Goodman, & the Committee on Pediatric Research, 2015). Poverty and adverse childhood experiences have been documented to have long-term negative effects on brain development and cognition (Black et al., 2017). Two longitudinal studies have also documented the effects of early childhood disadvantage on poorer cardiovascular function (Hardy, 2017). Childhood disadvantage was measured by annual family income and parent occupation. Poverty during childhood has also been linked with early adolescent behavioral problems (Mazza et al., 2017). The need for programs to address poverty in early childhood to prevent long-term negative consequences is clear.

Access to care can be measured by the proportion of a population that has health insurance. Because of their socioeconomic situation, racial and ethnic minorities are much more likely to be underinsured or to lack health insurance. When insurance is available, it is likely to be public insurance, primarily Medicaid. Health insurance contributes to the amount and type of health services obtained. Lack of health insurance has important implications for health promotion and prevention efforts, such as screening and access to wellness programs. Insurance status has also been correlated with self-reported health status. Those who rate their health as fair or poor are more likely to be uninsured than are those who rate their health as good or excellent. Individuals living in poverty also experience greater barriers in accessing care, have more difficulty getting an appointment, and wait longer during health care visits. These factors are compounded by the fact that many communities of poverty mistrust the government and government-controlled programs (Twenge, Campbell, & Carter, 2014). Socioeconomic barriers to accessing care exist for culturally, racially, and ethnically diverse populations. These barriers have been repeatedly documented.

PROMOTING EQUITY IN HEALTH

Achieving equity in health means that everyone has the opportunity to attain their full health potential, and no one is disadvantaged because of social, demographic, or geographic differences. The early literature on health disparities focused on racial/ethnic differences in health and "closing the gap"; however, "achieving health equity" is now more commonly discussed. Equity in health places emphasis on the multiple, avoidable influences on individual and population health and draws attention to the many challenges that must be addressed. Promotion of health equity moves health promotion to a political activity, as it moves from the individual level to a broader focus on strategies to change the distribution of social and economic resources.

Implement Multilevel Interventions

Achieving health equity is possible when multilevel interventions and programs are directed to individuals, communities, and social policies. Multilevel interventions address multiple factors to effect change in individuals and their socioeconomic context. Multilevel interventions go beyond individual-focused strategies to structural and socioeconomic influences to promote change. Multilevel interventions have been called *fourth-generation health disparities research* (Thomas, Quinn, Butler, Fryer, & Garza, 2011). These types of interventions incorporate both qualitative and quantitative methods to implement programs and evaluate outcomes. They are complex, pose many challenges, and require input from multiple sources, such as transdisciplinary health care teams, community organizations, and local and state governments.

Empower Communities

Community empowerment is a social action process that enables individuals, communities, and organizations to gain control over their lives within their social and political context to promote equity. It involves a shift in power between individuals and other social groups. Local community organizations empower individuals by working together to build trust and improve neighborhood programs. Individuals also work with community members to advocate for new programs and resources for their neighborhoods. For example, they may work together to advocate for after-school programs for youth, parks for leisure activities for families, or increased law enforcement presence; or they may work to bring affordable health screening services to the neighborhood for those without transportation. Community agencies can advocate for local school board participation. In addition, community members can be empowered to take an active role in promoting healthy and safe schools and neighborhoods.

Empowered communities believe in their capacity to change inequities and use that capacity to bring about change. Empowered community members feel a sense of community, which increases a sense of caring and support for each other and facilitates participation in change, such as working to obtain affordable housing, public transportation, safe walking places, and access to healthy foods. Empowered communities work with external powers to address community needs. For example, they may lobby and engage in policy decisions that impact the health of their communities. The ultimate goal of community empowerment is to create relationships and policies to promote health equity.

Focusing on working conditions, household and neighborhood hazards, and availability of community resources such as healthy foods and physical activity areas brings attention to environmental factors, including food deserts and food swamps described in Chapter 7, that can be changed within communities and worksites. Empowered community members can organize walking groups, community lectures, and health fairs. Community members should be able to participate in decisions that influence the health of their community. Empowerment means having a political voice to garner resources to change the community.

Community-based organizations (CBOs) are logical places to begin to bring about community change, as these organizations are enmeshed in the life of the community (Abrams, Davis, Ellison, Moseley, & Nowell, 2016). These nonprofit organizations are places where community members meet to socialize or address their concerns. CBOs can organize programs to teach individuals skills that empower them to address community issues. Leaders of CBOs can represent and advocate for the community. CBOs can empower members to establish new programs and use their collective power to advocate for policy changes. Empowered CBOs are able to build community capacity, as they know the strengths, weaknesses, and availability or lack of resources within their community.

Engage in Community-Based Participatory Research

Community-based participatory research (CBPR) is a collaborative approach in which all partners participate and are equally involved in the research process. The method builds on community strengths, offering an effective strategy to build community capacity (Frerichs, Hassmiller, Dave, & Corbie-Smith, 2016). It is a useful engagement approach in communities with health inequities, as it functions to transform power structures to create knowledge and promote actions for social change. CBPR has been successfully implemented to expose power inequities in disadvantaged communities, as the strategy enables community voices to be heard. CBPR acknowledges the need to involve and value diverse stakeholders and perspectives, making it an important strategy to address inequities in low-SES neighborhoods and communities.

Advocate for Upstream Policies

Public policies to promote health equity must address three key areas: early childhood development, employment, and income. Public policies that address these key areas have all been associated with lower rates of poverty and income inequities. There is a need to shift policy development from a focus on individual health risk behaviors to the redistribution of economic resources to promote a healthy society for all. In other words, the focus needs to change to upstream policies that target education, jobs, child development, community revitalization, housing, and transportation. Public policies can be enacted through legislation, fiscal measures, taxation, and organizational change.

Nurses and all other health professionals need to become knowledgeable about public policy to be able to advocate for policies that promote healthy communities and equitable socioeconomic conditions. In community settings, nurses may become spokespersons for the people living in poverty in order for their voices to be heard. At the individual level, strategies to alleviate poverty include helping families obtain available benefits, providing information about available services and how to access them, targeting those in greatest need, teaching life skills, and partnering individuals with community agencies to provide additional support. Programs that teach cognitive reappraisal and coping skills to buffer stress have had positive results in low socioeconomic status populations (Atal & Cheng, 2016; Troy, Ford, McRae, Zarolia, & Mauss, 2017). These strategies teach individuals to reframe their emotions in environments where they have little control, thereby decreasing anxiety and depression. At the community level, nurses can promote community dialogue between community members, CBOs, and persons in positions to influence policies. Membership in professional organizations that promote agendas to reduce health inequities is another avenue for action. Working in collaboration with all stakeholders enables nurses to raise awareness of health inequities, advocate for change, and take action, such as lobbying to promote change.

HEALTH LITERACY AND DIVERSE POPULATIONS

Health literacy, a concept introduced in the 1970s, has traditionally referred to the skills necessary to understand health information. Medical health literacy skills include basic reading and writing (*print literacy*), using quantitative information (*numeracy*), and speaking and listening effectively (*oral literacy*). These skills are considered necessary to be able to read and understand health information such as specific instructions or pre-scriptions and consents, to make appointments, to complete medical forms, and to self-manage chronic conditions.

Health literacy is considered a social determinant of health. Low health literacy has been associated with worse health status, poorer health knowledge and comprehension, increased hospitalizations and use of medical services, and decreased participation in preventive activities, such as mammogram screening and influenza immunizations. Low health literacy is associated with poor socioeconomic status. Diverse populations that are disproportionally affected include racial/ethnic minorities, older adults, individuals with less than a high school education, those who spoke another language prior to starting school, persons who do not speak English, and persons living in poverty.

The relationship of health literacy with poor health outcomes led the U.S. Department of Health and Human Services (USDHHS) to publish a national action plan to address health literacy issues (U.S. Department of Health and Human Services, Office of Disease Prevention and Health Promotion, 2010). This document has brought national attention to the problem of health literacy and has been important in the development of strategies and programs to decrease health literacy. Decreasing health literacy is included in the overarching goal addressing social determinants of health in *Healthy People 2020* (Healthy People 2020, 2010b). It is also an overarching goal in *Healthy People 2030*. Health literacy is an empowerment tool, as persons with higher health literacy are able to access and analyze information to make better health care decisions, which results in positive health outcomes.

Expanding Definitions of Health Literacy

The definition of health literacy has expanded to include a constellation of skills that an individual needs to function effectively in the health care environment and act appropriately on health information. The skills are reading, writing, arithmetic, listening, communicating, making decisions, navigating, and analyzing and applying information and skills to improve or promote health. Individuals with adequate health literacy are able to take responsibility for their health as well as the health of their families and communities (Guzys, Kenny, Dickson-Swift, & Threlkeld, 2015). One commonly cited definition of health literacy is provided by the Institute of Medicine (IOM), which describes health literacy as an individual's capacity to obtain, process, and understand basic information and services needed to make appropriate health care decisions (Nielsen-Bohlman, Panzer, & Kindig, 2004). The Healthy People 2020 definition describes health literacy as the ability of individuals to obtain, process, and understand health information needed to make appropriate decisions.

The World Health Organization defines health literacy as the cognitive and social skills that determine the motivation and ability of an individual to gain access to, understand, and use information in ways that promote and maintain good health (Kumaresan, 2013). This broader definition indicates that individuals must have the knowledge, skills, and self-confidence needed to take action to improve their personal health as well as the health of the communities in which they reside. The National Institutes of Health also expands the definition of health literacy to include the materials, environments, and challenges associated with disease prevention and health promotion.

Three levels of skills, first categorized by Nutbeam (2000), are commonly used to describe health literacy. *Functional* health literacy refers to basic level skills necessary to access information; *interactive* health literacy refers to communication skills needed to interact with health care professionals and the ability to understand information provided; and *critical* health literacy refers to advanced level skills needed to analyze and use information (Nutbeam, McGill, & Premkumar, 2017). *Medical* health literacy *has* traditionally been defined as *functional* health literacy, as noted in the IOM definition. *Interactive* health literacy has also been called *communicative* health literacy, as it focuses on being able to interact with health care professionals to obtain information and explanations that are understandable. These are summarized as follows:

- *Functional:* Basic level skills, such as reading and writing, to be able to obtain and apply information.
- *Interactive:* Communication skills to interact with health care professionals, and obtain and apply information.
- *Critical:* Advanced cognitive skills to analyze and apply information to control one's health.

These levels provide guidance on where to begin in teaching health literacy skills. For example, if a client needs to learn a specific task, such as making appointments, *functional* skills are a beginning point. If they need to learn specific skills, such as understanding a food label, *interactive* health literacy skills are needed. *Critical* health literacy skills need to be taught when clients need to learn, analyze, and apply health information, such as obtaining and evaluating health information from various websites. Both *interactive* and *critical* health literacy involve cognitive skills individuals need to take responsibility for their health. Unfortunately, most health literacy programs only teach functional literacy skills with less attention given to higher-level skills needed to use health information. In addition, until recently, measures of health literacy tended to focus only on functional health literacy skills.

Clients with low health literacy need many skills to manage their health effectively. In addition to reading, writing, and numeracy skills, the following are needed:

- When to seek health information and care
- Where to seek health care
- Verbal communication skills
- Skills to process information
- Skills to make choices
- Skills to use information

Health literacy involves an individual's cognitive, emotional, and social skills outside the control of the health care system. Assessing individuals' level of health literacy enables the nurse to identify factors that contribute to barriers to health and health promotion, to problem solve to improve access to health services, to plan appropriate strategies for educational programs, and to implement programs to improve health literacy (Batterham, Hawkins, Collins, Buchbinder, & Osborne, 2016).

HEALTH LITERACY STRATEGIES FOR DIVERSE POPULATIONS

Addressing health literacy needs is a basic component of designing health promotion programs for ethnically and culturally diverse populations. Many resources are available on federal, university, and nonprofit websites to assist in developing literacy and

TABLE 12–2 Health Literacy Oral Communication Strategies

- Begin with warm greeting and welcoming attitude
- Know appropriate eye contact
- Listen without interrupting
- Use plain, nontechnical, familiar language
- Use the client's words
- Slow down, speak at a moderate pace
- Clearly state what needs to be known
- Be specific and concrete
- Limit information
- Repeat key points, summarize
- Demonstrate, draw picture, and/or use models
- Invite participation
- Use teach-back to confirm understanding
- Use open-ended questions, avoid yes–no questions
- Encourage questions
- Highlight the positive

Source: From Brega et al., 2015.

culturally appropriate oral and written materials and online information. The federal plain language guidelines are also available online. These guidelines were written to support the U.S. Federal Plain Writing Law of 2010 that requires plain language usage in all public documents, presentations, and electronic communications. Nurses need communication and teaching skills to interact with clients with low health literacy and the knowledge necessary to develop literacy appropriate written materials.

Use Plain Language to Communicate Oral Messages

Strategies for delivering clear messages incorporate plain language principles. Some of the major strategies to keep in mind are listed in Table 12–2. Messages need to reflect the age, language, literacy level, and cultural diversity of the target individual or group. Messages must be relevant to the target group's key beliefs, attitudes, and values, using familiar and acceptable language and images. Messages may need to be presented multiple times using narratives and visual illustrations to capture attention and reinforce content. Tailored cultural messages that incorporate the client's personal information are more effective than standard communication. In addition, communication channels that are familiar to the client and are easily assessable are more effective.

Use Plain Language to Communicate Written Messages

Written information should be easy to read and understand, using plain language principles. Plain language makes information easier to understand. Plain language writing simply means writing clearly so that individuals understand the information the first time it is read. Strategies for communicating effective written messages are described in Table 12–3.

TABLE 12–3   Elements of Plain Language for Written Communication

Writing Clearly	Formatting
• Present most important message first	• Use generous amounts of white space
• Write in active (subject–verb) voice	• Use fonts that are familiar, such as serif
• Use simple, everyday words	• Use 11–13-point print size
• Define technical terms	• Emphasize words with bolding
• Keep sentences short	• Use meaningful headings
• Provide specific action steps	• Use short paragraphs
• Avoid abbreviations and acronyms	• Use bullets and numbered lists
• Use positive, encouraging tone	• Use culturally appropriate pictures
• Avoid authoritarian, intimidating tone	

Source: Information available at the National Institutes of Health, Office of Communications and Public Liaison and Brega et al. (2015).

Nonprint materials also can be used to communicate information. For example, videos are helpful to demonstrate procedures such as how to wear a pedometer. Pictures can supplement written or verbal information.

Apply Teach-Back Method to Confirm Understanding

The "teach-back" technique is an effective method to assess and verify an individual's understanding of information provided during an interaction. This method goes beyond asking clients if they understand. Instead, they are asked to state or demonstrate how they will use the information. For example, after a demonstration that shows how to wear a pedometer and reset the steps, the client is asked to perform the procedure. If it is not performed correctly, the information is clarified or another approach is implemented to teach the information. The client should practice until the skill is mastered, or the instructions are understood.

It is important not to rush, to remain patient, and to provide positive feedback with each step of the procedure or activity being demonstrated. Statements such as "Do you understand?" or "Do you have any questions?" are replaced with statements such as "Show me how you will do it when you get home" or "Tell me what you understand." Open-ended questions should be asked to avoid yes or no answers. Steps and strategies in the teach-back process are outlined in Table 12–4.

Incorporate Culture and Language

Culture influences how individuals understand and respond to information. For low-literacy, culturally diverse populations, only terms that the individuals or groups are comfortable with should be used. Do not assume that all minority groups are alike. Consider the subpopulation and geographic location. Mexican Americans in the Southwest, for example, may respond differently to the same terminology based on their different contexts from Puerto Rican Americans in the Northeast. Differences also exist within the same culture or ethnic group, depending on the age, gender, class, or religious practices. When working with an individual or group from a specific cultural

TABLE 12–4   Teach-Back Process: Steps and Strategies

1. Convey a caring voice and positive attitude
2. Plan your approach ahead
3. Use plan language and conversational style
4. Chunk information in small segments
5. Use handouts and demonstrations
6. Ask clients to explain back, using their own words
7. Use "show me" approach to ask clients to demonstrate a skill
8. Use noncritical, open-ended questions
9. Clarify and explain again
10. Have client explain back or demonstrate again and recheck

Source: Adapted from Brega et al. (2015).

background, begin with an assessment of their beliefs about health and illness, religious beliefs, food customs, and family patterns, including decision-making. This information may influence how clients respond to information and recommendations. Nurses should ask clients what is important to know about their health beliefs and customs so that the information can be used in the health promotion or prevention plan. Learning the role of family members in the client's health is also important to the planning process. In addition, norms about eye contact and body language enable the nurse to understand the client's responses to communication.

Language preferences should be assessed to document any language assistance that might be needed in the teaching or counseling process. Questions such as "What language are you most comfortable speaking?" and "Would you like an interpreter?" should be asked. If an interpreter is needed, someone from the same community who has been trained and has experience in translating and knows the local language should be chosen (Vander-Wielen et al., 2014). Untrained persons, family and friends, and minor children are unacceptable in most situations, as they make errors or impose their views on the client. Using minors may place children in a vulnerable position. When translating written materials, word-for-word translation is not always accurate due to cultural nuances.

Address Internet Access and eHealth Literacy Messages

Electronic health (eHealth) literacy is defined as a set of skills and knowledge necessary to successfully interact with health technology tools (Kim & Xie, 2017). Persons with limited health literacy are less likely to use the Internet and online health information, and may have difficulties interacting with eHealth. However, mobile technologies, including eHealth, have the potential to reduce health disparities as they address individual barriers, such as access to hard-to-reach populations, flexible and frequent communication, and provision of low-cost interventions using multiple strategies, such as audio, video, and graphic information. In addition, mobile applications may provide a sense of support, which is often missing in the health care system for groups that experience health disparities and low health literacy (Peek, 2017). Ownership of a home personal computer and Internet access remain the major barriers defining the digital divide (Lin et al., 2015). Limited Internet use is also linked to lack of computer training, lack of skills or family support for skill building, older age, limited income, and lower education.

Literature supports the use of digital technologies to reduce health disparities, and studies of mobile health interventions in diverse populations confirm its potential to improve health. However, interventions to eliminate the digital divide and promote eHealth literacy need to be developed and implemented. Strategies should address the following:

- How to access online resources for health information
- How to search for information effectively
- How to evaluate the quality of online information

Addressing the eHealth literacy of older adults is important, due to the potential benefits for this group. In addition, the lack of Internet access in disadvantaged neighborhoods continues to be a major barrier for nonuse. Public policy should focus on extending affordable Internet access to disadvantaged communities as well as rural areas with limited access.

Design features that facilitate navigation of the Internet and understanding of the content have been published by the Office of Disease Prevention and Health Promotion. The online research guide provides information to design digital health information tools and health websites for persons with low health literacy (U.S. Department of Health and Human Services, Office of Disease Prevention and Health Promotion, 2015). Plain language is an underlying strategy to engage users. Persons with limited literacy skills need opportunities to learn the skills needed to obtain online health information. Challenges with the communication technologies remain and require attention to health literacy and digital health literacy to be effective for diverse populations.

HEALTH LITERACY TRAINING FOR HEALTH PROFESSIONALS

Health literacy is a key component of effective communication between individuals and health professionals. In order for health literacy to become an effective component of all health promotion activities, nurses and other health professionals need to understand and apply health literacy principles and strategies in their communication and in the design of written health information and websites. However, health literacy is not being adequately addressed in many nursing and health professional schools and continuing education programs.

An assessment is the first step to identify health literacy training needs. This should be followed by training, which can be incorporated into orientation programs, didactic courses, and ongoing staff meetings. One successful strategy with health professional students is to develop interdisciplinary international programs that combine service learning with cultural immersion. These programs provide opportunities for students to learn how to work with diverse cultures.

At the national level, the U.S. Department of Health and Human Services, Office of Disease Prevention has developed a website that provides information and resources to learn about health literacy and how to implement health literacy strategies in practice. In addition, videos highlighting interviews with individuals illustrate how to approach health literacy issues. PowerPoint presentations can be downloaded to teach health literacy skills. The Centers for Disease Control (CDC) has an online course to teach health professionals and students about health literacy. Resources available on the CDC website can be used for teaching individuals or groups.

The Health Literacy Universal Precautions Toolkit is an excellent resource for nurses (Brega et al., 2015). It is available on the Agency for Healthcare Research and Quality (AHRQ) website. Health literacy universal precautions are used to draw attention to the difficulty in recognizing limited health literacy, thus the need to use a universal approach. The purpose of the kit is to provide evidence-based guidance to enable professionals to address spoken and written communication, self-management and empowerment, and supportive systems to promote health literacy. It contains many resources, including Power-Point presentations, worksheets, and sample forms. Over 20 topics are addressed with concrete information and strategies to address health literacy issues. The toolkit also offers additional resources and access to other helpful websites to educate health professionals.

HEALTH CARE PROFESSIONALS AND CULTURAL COMPETENCE

Expertise in cultural competence and sensitivity to differences among cultures is a needed skill, considering the racial, ethnic, and cultural diversity of populations and the number of factors operating to create health disparities in these groups. *Cultural competence* is defined as appropriate and effective communication that requires one to be willing to listen and learn from members of diverse populations. It also includes the provision of information and services in appropriate languages, at appropriate comprehension and literacy levels, and in the context of the individual's health beliefs and practices. In culturally competent health promotion programs, the beliefs, interpersonal styles, attitudes, and behaviors of individuals and families are respected and incorporated into all program activities. Culturally competent nurses continually adapt their practice to understand the cultures of their clients. Culturally competent health professionals are aware of their own cultural values and beliefs and recognize how these influence their attitudes and behaviors toward another group.

Continuum of Cultural Competence

Cultural–linguistic competence has been described by various authors, using a continuum of interpersonal behaviors. Bushy's (1999) classic continuum, which addresses individuals, ranges from *ethnocentrism* at one end to *enculturation* at the other end of the spectrum. Enculturation is not a discrete endpoint, as development of cultural competence is a life-long process (Isaacson, 2014; Tervalon & Murray-Garcia, 1998). The continuum is highlighted in Figure 12–3.

> *Ethnocentrism* refers to assumptions or beliefs that one's own way of behaving or believing is most preferable and correct and the standard by which all cultural groups will be judged. This view devalues the beliefs of other cultural groups or treats them as inferior.

> *Cultural awareness*, the next stage on the continuum, refers to an appreciation of and sensitivity to another person's values, beliefs, and practices. At this stage, one acknowledges the need for cultural information and skills.

> *Cultural knowledge* refers to gaining understanding of and insight into different cultures.

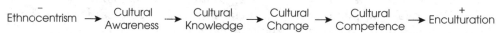

FIGURE 12–3 Continuum of Cultural Competence

Source: From Bushy (1999).

Cultural change occurs.

Cultural competence, the next stage, is the level at which nurses are aware, sensitive, and knowledgeable about another's culture and have the skills to conduct culturally competent programs.

Enculturation, the final anchoring point, refers to fully integrating the values of the other culture. Enculturation is evident when the nurse develops culturally sensitive health promotion programs in collaboration with individuals in the cultural group and incorporates members of the culture to deliver and evaluate the intervention.

Developing cultural competence is not a linear process. Progress depends on attitudes, life experiences, exposure to other cultures, and receptivity to learning about new cultures. Progress also depends on institutional policies and practices. Acquisition of cultural competence skills is an ongoing process to ensure delivery of health promotion interventions that are appropriate, acceptable, and meaningful for persons of diverse backgrounds. Diversity is embedded in cultural competence, but it is just one component. Accepting and understanding differences in customs and patterns of thinking are ways in which diversity is valued.

Cultural humility refers to an ongoing commitment to self-evaluation and self-critique when interacting with diverse populations (Isaacson, 2014). Cultural humility includes equalizing the power imbalance between health care professionals and clients and developing collaborative partnerships with communities on behalf of diverse populations (Foronda, Batiste, Reinhold, & Ousman, 2016; Tervalon & Murray-Garcia, 1998). Cultural humility goes beyond cultural competence, as it requires that health care professionals take responsibility for interactions with clients through active listening and ongoing self-reflection of their own attitudes and feelings toward diverse cultures. In other words, nurses learn to view individuals' cultures from their point of view and to recognize their biases. Cultural humility requires a life-long commitment, as cultures are dynamic and change over time (Yeager & Bauer-Wu, 2013).

Cultural competency programs have three essential components: awareness, knowledge, and skills. First, nurses must become aware of their own cultural beliefs, values, and biases. This can be accomplished through a self-assessment. Measures to assess cultural competence are widely available. Second, cultural knowledge and life experiences of the other culture are learned along with cross-cultural communication strategies. The third component focuses on developing skills needed to become culturally competent and making a commitment to developing cultural humility. These skills, including verbal and nonverbal communication strategies, need to be practiced under supervision.

Strategies for Culturally Competent Communication

Culturally competent communication skills build trust relationships with diverse clients. Trust is necessary to obtain valid information to develop interventions or manage issues of concern. Culturally competent communication includes skills in verbal and nonverbal communication, recognition of potential cultural differences, incorporation of cultural knowledge, negotiation and collaboration, and shared decision-making (Teal & Street, 2009) (see Figure 12–4). *Verbal skills* should reflect respect and empathy, nonjudgmental concern and interest, reflections, and follow-up questions. *Nonverbal communication skills*

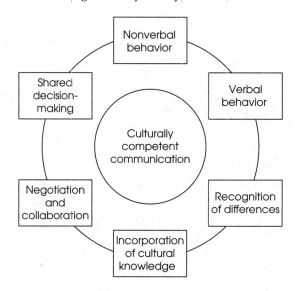

FIGURE 12–4 Components of Culturally Competent Communication

should also reflect respect, concern, and interest in the client's well-being. Skills include active listening and focusing on the client. *Recognizing cultural differences* involves monitoring potential cultural misunderstanding to prevent crossing cultural boundaries. Observing the client's reactions, asking for their perceptions, and exploring their understanding are useful strategies. Differences are acknowledged, and information and priorities are based on client input and preferences. *Communication skills* for negotiation *and* collaboration require awareness and adaptability to come to a shared understanding and agreed-upon priorities. *Shared decision-making* ensures client engagement in the communication process. Communication skills that promote cultural awareness and sensitivity prevent health care professionals from stereotyping clients and ignoring cultural issues.

An additional layer of complexity is added when working with a translator. Translators must be both content and contextual experts. They should be immersed in the same native language and community as the client, if possible, and understand the dialect and context in which the words are being used.

Considerations in Planning Culturally Competent Programs

Assessment of characteristics of diverse populations that may affect the success of health promotion programs is the first step to achieving goals. These factors include demographic, cultural, and health care system variables. The culturagram is a family assessment tool that was originally developed for social workers to improve their understanding of culturally diverse families (Congress, 1994, 2005). The tool assesses the cultural norms, values, beliefs, and practices of families, so it is relevant for all health care professionals to understand culturally diverse families in their practice. As seen in Figure 12–5, the assessment includes 10 areas to consider to learn about the client's culture as well as the family context. It can be used as an interactive tool when meeting with clients by giving them a copy during the interview. Relevant questions should be generated for each domain for family discussion (Substance Abuse and Mental Health Services Administration, 2014).

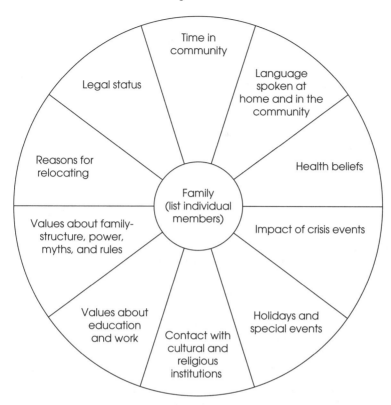

FIGURE 12–5   A Culturagram for Cultural Assessment

Source: From Congress (2005).

Knowledge of the *language spoken* is a key feature in the delivery of programs. Inability to communicate in the dominant language creates barriers to accessing programs and health care. It may also result in errors and/or inappropriate care. Even in some non-native English speaking clients, communication may be problematic, as clients may not fully understand the information and may avoid further verbal communication to get their questions answered. Health promotion programs are more successful when they are delivered in the language of the participants. Persons who represent the target culture and speak the same language should be involved in developing and implementing the intervention. In addition, culturally specific newspapers and radio and television stations can be targeted to deliver health messages in the appropriate language.

Geographic location is another major factor to consider in designing programs, as the physical environment plays a significant role in promoting healthy behaviors. Low-income urban neighborhoods are associated with areas that are unsafe. Research on "walkability" indicates that attractive, aesthetically pleasing settings are more conducive to physical activity (Wasfi, Steinmetz-Wood, & Kesterns, 2017). Fear due to drug sales or violence may be a major factor in limiting outside activities. Low-income neighborhoods have fewer services available, such as clinics or community centers, and experiences disadvantages in access to private transportation. In addition, limited grocery stores result in higher prices paid for fresh fruits and vegetables that may be scarce and of poor quality. These issues need to be considered when the behaviors that need to change include physical activity or healthy eating.

The concept of *family* also differs across cultures. In some cultural groups, the family is an extension of the individual. The family may include more than the immediate relatives. The needs of the family may have priority over the needs of the individual in some cultures, as seen in many Asian and Hispanic cultures. In these groups, support from family members is more important than external support; so family members should be intimately involved with the individual and participate in the learning process. Family-oriented approaches, using family and extended family networks, are more likely to be successful in behavior change in African American and Hispanic cultures. In cultures with high levels of familism, obligation to one's family is valued and take priority over concerns for oneself (McLaughlin et.al, 2017). When this value is emphasized, the value of the behavior change of the woman for the entire family should be emphasized. Family networks may also include church relationships, as they offer social support and communication networks. Educational strategies should capitalize on the powerful effects of family networks to promote behavior change.

Time orientation refers to the differing perception of time among cultures. A present orientation is common in populations experiencing health inequities, as the focus is on living in the present; the future may have less meaning (Keefe, 2015; Gennetian & Shafir, 2015). Persons with a present orientation have more difficulty changing behaviors, as current, day-to-day needs take priority. Knowledge of an individual or culture's dominant time orientation as well as values related to "clock" time helps to eliminate misunderstandings, such as missed appointments or tardiness.

Health care system factors also are important to assess prior to health promotion efforts. Disadvantaged populations have problems accessing care and participating in health-promoting programs due to costs, distance, transportation, and language. Missed appointments or program sessions may not mean that the individual is not interested. Transportation or childcare may not be available, or bilingual support may be inadequate. Program acceptance depends on multiple factors, including lack of trust, prior interactions with health care providers, and a failure to incorporate the client's cultural values.

Culturally sensitive approaches enhance access and acceptance of health promotion programs. Focus group or individual interviews in the target community may reveal culturally relevant information on which to base interventions. Community priorities and availability of community resources also should be identified. Churches or other sites within the community should be used whenever possible to facilitate easy access as well as offer a familiar environment.

Strategies for Developing Culturally Appropriate Programs

Health promotion programs and materials need to integrate elements of the client's culture to facilitate acceptance, understanding, and adoption of the information and skills taught. Successful strategies incorporate the recommended written and oral communication for low-literacy populations described in Tables 12–2 and 12–3. Strategies for developing culturally sensitive health promotion messages and written information incorporate both "structure surface" and "deep surface" elements (Resnicow, Soler, Braithwaite, Ahluwalia, & Butler, 2000). In addition, strategies that promote culturally appropriate health promotion program development include (1) *peripheral*, (2) *evidential*, (3) *linguistic*, (4) *constituent-involving*, (5) *sociocultural*, and (6) *cultural tailoring* (Kreuter, Lukwago, Bucholtz, Clark, & Sanders-Thompson, 2002).

"Structure surface" refers to matching messages and materials to *observable* social and behavioral characteristics of the group's culture. For example, language, food preferences, clothing, product brands, or music is incorporated in written or visual media. In addition, the program is implemented with ethnically similar persons in settings familiar to or preferred by the cultural group. *Structure surface* elements are similar to *peripheral* strategies, as these are efforts to package the program content to visually appeal to the cultural group. Colors, images, pictures, or titles are used to reflect the social and cultural world of the targeted group. Thus, the information is viewed as familiar and comfortable. *Structure surface* elements or *peripheral* strategies integrate the client's culture preferences and behavior patterns into the program. Materials that are matched to an individual's culture help establish credibility and create interest, increasing acceptance and receptivity of the information.

"Deep structure" refers to incorporating cultural, social, environmental, and historical factors that influence health behaviors in racially and culturally diverse populations. Inclusion of deep structure elements is more complex, as the influence of cultural norms, customs, religion, family, economic situation, and society on the client's beliefs and health behaviors is taken into account when designing the program components. The culturagram described earlier can be helpful in assessing the information needed to ensure a culturally appropriate program. Understanding family, culture, and societal influences from the client's perspective also produces a culturally relevant program and increases the likelihood of its effectiveness.

Evidential strategies are those used to present information in a way that increases the perceived relevance of the health topic for the specific cultural group. For example, provision of information on the prevalence of diabetes in Mexican Americans has been used to raise awareness and promote lifestyle change in this high-risk group. The message becomes more meaningful when it is perceived to be directly applicable to those receiving the message.

Linguistic strategies are implemented to translate materials and programs into the cultural group's dominant or native language. Strategies such as translating materials or delivering the program in the target culture's native language are essential. Verbatim translation is not sufficient. *Linguistic* strategies are used to retain original meaning while using language understood by the target cultural group. Cultural equivalence, which ensures cultural, conceptual, and contextual relevance, is achieved by forward and backward translation and independent bilingual translators who are familiar with the language and idioms of the target group.

Constituent-involving strategies are those that seek input and capitalize on the experiences of the target population. Strategies include using peers or lay helpers from the clients' cultural group and involving community members in planning and implementing the health promotion program. Community participation assists in successfully incorporating both surface and deep structure into program materials and content.

Sociocultural strategies recognize, reinforce, and build on the group's values, beliefs, and behaviors to provide context and cultural meaning to the programs. *Sociocultural* strategies address *deep structure* elements. For example, program sites to change dietary behaviors for African Americans may be more successful when the beauty salon or barber shop is used, as these places have meaning and familiarity. Programs that are culturally meaningful and relevant are more effective for changing behaviors in culturally diverse populations. They are more complex and time consuming to implement.

Cultural tailoring strategies are any combination of change strategies intended to reach an individual based on characteristics unique to that person. Targeted strategies are distinguished from tailored strategies as the group is the focus with targeted strategies. Both targeted and tailoring strategies are important. When individual differences are small, the group can be the major target. When unique individual differences are evident, cultural tailoring strategies that focus on the individual are needed. Although culture is a shared group characteristic, individuals within cultures differ on cultural characteristics, so cultural tailoring is considered an appropriate strategy.

In summary, multiple strategies facilitate the development and implementation of culturally appropriate interventions. Effective communication is a core concept. Incorporating community members of the target group, including bilingual staff and lay health advisors; integrating the cultural beliefs and values of the family and community; and attending to health literacy issues are key strategies to promote relevant, culturally appropriate programs.

CONSIDERATIONS FOR PRACTICE IN DIVERSE POPULATIONS

Nurses have multiple health promotion opportunities and challenges with diverse populations because of the prevalence of health inequities that increase their risks for diseases and chronic illnesses. Nurses must first examine their own attitudes and values and how these may either facilitate or impede culturally appropriate client encounters. A commitment to becoming culturally competent is necessary to effectively promote healthy behaviors with culturally diverse groups. Culturally competent communication skills and knowledge are necessary to design culturally and literacy appropriate programs. These skills can be learned through courses and practice. Factors such as potential language difficulties, educational level, poverty, unsafe housing or neighborhoods, and different cultural beliefs are challenges that need to be confronted to change lifestyles. Collaborative partnerships with other health care professionals and organizations within the community are critical. Nurses need to learn policy analysis and advocacy skills to be able to represent the voices of racial and culturally diverse groups and lobby for policies and changes to promote health equity for all.

OPPORTUNITIES FOR RESEARCH IN DIVERSE POPULATIONS

Although evidence documents the adverse health outcomes caused by health inequities, research to promote health equity is limited due to the multiple determinants and the complex, multilevel interventions needed. Multiple methodologies, including community-based participatory research, and many stakeholders are needed to support multilevel interventions that target sociocultural, behavioral, and environmental systems. The effects of changing policies that increase socioeconomic status and access to quality services and care need rigorous investigation. Appropriate health literacy interventions that target subpopulations such as children and adolescents, older adults, and rural residents should be designed and tested, as these subgroups have received less attention.

Transdisciplinary research teams are crucial in research to address the complex social determinants of health inequities. Community interventions that partner with stakeholders should be implemented to evaluate changes that focus on living conditions within the community. Health policy research also is a priority, and the effects of policy in achieving health equity must be evaluated.

Digital technologies, including mHealth and eHealth, offer great potential for addressing health inequities. Research is needed in low-literacy and rural populations and the elderly to test interventions that address literacy and user issues.

Culturally diverse racial and ethnic groups traditionally have been underrepresented in research for many reasons, including unsuccessful recruitment and retention strategies, lack of culturally sensitive interventions and measures, literacy levels, and lack of trust. Recruitment of communities for interventions that evaluate large-scale changes is an even bigger challenge. However, research is needed to evaluate large-scale change in order to influence policy.

Summary

Although progress has been made in the health of the American people due to basic improvements—such as safe drinking water, sanitation, the availability of nutritious food, and advances in medical care—evidence shows that, in addition to these improvements, structural factors that define a person's social class and socioeconomic position in society are powerful predictors of health. At all levels of income, health and illness follow a social gradient, with lower socioeconomic levels associated with poorer health. Ethnically, racially, and culturally diverse populations have multiple threats to health that require attention from practitioners, researchers, and policy makers. Although the multiple, contributing factors are complex, they are amenable to change. Nurses, as primary care providers, are well positioned to take a leadership role in designing and implementing culturally competent health promotion programs and advocate for public policies that promote health equity for all.

Learning Activities

1. Using the culturagram in Figure 12–5, perform a cultural assessment with an immigrant family with young children. Write down all of the questions that you will need to answer for each domain. Summarize your assessment. What did you learn about the family? Reflect on your biases, prejudices, and stereotype about your own group and others different from you.
2. Choose a health pamphlet or brochure and critique it using the strategies for effective written communication in Table 12–3. Revise the pamphlet or brochure, based on your critique, using plain language principles, to make it literacy appropriate.
3. Choose a health topic or skill and perform a teach-back with a peer (colleague or student), using the steps in Table 12–4. Develop a checklist for your peer to evaluate your implementation of the teach-back method.
4. Identify an issue in a disadvantaged community, such as unsafe housing. Describe how you would advocate at local and state levels to promote policies to address the issue in the community.
5. Using the guidelines found in the Making Health Literacy Real Toolkit (see the CDC.gov website), conduct a health literacy assessment on an organization, such as the county health department. Identify potential barriers and strategies to overcome in improving health literacy in the organization.

References

Abraido-Lanza, A. F., Echeverria, S. E., & Florez, K. R. (2016). Latino immigrants, acculturation, and health: Promising new directions in research. *Annual Review of Public Health*, 37, 219–236.

Abrams, J., Davis, E. M., Ellison, A., Moseley, C., & Nowell, B. (2016). *Community-based organizations in the U.S. West: Status, structure, and activities.* Ecosystem Workforce Program Working Paper #67. Eugene, OR: University of Oregon.

Alba, R., & Barbosa, G. Y. (2016). Room at the top? Minority mobility and the transition to demographic diversity in the USA. *Ethnic and Racial Studies*, 39(6), 917–938.

Atal, S., & Cheng, C. (2016). Socioeconomic health disparities revisited: Coping flexibility enhances health-related quality of life for individuals low in socioeconomic status. *Health and Quality of Life Outcomes, 14*(7), 1–7. doi:10.1186/s12955-016-0410-1

Batterham, R. W., Hawkins, M., Collins, P. A., Buchbinder, R., & Osborne, R. H. (2016). Health literacy: Applying current concepts to improve health services and reduce health inequities. *Public Health, 132,* 3–12. doi:10.1016/puhe.2016.01.001

Black, M., Walker, S., Fernald, L., Anderson, C., DiGirolamo, A., Lu, C., . . . Grantham-McGregor, S. (2017). Early childhood development coming of age: Science through life course. *The Lancet, 389,* 77–90. doi:10.1016/S0140-6736(16)31389-7

Bradley, E. H., Canavan, M., Rogan, E., Talbert-Slagle, K., Ndumele, C., Taylor, L., & Curry, L. A. (2016). Variation in health outcomes: The role of spending on social services, public health, and health care, 2000–09. *Health Affairs, 35*(5), 760–768. doi:10.1377/hlthaff.2015.0814

Bradley, E. H., Sipsma, H., & Taylor, L. A. (2017). American health care paradox—High spending on health care and poor health. *QJM: An International Journal of Medicine, 110*(2), 61–65. doi:10.1093/qjmed/hcw187

Braveman, P. (2014a). What are health disparities and health equity? We need to be clear. *Public Health Reports, 12*(1 Suppl 2), 5–8. doi:10.1177/00333549141291S203

Braveman, P. (2014b). What is health equity: And how does a life-course approach take us further toward it? *Maternal and Child Health Journal, 18*(2), 366–372. doi:10.1008/s10995-013-1226-9

Brega, A. G., Barnard, J., Mabachi, N. M., Weiss, B. D., DeWalt, D. A., Brach, C., . . . West, D. R. (2015). *AHRQ Health Literacy Universal Precautions Toolkit* (2nd ed.). AHRQ Publication No. 15-0023-EF. Rockville, MD: Agency for Healthcare Research and Quality.

Bushy, A. (1999). Resiliency and social support. In J. G. Sebastian & A. Bushy (Eds.), *Special populations in the community: Advances in reducing health disparities* (pp. 189–195). Gaithersburg, MD: Aspen Publications, Inc.

Chen, T. L., Goodman, E., & the Committee on Pediatric Research. (2015). Race, ethnicity, and socioeconomic status in research on child health. *Pediatrics, 135*(1), e225–e237. doi:10.1542/peds.2014-3109

Commission on Social Determinants of Health. (2008). *Closing the gap in a generation: Health equity through action on the social determinants of health.* Final Report of the Commission on the Social Determinants of Health. Geneva, Switzerland: World Health Organization.

Congress, E. (1994). The use of culturagrams to assess and empower culturally diverse families. *Families in Society, 75*(9), 531–540.

Congress, E. P. (2005). Cultural and ethical issues in working with culturally diverse patients and their families: The use of the culturagram to promote cultural competence practice in health care settings. *Social Work in Health Care, 39*(3–4), 249–262.

Foronda, C., Baptiste, D., Reinhold, M., & Ousman, K. (2016). Cultural humility: A concept analysis. *Journal of Transcultural Nursing, 27*(3), 201–217. doi:10.1177/1043659615592677

Frerichs, L., Hassmiller, K., Dave, G., & Corbie-Smith, G. (2016). Integrating systems science and community-based participatory research to achieve health equity. *American Journal of Public Health, 106*(2), 215–222. doi:10.2015/AJPH.2015.302944

Gennetian, L. & Shafir, E. (2015). The persistence of poverty in the context of financial instability: A behavioral perspective. *Journal of Policy Analysis and Management, 34*(4): 904–936.

Guzys, D., Kenny, A., Dickson-Swift, V., & Threlkeld, G. (2015). A critical review of population health literacy assessment. *BMC Public Health, 15,* 215. doi:10.1086/s12889-015-155-6

Hardy, R. (2017). The persisting challenge of socio-economic inequalities in health across the life course. *JAMA Pediatrics,* E1–E3.

Healthy People 2020. (2010a). Revised definitions for health disparities and health equity. Retrieved from http://www.healthypeople.gov/2020/minutes-sixth-meeting-october-15-2008/page/0/1

Healthy People 2020. (2010b). Social determinants of health. Retrieved on July 20, 2017, from http://www.healthypeople.gov

Irwin, A., Solar, J., & Vega, J. (2017). The United Nations Commission on Social determinants of health. In S. Quah (Ed.), *International encyclopedia of public health* (2nd ed., Vol. 6, pp. 557–561). New York, NY: Elsevier.

Isaacson, M. (2014). Clarifying concepts: Cultural humility or competence. *Journal of Professional Nursing, 30*(3), 251–258. doi:10.1016/profnurs.2013.09.011

Keefe, S. (Ed.) (2015). *Appalachian Mental Health.* University Press of Kentucky

Kids Count Data Center. (2015). *Children in poverty by race and ethnicity.* The Annie E. Casey Foundation. Retrieved on July 25, 2017, from http://datacenter.kidscount.org

Kim, H., & Xie, B. (2017). Health literacy in the eHealth era: A systematic review of the literature. *Patient Education and Counseling, 100*(6), 1073–1082. doi:10.1016/j.pec.2017.015

Kreuter, M. W., Lukwago, S. N., Bucholtz, D. C., Clark, E. M., & Sanders-Thompson, V. (2002).

Achieving cultural appropriateness in health promotion programs: Targeted and tailored approaches. *Health Education & Behavior, 30*(2), 133–146. doi:10.1177/1090198102251021

Kumaresan, J. (2013). Health literacy perspectives. In L. M. Hernandez (Rapporteur), *Health literacy: Improving health, health systems, and health policy around the world: Workshop summary* (pp. 9–36). Washington, DC: National Academies Press.

Lin, C., Atkin, D., Cappotto, C., Davis, C., Dean, J., Eisenbaum, J., . . . Vidican, S. (2015). Ethnicity, digital divides and uses of the Internet for health information. *Computers in Human Behavior, 51*, 216–223. doi:10.1016/j.chb.2015.04.054

Mazza, J., Lambert, J., Zunzunegui, M., Tremblay, R., Boivin, M., & Cote, S. (2017). Early adolescence behavior problems and timing of poverty during childhood: A comparison of lifecourse models. *Social Science & Medicine, 177*, 35–42. doi:10.1016/socscimed.2017.01.039

McLaughlin, E., Campos-Melady, M/. Smith, J., Serier, K., Belon, K., Simmons, J., & Kelton, K. (92017). the role of familism in weight loss treatment for Mexican American women. *Journal of Health Psychology.* 22(2): 1510–1523. doi:10.1177/1359105316630134

Nielsen-Bohlman, L., Panzer, A. M., & Kindig, D. A. (Eds.). (2004). *Brief report: Health literacy: A prescription to end confusion*, Washington, DC: National Academies Press.

Nutbeam, D. (2000). Health literacy as a public health goal: A challenge for contemporary health education and communication strategies into the 21st century. *Health Promotion International, 15*(3), 259–267. doi:10.1093/heapro/15.3.259

Nutbeam, D., McGill, B., & Premkumar, P. (2017). Improving health literacy in community populations: A review of progress. *Health Promotion International*, 1–11. doi:10.1093/heapro/dax015

Peek, M. (2017). Can mHealth interventions reduce health disparities among vulnerable populations? *Diversity and Equality in Health and Care, 14*(2), 44–45.

Resnicow, K., Soler, R., Braithwaite, R., Ahluwalia, J., & Butler, J. (2000). Cultural sensitivity in substance use prevention. *Journal of Community Psychology, 28*(3), 271–290. doi:10.1002/(SICI)1520-6629

Robinette, J., Charles, S., & Gruenwald, T. (2017). Neighborhood socioeconomic status and health: A longitudinal analysis. *Journal of Community Health*, 1–7. doi:10.1007/s10900-017-0327-6

Solar, O., & Irwin, A. (2010). *A conceptual framework for action on the social determinants of health.* Social Determinants of Health Discussion Paper 2. Geneva, Switzerland: World Health Organization Press.

Substance Abuse and Mental Health Services Administration. (2014). *Improving cultural competence.*

Treatment Improvement Protocol (TIP) Series No. 59, HHS Publication No. (SMA) 14-4849. Rockville, MD: Substance Abuse and Mental Health Services Administration.

Teal, C. R., & Street, R. L. (2009). Critical elements of culturally competent communication in the medical encounter: A review and model. *Social Science & Medicine, 68*(3), 533–543. doi:10.1016/j.socscimed.2008.10.015

Tervalon, M., & Murray-Garcia, J. (1998). Cultural humility versus cultural competence: A critical distinction in defining physician training outcomes in multicultural education. *Journal of Healthcare for the Poor and Underserved, 9*(2), 117–125. doi:10.1353/hpu.2010.0233

Thomas, S. B., Quinn, S. C., Butler, J., Fryer, C. S., & Garza, M. A. (2011). Toward a fourth generation of disparities research to achieve health equity. *Annual Review of Public Health, 32*, 399–416.

Troy, A., Ford, B., McRae, K., Zarolia, P., & Mauss, I. (2017). Change the things you can: Emotion regulation is more beneficial for people from lower than from higher socioeconomic groups. *Emotion, 17*(1), 141–154. doi:10.1037/emo0000210

Twenge, J., Campbell, W., & Carter, N. (2014). Declines in trust in others and confidence in institutions among American adults and late adolescents, 1977–2012. *Psychological Science, 25*(10), 1914–1923. doi:10.1177/0956797614545133

U.S. Department of Health and Human Services, Office of Disease Prevention and Health Promotion. (2010). *National action plan to improve health literacy.* Washington, DC: Author. Retrieved from https://health.gov/communication/initiatives/health-literacy-action-plan.asp

U.S. Department of Health and Human Services, Office of Disease Prevention and Health Promotion. (2015). *Health literacy online: A guide to simplifying the user experience.* Retrieved from http://health.gov/healthliteracyonline/

Vander-Weilen, L., Enurah, A., Rho, H., Nagarkatti-Guide, D., Michelsen-King, P., Crossman, S., & Vanderbilt, A. (2014). Medical interpreters: Improvements to address access, equity, and quality of care for limited-English proficient patients. *Academic Medicine, 89*(10), 1324–1327. doi:10.1097/acm.0000000000000296

Wasfi, R., Steinmetz-Wood, M., & Kestens, Y. (2017). place matters: A longitudinal analysis measuring the association between neighborhood walkability and walking by age group and population center size in Canada. *PLoS ONE, 12*(12),:e0189472. doi:10.1371/journal.pone.0189472

Yeager, K., & Bauer-Wu, S. (2013). Cultural humility: Essential foundation for clinical researchers. *Applied Nursing Research, 26*(4), 251–256. doi:10.1016/apnr.2013.06.008

CHAPTER 13

Health Promotion in Community Settings

OBJECTIVES

This chapter will enable the reader to:

1. Describe the difference between promoting individual health and family health.
2. Describe the health-promoting school concept.
3. Discuss the renewed focus on integrating health into the school curriculum.
4. Summarize the advantages of offering health promotion programs in workplaces.
5. Discuss the cost-effectiveness of health promotion programs in the workplace.
6. Justify the rationale for emphasizing health promotion in nurse-led clinics and health centers.
7. Describe factors that facilitate successful community-based health promotion programs.
8. Discuss the principles of community engagement for developing successful community partnerships.

Promoting health in all settings has increased globally. People of all ages benefit from gender and culturally sensitive health-promoting programs delivered in places where they spend the majority of their time: home, school, work, and community. Demonstrated success and cost-effectiveness of health promotion programs have increased program offerings in schools, worksites, and communities. This chapter presents an overview of settings for health promotion and the roles each plays in developing healthy behaviors. Included are strategies to foster healthy lifestyles by integrating health and wellness programs in schools and workplaces, and developing partnerships to promote healthy communities.

HEALTH PROMOTION IN FAMILIES

The family plays a critical role in the health of its individual members. Families provide the environment in which health values, attitudes, and behaviors are learned. Factors influencing values, attitudes, and behaviors in families include:

1. Family structure
2. Finances
3. Gender and age of members
4. Parenting practices
5. Communication styles
6. Power relations
7. Education
8. Decision-making patterns (Wright & Leahey, 2012)

    Just as individuals have overall responsibility for their health decisions, families must assume similar responsibility for the health behaviors of their members. The essential role of the family is to build human capital by investing in the health, education, values, and skills of its members so that they can assume productive roles in society. The family is the *major* unit responsible for the socialization of children; thus, families are ideal targets for health promotion and prevention planning efforts.

    Various family forms are common in contemporary society. Family units may be traditional two-parent families, one-parent families (often mother-only families, although the number of father-only families is growing), blended families (combination of two preexisting families), extended families (nuclear plus one or more relatives, often older), augmented families (additional members, not blood relations), married same-sex adults with children, and unmarried adults (blood and nonblood relations). The nurse must be sensitive to both the commonalities and differences across family types. Understanding the milieu in nontraditional families is essential to successful health promotion planning. The responses to the questions in Table 13–1 will enable the nurse to assist the family in developing a health promotion plan based on information about family values, beliefs, and lifestyle.

TABLE 13–1   Questions to Generate Information about Family Values, Beliefs, and Lifestyles

---

1. How does the family define health?
2. What health-promoting behaviors does the family engage in regularly?
3. What health-promoting behaviors are particularly enjoyable to family members?
4. Do all family members engage in these behaviors, or are patterns of participation highly variable in the family?
5. Is there consistency between stated family health values and their health actions?
6. What are the explicit or implicit health goals of the family?
7. What factors are operating to prevent health-promoting behaviors?
8. What resources are available to facilitate health-promoting behaviors?

Families demonstrate a range of abilities, insights, and strengths, and they exert significant influence on its members that include:

- *Cultural/attitudinal*, such as church attendance, school engagement, and community involvement
- *Social/interpersonal* and *social support*, such as family activities, family meetings and gatherings, and communication styles
- *Intrapersonal/psychological concepts*, such as self-esteem, coping, and depression

Health promotion in families places special emphasis on the parents, as they have a major influence on children's lifestyle (Vedanthan et al., 2016). Effective communication and coping styles of parents and a healthy home environment promote healthy behaviors. Parents/guardians role model their eating habits and sedentary or physical activity behaviors. Many studies have documented an association between obesity in adults and obesity in their children. The quality of parenting styles also shapes future health behaviors of children. Parents who are supportive and encouraging and reduce their screen time increase children's physical activity and decrease the children's screen time as well (Xu, Wen, & Rissel, 2015). Parenting characteristics, such as permissiveness, neglectfulness, controlling, punishing, demanding, or nonsupportive, should be assessed. The type of parenting style should alert the nurse to teach parents appropriate parenting skills so that the parents learn to change their parenting style and model healthy behaviors for their children.

Nurses are challenged to assist families to identify relevant health goals, plan positive lifestyle changes, and capitalize on family members' strengths to achieve desired health outcomes. Family-based health promotion programs are more successful than individual-focused programs when either the parents or the children are targeted. Changes in children influence parents, and changes in parents enable them to promote healthy behaviors in their children. The shared family environment can become a health-promoting one for all members.

HEALTH PROMOTION IN SCHOOLS

More than 50 million U.S. children are enrolled in K–12 private or public schools (Centers for Disease Control and Prevention, 2014a). Based on these numbers, schools are the most efficient system to offer programs to increase healthy behaviors among children and adolescents. However, they remain largely an untapped resource (Kolbe, Allensworth, Potts-Datema, & White, 2015).

School years are a critical time to establish lifelong healthy habits. Improving students' physical and mental health

- Increases learning capacity
- Improves mental alertness
- Decreases absenteeism (Centers for Disease Control and Prevention, 2014a)

Over the last four decades, many school systems have engaged in building health-enhancing environments. In the *earliest phase*, health promotion programs were implemented to provide information to enhance health and avoid or reduce health risks. The *second phase* of program development focused on the influence of teachers, parents, and peers. Teachers and school health personnel set the expectation for healthy behaviors

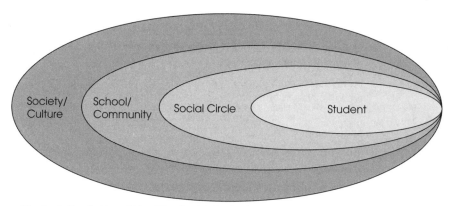

Student: The first level identifies the biological and personal history factors such as age and education

Social Circle: Student's peers, family members, and others who influence one's behavior and experiences

School/Community: Settings that influence the student and where social relationships form

Society/culture: Broad societal factors such as health, economic, and educational policies, and social and cultural norms that influence the student's environment

FIGURE 13–1   Social-Ecological Model

Source: Adapted from the Centers for Disease Control and Prevention. http://www.cdc.gov/violenceprevention/overview/social-ecologicalmodel.html

and served as role models for health-enhancing lifestyles. The assumption in both phases was that *individuals determine their lifestyle behaviors*. Individual-level theories such as social cognitive theory (see Chapter 2) provided the framework, and most school-based interventions covered specific topics, for example, physical activity, smoking cessation, or dietary habits. These programs usually provided health education courses within the school curriculum and health content was limited to these specific health courses.

Recognition of the value of families and communities in health promotion and learning led to the adoption of a social-ecological model in the *third phase* of health promotion program development. The social-ecological model describes the interrelationship of individuals with their social and physical environments. The social-ecological framework, shown in Figure 13–1, presents a clear understanding of the relationship between the student, family, school, community, and the society and culture at large.

School Curricula and Healthy Environments

The Centers for Disease Control and Prevention (CDC) developed the National Health Education Standards and the School Health Guidelines to Promote Healthy Eating and Physical Activity to promote healthy schools. Both sets of guidelines promote health education and healthy lifestyles for children from pre-kindergarten through grade 12. The National Health Education Standards, shown in Table 13–2, were developed to support health-enhancing behaviors at all grade levels and provide a framework for designing curricula, allocating teaching resources, and assessing student achievement

TABLE 13–2	National Health Education Standards
Standard 1	Students will comprehend concepts related to health promotion and disease prevention to enhance health.
Standard 2	Students will analyze the influence of family, peers, culture, media, technology, and other factors on health behaviors.
Standard 3	Students will demonstrate the ability to access valid information, products, and services to enhance health.
Standard 4	Students will demonstrate the ability to use interpersonal communication skills to enhance health and avoid or reduce health risks.
Standard 5	Students will demonstrate the ability to use decision-making skills to enhance health.
Standard 6	Students will demonstrate the ability to use goal-setting skills to enhance health.
Standard 7	Students will demonstrate the ability to practice health-enhancing behaviors and avoid or reduce health risks.
Standard 8	Students will demonstrate the ability to advocate for personal, family, and community health.

Source: CDC National Health Education Standards-SHER-Adolescent and School Health. Accessed at http://www.cdc.gov/healthyyouth/sher/standards

and progress (Centers for Disease Control and Prevention, 2005). The current guidelines have become an accepted reference for school health education. Schools that have incorporated the National Health Education Standards into their curriculum have reported healthier learners, improved academic scores, and higher graduation rates (Bradley & Green, 2013).

The School Health Guidelines to Promote Healthy Eating and Physical Activity were developed to serve as a basis for developing, implementing, and evaluating school policies to promote healthy eating and physical activity for students (Centers for Disease Control and Prevention, 2011). These guidelines are based on research and best practices that have shown that meeting nutritional and fitness goals results in improved attendance, fewer behavioral problems, and higher academic achievement. The document incorporates the federal dietary and physical activity guidelines for Americans and *Healthy People 2020* objectives. These guidelines contain strategies to assist in the implementation and provide resources for teachers and students. They are available on the CDC website.

School health promotion programs provide health knowledge and promote healthy lifestyles (Patton et al., 2016). Programs that incorporate the educational standards and guidelines not only build resilience, but also assist children and adolescents in developing lifelong healthy behaviors. The support of children early in life has a long-term effect on their health as well as the health of society.

Health-Promoting Schools

The health-promoting school approach, inspired by the World Health Organization (WHO) Ottawa Charter for Health Promotion, was introduced in the 1980s. The WHO

Health Promoting Schools framework defines a *health-promoting school* as one that is constantly striving to promote healthy living, learning, and working conditions of students, faculty, and members of the community (World Health Organization, 2017). The *health-promoting school framework* is an ecological model that combines traditional health education in the school curriculum with actions to improve health through changes in the student's social and physical environments, and engaging families and communities to reinforce health education and health behaviors (Langford et al., 2017). The health-promoting school approach has been adapted in the United States, Canada, Australia, New Zealand, and many European countries, under different nomenclature, such as comprehensive school health programs or the whole school approach. In Europe, almost two-thirds of the countries have a formal health-promoting school policy.

The contribution of schools to a student's health has been well substantiated (Turunen, Sormunen, Jourdan, von Seelen, & Buijs, 2017). School health promotion programs that account for social and environmental factors are also more successful. Evidence for health-promoting schools in high-income countries is positive. However, information is lacking for low-income countries. Further research is needed to identify the factors that promote success. In addition, there has been a call for more tailoring and greater rigor in evaluating the multilevel program outcomes.

The health promotion school approach is complex as implementers must take into account the factors considered essential for health-promoting schools (Penny et al., 2017). Administrative support and leadership, teacher support, school connectedness and stability in the community, and financial and human resources are components of the social and physical environments necessary for successful implementation.

The Whole School Collaborative Approach to Learning and Health

The health-promoting school approach in the United States is the whole school approach, which is described as the Whole School, Whole Community, Whole Child (WSCC) model. The WSCC model is a result of collaboration between the CDC and ASCD (formerly, the Association for Supervision and Curriculum Development). It is a social-ecological model that expands the CDC's coordinated school health approach, which had been the foundation for health promotion in schools for many years, and the ASCD's education-focused Whole Child Model. The new model, shown in Figure 13–2, is designed to support an integrated, collaborative approach by linking health with learning (Lewallen, Hunt, Potts-Datema, Zaza, & Giles, 2015). The five tenants (being healthy, safe, engaged, supported, and challenged) that surround the student in the model stress the need to make the student the focal point in health and education. The white band stresses the integration and collaboration among the school, health, and community; and the outer ring of the model reflects the range of learning and health support systems needed to support the health of the whole child (Centers for Disease Control and Prevention, 2014b).

Although there has been renewed interest in school health, it is still not a primary focus or the central mission in many schools in America. Two major reasons are the lack of infrastructure and financial resources to implement models such as the WSCC model (Rasberry, Slade, Lohrmann, & Valois, 2015). Necessary personnel, including school health coordinators and school health advisory or coordinating councils and teams, may not be available. In addition, strong leadership and administrative support may be

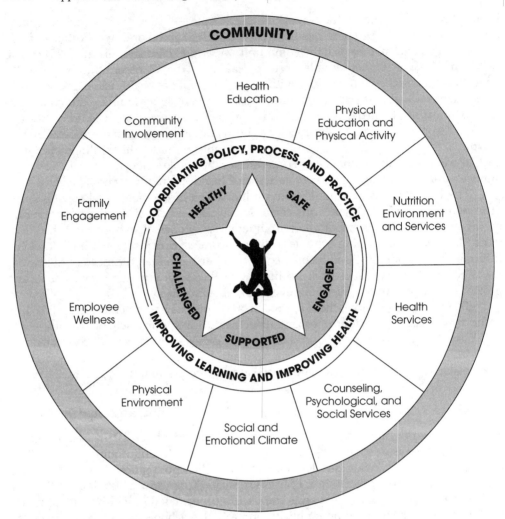

FIGURE 13–2   Whole School, Whole Community, Whole Child Model

Source: Courtesy of Association for Supervision and Curriculum Development.

missing due to lack of buy-in. The school principal has to be supportive and take a leadership role, and the model should be integrated into the school's mission. Financial concerns are a major barrier in many school districts. Community collaboration is a key to promoting whole child health. Community stakeholders and parents need to be active participants. Community building has to be a priority to get community buy-in and resources for schools to implement health programs.

Health-Promoting Interventions in Schools

Developmentally appropriate and effective evidence-based health programs are necessary to integrate health education into schools. Although research on health promotion interventions in children and adolescents is abundant, many programs have not been shown to be effective because of issues such as low participation or high dropout rates or inadequate implementation. Programs that have been tried in schools often are not rigorously evaluated to understand reasons for success or failure to change behaviors (Naylor et al., 2015). Many studies target physical activity due to the high prevalence of overweight and obesity in these groups. Current evidence, while limited, documents the value of physical activity in learning, healthy habit formation, and reducing weight in children, providing a mandate for incorporating physical activity into schools, using novel strategies, as described in the following research.

Walking school buses are considered a positive strategy to increase physical activity in children by getting them to walk to school. The concept was introduced in 1992, but it has only recently been implemented in the United States and Great Britain. The walking school bus builds on research documenting that school-based walking interventions increase physical activity in children (Carlin, Murphy, & Gallagher, 2016). Results of a review of studies conducted between 2002 and 2012 in the United States, Australia, and New Zealand found that the program increased the number of children walking to school, and activity levels improved (Smith et al., 2015). One study showed a decrease in body mass index, and there was evidence that children learned road safety skills. Barriers to walking reported were safety concerns of the parents, recruitment of people to lead the walking school bus, and time. Facilitators included the children's enjoyment of walking and interactions with other students. The walking school bus program was found to be a positive strategy to increase activity levels in children and a potential step to forming a healthy physical activity habit. School nurses have opportunities to promote the program or engage with communities to take leadership for the program, instead of expecting parents, who usually work, to do so.

A *before-school running/walking club* has been investigated as a way to increase physical activity and improve readiness to learn in elementary school children (Stylianou et al., 2016). Findings documented a positive impact on classroom behavior and readiness to learn on the 2 days a week that children participated in the running/walking club before school. The results are consistent with studies that have implemented physical activity at recess and in the classroom. A proposed mechanism is that physical activity may be linked to improvements in cognitive processes. The results of these types of studies have implications for the timing of physical activity in schools, as morning physical activity may be more beneficial than after-school physical activity for learning and classroom behavior.

Physically active academic lessons have also been tested as a mechanism to decrease the amount of time children spend in sedentary activity during the school days, which is currently over 90% (Grieco, Jowers, Errisuriz, & Bartholomew, 2016). These types of activities target regular classroom education, so they do not take additional time from the curriculum. Results have documented the benefits of adding physical activity to lessons during the school day. Time-on-task, a measure of attention and behavioral control, or student engagement, has been shown to increase following physical activity. These results are consistent with the before-school physical activity programs, reinforcing the benefits of physical activity on learning and classroom behavior in children.

Health-promoting behaviors acquired in the school years are more likely to become an integral part of one's life. Development of healthy behaviors in school-aged children and adolescents is critical to increasing healthy lifestyles across all life stages.

HEALTH PROMOTION IN THE WORKPLACE

The structure and nature of work, as well as the profile of the American worker, continue to evolve. America's workforce is older and more racially and ethnically diverse, with proportionally more women. Racial and ethnic minorities disproportionately work in low-paying jobs and have higher risks of work-related health problems. The primary categories of jobs in today's workforce are (1) *knowledge work*, requiring a relatively high level of education or technical training, and (2) *service* jobs (Bureau of Labor Statistics, 2017).

Most large companies (251–1,000 full-time equivalent employees [FTEs]) offer employees wellness and health promotion programs, and health insurance for nonelderly employees. Midsize companies (100–250 FTEs) usually offer nonelderly employees health insurance coverage but are less likely to offer health promotion programs. Nonelderly employees in small companies (≤100 FTEs) are unlikely to have health insurance coverage through their employer, and small companies are unlikely to provide health promotion programs. Small and midsize companies employ most of the workers in the United States, so the gap in health program offerings and health insurance coverage is significant for the majority of workers in America. Many small business employees are at risk for injury, illness, and death, and the type of work may contribute to unhealthy lifestyles, stress, and chronic diseases. Unhealthy workers are more likely to be absent, less productive, and use more health care resources compared to healthy workers. Therefore, small and midsize businesses have one of the greatest opportunities to improve the health of their employees and prevent illness and injury through workplace health programs and health insurance (Lang, 2017; Terry, 2017).

Changes in Work and Workplaces

Changes in work and workplaces have many implications for health. Figure 13–3 addresses how work shapes the health of workers and their families, including exposing workers to physical and psychological risks as well as offering work-related resources and opportunities. The risks and resources result in both positive and negative outcomes, which have an effect on physical and mental health.

Average American adults spend about half their waking hours at work. When they have untreated health problems, they do not perform effectively. Poor employee health results in absenteeism, accidents, and high health care and related costs. In 2015, American businesses lost more than $225 billion dollars due to lost productivity from worker illness and injury (Centers for Disease Control and Prevention Foundation, 2015). Employees who are above normal weight, or have at least one chronic health problem, take an extra 450 million sick days compared with healthy workers. Employers, employees, and society collectively bear the cost of poor workforce health (McLellan, 2017).

A relatively new concept in workplace health is *presenteeism*. Presenteeism is being present at work, in spite of being ill due to a health problem. Presenteeism results in a decrease in overall work performance. It is a serious problem for the employee as well as the employer, as it has been estimated to be much costlier than absenteeism in terms of revenue due to loss of job productivity (Pohling, Buruck, Jungbauer, & Leiter, 2016). *Presenteeism* may occur as a result of job pressures, including job uncertainty or insecurity, understaffing, insufficient staffing, high time pressure, and high team responsibilities.

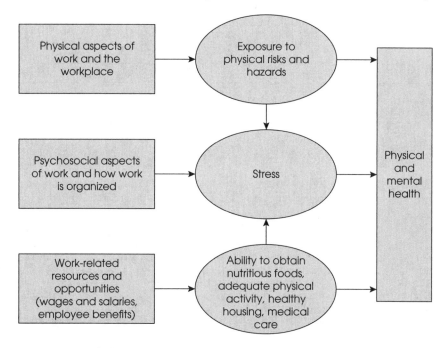

FIGURE 13–3   How Work Shapes Health for Workers and Their Families

Source: Robert Wood Johnson Foundation Commission to Build a Healthier America. Issue Brief 4: Work Matters for Health, December 2008. Accessed at http://www.commissiononhealth.org/ PDF/0e8ca13d-6fb8-451d-bac8-7d15343aacff/Issue%20Brief%204%20Dec%2008%20-%20Work%20 and%20Health.pdf

Figure 13–4 describes work-based strategies to improve the health of employees and their families and reduce both *presenteeism* and absenteeism. Employers need to be alert to work-related risks and stressors and provide a supportive environment with the resources and services needed to reduce stress and other health risks.

Workplaces offer access to large numbers of adults and serve as a vehicle for delivering interventions at multiple levels: individual, interpersonal, environmental, and organizational. Workplace programs have the potential to (1) increase healthy behaviors, (2) increase productivity, (3) decrease presenteeism and absenteeism, (4) decrease health care and disability expenditures, and (5) increase employee morale (Harris, 2016). These outcomes ultimately result in a more productive and competitive workforce.

Workplace programs have access to employees over an extended period and have the ability to modify policies and promote environmental change to enhance healthy behaviors. Also significant is the potential to modify social norms and increase interpersonal support for coworkers who are motivated to change.

Workplace programs increase employee awareness of the need to adopt healthy behaviors, facilitate change, and create supportive environments for change (Harris, Hannon, Beresford, Linnan, & McLellan, 2014). Awareness occurs through health newsletters and posters and signs in the workplace. Programs may be offered as annual

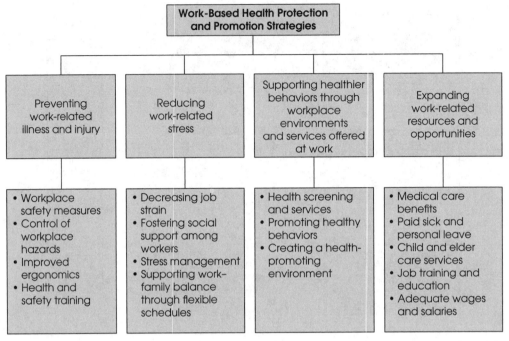

FIGURE 13–4 Work-Based Strategies to Improve Health

Source: Robert Wood Johnson Foundation Commission to Build a Healthier America. Issue Brief 4: Work Matters for Health, December 2008. Accessed at http://www.commissiononhealth.org/ PDF/0e8ca13d-6fb8-451d-bac8-7d15343aacff/Issue%20Brief%204%20Dec%2008%20-%20Work%20 and%20Health.pdf

events, such as health fairs or health screening, or comprehensive multilevel programs. They may also be offered individually through interactive programs on computers or mobile apps. Membership fees may be subsidized to encourage workers to join an off-site exercise facility. Environments can be changed to be more supportive of healthy behaviors, such as offering healthier food choices in the cafeteria or a walking path near the workplace. Programs may include an on-site exercise facility as well as classroom and/or online resources that address topics such as nutrition/weight control, smoking, control substance use, and stress (see Chapters 6, 7, and 8). Mobile health applications (apps) that supplement classroom programs enable employees to self-monitor their behaviors and minimize face-to-face interactions, potentially decreasing program costs.

A multifaceted on-site program is likely to attract and retain a broader spectrum of workers. It is also more cost-effective. These types of programs also are more likely to have successful long-term results if they include risk reduction counseling, modify workplace policies, and make changes in the physical work environment. For example, *smoke-free* workplaces made a major contribution to the decline of cigarette smoking in the United States. This policy change also resulted in a decrease in exposure of non-smokers to environmental tobacco smoke.

Workplaces create a cultural milieu that either supports or discourages participation in health promotion programs. The leadership and attitudes of executives and managers influence participation rate and engagement in health-promoting activities. Offering a variety of health promotion programs, using different approaches, increases the appeal of programs to employees of diverse cultural backgrounds, skills, and ages (Marzec, 2017).

Programs are more likely to succeed when they not only address multiple risk factors, but also integrate family members and the community. Including families in health promotion programs lowers health care costs, as many large employers pay the health care costs for family members as well as employees. Smokers are more likely to have spouses/family members who also smoke, and employees with physically active spouses and children are more likely to be active themselves.

Changing the workplace culture, or creating new social norms, is central to long-term change. Another strategy that is gaining in popularity is offering incentives, such as paid time off or gift cards. Other successful strategies include setting and monitoring goals for change, providing the resources needed to change, such as exercise facilities, offering tailored programs that meet individual needs, and marketing the program to increase awareness and motivation to participate (Harris, 2016).

Community involvement can begin by tapping the expertise of teachers and school nurses. Their collaboration with leaders of workplace programs can promote consistency and integration of health promotion concepts across the workplace and schools. In addition, other community organizations can be recruited to share exercise facilities and programs. These strategies will facilitate "seamless" health promotion programming in communities, which has the potential to increase behavior change efforts across the life span.

Costs and Benefits of Workplace Health Promotion Programs

A growing body of evidence indicates that health promotion programs are effective in promoting behavior change (Lang, Cluff, Payne, Matson-Koffman, & Hampton, 2017; Ostbye, Stroo, Eisenstein, & Dement, 2016; Terric & Winslow, 2015). However, some employers still question the cost-effectiveness of implementing wellness programs in the workplace, even if the return on investment (ROI) justifies their cost. Wellness programs include lifestyle management and disease management. Lifestyle management programs focus on employees with health risks, such as smoking, obesity, and poor physical activity habits, and implement programs to reduce these risks and prevent the development of chronic diseases. The goal of disease management programs is to assist employees who have a diagnosed chronic health problem, such as type 2 diabetes or hypertension, successfully manage the disease. In 2014, the RAND Corporation completed a review of employee wellness programs and reported that they reduced overall health care costs by about $30 per member per month. Disease management programs accounted for 87% of these savings, driven by fewer hospital admissions and emergency room visits. However, more employees participated in lifestyle management programs (87%) than disease management programs (13%), and the ROI differed significantly between the two components: $3.80 for disease management and $0.50 for lifestyle management for every dollar invested (Mattke et al., 2013).

Changes did occur in the lifestyle management programs. A review of the health behaviors targeted showed positive changes in physical activity, smoking, weight and body mass index, and cholesterol. However, the health outcomes (the potential to prevent chronic diseases) related to these changes take many years to evaluate. Also, the study did not measure absenteeism, productivity, or retention, so the potential cost saving related to these outcomes was not considered. In addition, employee morale and changes in workplace culture were not measured.

The RAND study points to the complexity of measuring ROI in health promotion and wellness programs. Employers want to improve employee health in the most cost-effective way and improve productivity. However, evaluation of costs is complex as so many factors are involved. The health outcomes for changing lifestyles may not be seen for many years. In addition, program participation and success depends on many factors, including marketing, communication, support, resources, program type and intensity, and perceived benefits (O'Donnell, 2015). In spite of the complexity of measuring cost outcomes, some employers may misinterpret published results of cost-effectiveness research and decrease their financial investment, replacing higher cost programs with less costly, less comprehensive interventions. Workplace wellness programs offer both short- and long-term benefits; however, reducing health care coverage and increasing employee insurance costs are sure to have a negative effect on the workforce.

A growing body of research indicates that the presence of health and safety programs in companies is associated with higher financial performance in the marketplace (Fabius et al., 2016). Companies that have effective wellness and safety programs have higher stock values and outperform companies that have not been recognized for excellence in these programs (Grossmeier et al., 2016). Although other factors play a role in a company's financial performance, current evidence substantiates the value of investing in employee health, as good employee health is good business.

Worksite programs are common in larger corporations. However, companies that employ fewer than 50 FTEs have not committed to these programs due to financial and human resource constraints. Programs in small workplaces are easier to communicate as they have a smaller numbers of employees who are more likely to be familiar with each other. Familiarity may facilitate mutual support for change (Wollesen, Menzel, Drogemuller, Hartwig, & Mattes, 2017). Factors that promote successful implementation of programs in small and midsize companies are similar to those in larger companies. Smaller companies can also take advantage of mobile health application or Web-based programs and develop collaborative relationships with the community to share facilities and program expertise.

Participation in Workplace Programs

Participation is the critical component of worksite health programs. It is also the major *weakness*, as the average attendance is consistently less than 50% (McCleary et al., 2017). In the National Healthy Worksite Program, smaller companies reported the greatest attrition rates (Lang et al., 2017). Many workers hesitate to identify health problems that may not be evident, as they fear loss of their job and/or privacy. Other barriers to participation include lack of time, use of off-site facilities and programs, and lack of intrinsic motivation. Lower participation rates may also be due to lack of social support, low job control, fatigue due to job demands, and programs conducted during leisure time (Jorgensen, Villadsen, Burr, Punnett, & Holtermann, 2016). Attention to these barriers will result in greater participation and potentially positive outcomes.

Some of the most *effective practices* to increase participation in worksite health programs include (1) management support, (2) employee involvement in program planning, (3) incentives/rewards, (4) marketing and communication activities, and (5) workplace policy and environmental changes. Incentives have become more popular in recent years, as research has shown greater changes in persons who receive incentives, such as reduced health insurance costs (Schneider, Bassett, Rider, & Sanders, 2016).

Innovative strategies continue to be implemented to improve the work environment. The nature of many work settings involves sitting for long periods, and sedentary behavior is associated with increased health risks. To reduce prolonged sitting, employees are using treadmill desks, stand-up desks, or other moving workstations, as well as large exercise balls in place of chairs. Other strategies include incorporating prompting software on the work computer or mobile or wearable technology to remind employees to stand at certain time periods to decrease uninterrupted sedentary periods (Stephenson, McDonough, Murphy, Nugent, & Mair, 2017). These efforts demonstrate companies' concern for their employees' health, and promote a health-promoting culture. Health is a business issue and an essential component of the business plan.

Nurses play a significant role in promoting healthy workplaces for their clients. Employers are responsible for ensuring that workplace demands are reasonable, expectations are clear, and goals are achievable. However, employees are ultimately responsible for achieving their own work–life balance. The nurse needs to assess the workplace environment and encourage the integration of health promotion programs that promote adequate rest, nutritious food, regular exercise, and stress reduction. The nurse can also serve as a role model and provide leadership in making positive changes in the workplace.

THE COMMUNITY AS A SETTING FOR HEALTH PROMOTION

Communities play a major role in promoting the health of its members. Community-centered approaches promote health and health equity and increase people's control over their health. Active involvement of individuals in the community is essential to bring about community change. Basic concepts in the community approach to health promotion are (1) self-determination, (2) shared decision-making, (3) bottom-up planning, (4) community problem solving, and (5) cultural relevance. Community-centered approaches to health promotion use participatory methods to involve members to make change. These approaches build community capacity to engage members of the community to create successful partnerships. The philosophy underlying the community-based approach is that health promotion is likely to be more successful when the community at risk identifies its own health concerns, develops its own programs, forms a board or other structure to make policy decisions, and identifies resources for program implementation.

Partnerships play a significant role in promoting the health of the community. A successful community partnership requires that all participants have ongoing knowledge of the community and view the community as a true partner. Community programs are developed through an ongoing negotiation process among all members. A community partnership, based on honesty and respect, requires time, people, and financial resources.

In community capacity building for health promotion, community members develop the knowledge and skills to address health problems within the community.

Community members assume leadership to bring about change by promoting participation of community members, collaborating with community organizations, negotiating for resources, and sharing control in decision-making. Community capacity building and ownership of health promotion projects are successful when community members are equal partners in planning, implementing, and evaluating the program. Community capacity building occurs through engaging the community and building partnerships to promote change.

Health Promotion in Low-Income, Culturally Diverse Communities

Community-based health promotion programs offer an ideal approach to reach communities with limited resources. Community-based health promotion interventions in low-income, racially and ethnically diverse communities have targeted obesity, physical activity, and healthy eating (Bernstein et al., 2017; Chuang, Sharma, Perry, & Diamond, 2017; Sato et al., 2016). The positive results of many programs provide evidence of the need to implement programs to promote change in communities with limited resources. Mobile health apps also have potential to supplement on-site programs conducted with low-income diverse samples, as they promote self-monitoring of behaviors (Peek, 2017). Community-based organizations (CBOs) also play a role in promoting health in diverse communities (Bloemraad & Terriquez, 2016). CBOs have the capacity to engage members of these communities, helping them build networks and a sense of empowerment to engage in healthy behaviors. They offer a place to meet, leadership, training, and resources.

Community health workers have been successful around the world working with low-income or diverse communities to improve and promote health and prevent diseases. They have increased in popularity in the United States because of rising health care costs and their success working with culturally diverse populations. Community health workers with adequate training and supervision have the potential to play an important role in community health promotion, supplementing the role of health care professionals (Perry, Zulliger, & Rogers, 2014).

When integrating community health workers into health promotion and disease prevention roles in the community, the nurse needs to lay the groundwork, using the following steps:

- Establish rapport with the community
- Hire workers from the targeted community to gain the trust and participation of community residents
- Share program ownership and decision-making with community health workers
- Closely link health workers with community health and social service agencies for professional backup

Health promotion services that are provided where people live, work, worship, and play are likely to be more successful than those offered *outside* the community. For example, creating awareness and offering programs in churches or health screenings in malls enable people to remain in their communities where they spend their leisure time. The synergy of bringing community strengths and resources together, and the empowerment that results from early successes, warrants continued attention to designing and planning community-wide, culturally sensitive health promotion programs.

CREATING HEALTH PARTNERSHIPS

A major strategy to optimize the health of communities is to establish health partnerships across settings. *Community health partnerships* are collaborative relationships between people and organizations that are committed to work together to achieve a common purpose. Community health partnerships recognize the value of community members, corporate leaders, and health care providers, who work together to create programs that address the health needs of the community. Partnerships optimize the combined resources of all partners to achieve mutual goals to empower individuals and families to improve their health as well as the health of the community. Initially, the following questions assess the community's readiness for participation:

1. Is current community problem solving an individual or collective effort?
2. How in touch are individuals in the community with each other?
3. What are the units of interaction (e.g., neighborhoods, townships, or housing complexes)?
4. Does crime or other factors prevent individuals from interacting?

An important goal of community partnerships for health promotion is *empowerment*. Community empowerment is a social action process in which individuals and groups act to gain control over their lives by changing their social and political environments (Minkler, 2012). Partnerships create conditions that empower the community. Partnerships for health promotion have the potential to bring about institutional and policy changes that affect many people. The commitment of partnerships to the broader goals of positive social, structural, and individual change is essential to improving the overall health of communities. Strategies for building successful partnerships include the following:

- Develop trusting and equitable relationships before beginning program
- Be physically present in the community
- Include all stakeholders in recruitment of partnership members
- Encourage diversity by recruiting multiple stakeholders
- Recruit community leaders
- Conduct a community event
- Understand and address partner motives for participating
- Establish ground rules (codes of conduct)
- Agree on a common vision
- Choose a respected, trusted leader
- Create decision-making protocols that are fair and open
- Ensure follow through on goals
- Anticipate and manage conflict and frustration among members (Centers for Disease Control and Prevention, Division of Tuberculosis Elimination, 2007; Matthew, 2017)

Effective interviewing and communication skills are essential. Strategies include asking open-ended, nonleading questions, listening to members, being neutral and calm, being clear about limitations, and using plain or simple language (Matthew, 2017).

TABLE 13–3 Principles of Community Partnerships

Find the right mix of ownership and control among partners

Recognize the assets of all partners

Develop relationships based on mutual trust and respect

Acknowledge the difference between community input and active community involvement

Resolve ethnic, cultural, and ideological differences between and among partners

Building partnerships requires substantial time and effort. Putting collaborative partnerships into practice is complex and represents a challenge for all the stakeholders. It is important for all stakeholders to both acknowledge their diverse interests in the early stages of the partnership and implement strategies to address any cultural barriers that exist. Partnership principles are described in Table 13–3. These principles enable stakeholders to learn to respect the diversity and strengths of all members and create a shared vision for community change.

Health partnerships address health care expenditures by advocating for funding, prevention, and health promotion services. Politically active partnerships can redirect public and private health care dollars to allocations that emphasize population-based health care services and clinical preventive services. Nurses are valuable members of community health partnerships. Knowledge of health promotion, community health, community engagement, and partnership building will enable nurses to take a leadership role in promoting community health.

The Role of Partnerships in Educating Health Professionals

Collaborative partnerships between communities and universities are critical for teaching nursing and other health care professional students how to engage communities to address health inequities and promote health. Opportunities to become immersed in the community enable students to experience diverse cultures; learn how conditions in communities influence the health of its members; participate with community members to identify and prioritize community health issues; and implement strategies to empower communities to solve their health issues. In addition, partnerships offer opportunities for students to practice in diverse settings, enhancing their skills and providing quality health care and counseling. Collaborative partnerships opportunities include experiences working with community organizations, community members, other health professionals, and policy makers to address community needs. These opportunities should also be available to professional nurses through continuing professional development.

Common characteristics of successful health professional programs that promote community partnerships have been identified (National Academies of Science, Engineering, & Medicine, 2016). Community-based learning experiences are a core component, as well as learning to work collaboratively with other professionals to address local needs. Learning to advocate for public policy to address community needs is also considered essential. Community partnership building, as discussed above, will facilitate community engagement and empowerment to address health inequities and the social determinants of health.

Multiple strategies can be implemented to provide student opportunities to engage in the community. Beginning students in a baccalaureate nursing education program can experience various aspects of the role of community health worker by distributing health education materials in a community, participating in screening programs, helping to organize health fairs, and collecting data such as surveying vending machines and fast-food stores to assist in community health assessments.

Advanced baccalaureate students with a greater understanding of the role of culture and socio-ecological principles might promote physical activity programs at schools and workplaces, assist community residents in identifying environmental health risks, and provide educational programs in the community to groups of individuals who have similar health risk profiles.

Master's and doctoral level students can collaborate with faculty and community member representatives to form teams to train and supervise community health workers in underserved communities or teach leadership skills to community members. They can also learn and apply effective communication skills to assist in developing community partnerships.

Community partnerships have played an important role in improving the health of many communities by creating community capacity and empowerment. In addition, partnerships set expectations that the university will function as a partner with other systems in the community to shape public policy that will promote healthy living in a safe environment.

HEALTH PROMOTION IN COMMUNITY NURSE-LED CLINICS AND PRACTICES

Ongoing changes in the U.S. health care system, including persistent health inequities, an expanding elderly population with chronic diseases, and large numbers of uninsured persons, have resulted in increased health care needs and greater demands on health care resources. The need to limit and decrease health care costs is shifting health care from the hospital setting to the community where people live and work. Primary care, an early element of health care delivery system reform, has been expanded, based on early evidence that primary care practitioners provided higher quality care at lower costs.

Nursing roles have also expanded to help meet the health care system demands. Advanced practice nurses, including nurse practitioners and advanced practice nurses with doctorates of nursing practice (DNP) degrees, are now playing major roles to promote health, prevent disease, and manage health problems cost-effectively in community-based nurse-led clinics and primary care settings (Wallace & Daroszewski, 2015). Evidence has documented the benefits of nurse-led clinics on patient outcomes, satisfaction, and cost-effectiveness, paving the way for nurses to play even greater roles in health care and health promotion (Randall, Crawford, Currie, River, & Betihavas, 2017).

The hallmark of nurse-led community clinics and nurse-led practices is primary care, where the focus is on "the individual and family" rather than "the presenting illness." Many families prefer health care from nurse practitioners in a client-friendly setting within their community that is respectful of their unique needs. Community-based, nurse-led clinics and practices offer multiple services, including health promotion and prevention counseling, behavioral interventions to promote healthy lifestyles, and screening to detect health risks.

An example of a long-term, successful nurse-led community-based practice is the University of South Carolina Children and Family Healthcare Practice. The center opened in 1998 to provide primary health care for children placed in the foster care system. The practice has expanded to offer comprehensive services to children and families in the surrounding community. Nurse practitioner faculty members are the primary care providers. In addition, they mentor nursing, pharmacy, and social work students who participate in the clinic as part of their clinical experience. A major focus of the nurse-led practice is education and prevention to teach patients and their families healthy lifestyle habits. Reimbursement is mainly from Medicaid, as three-fourths of the clients are Medicaid recipients. In 2016, the practice served over 7,000 patients.

Nurse-led community-based practices are usually located in diverse communities, accessible to the populations they serve; they may be close to schools to meet the health and illness needs of children and adolescents, in malls, and in low-income housing developments. Nurse-led retail clinics are located in pharmacies and operated by large businesses, such as Walgreens and CVS pharmacies. Nurse-led convenient care clinics are located in grocery stores and "big box" stores. These clinics emphasize convenience, no appointments, and short wait times (Wallace & Daroszewski, 2015). They provide health education as well as chronic disease management services that are usually more cost-effective and result in greater client satisfaction.

Nurses practice collaboratively with other health care professionals to promote health in culturally diverse ethnic/racial populations in low-income, urban and rural settings. As members of interdisciplinary teams and in leadership or independent roles, advanced practice nurses have the opportunity to address both individual- and community-level health problems. Community-based nurse-led clinics offer a unique way to gain familiarity with the community and its health problems. Nurses' unique knowledge and practice place them in positions to engage in policy advocacy to address care access issues and health inequities in communities (Xue & Intrator, 2016).

CONSIDERATIONS FOR PRACTICE TO PROMOTE HEALTH IN COMMUNITY SETTINGS

Multiple settings offer opportunities to provide health promotion programs. Knowledge of community health issues enables nurses to provide leadership in the design, development, implementation, and evaluation of health promotion programs in schools, workplaces, nurse-led practices, and primary care settings. Today's health problems are best solved by many sectors coming together in partnerships to address social and environmental conditions that compromise health. Community partnerships offer a way to communicate, collaborate, and empower to achieve solutions not attainable by single groups or organizations.

Nurses' holistic view promotes collaborative practice and enables them to empower communities to accomplish their health goals. The need for health care reform and the economic pressures for cost-effective, multidisciplinary, high-quality care places nurses in a unique position to provide leadership in multiple settings in the community. Community engagement, team building, and partnership building are concepts nurses need to understand to promote community health.

OPPORTUNITIES FOR RESEARCH IN COMMUNITY SETTINGS

The increased demand for health care resources has placed greater emphasis on the role of evaluation of community-based health promotion programs. Knowledge of the cost-effectiveness and both short- and long-term health outcomes will provide valuable information to advocate for resources and policies to promote healthy schools, workplaces, and communities. Suggested opportunities for research include the following:

1. Describe health promotion and disease prevention beliefs and practices in racially and culturally diverse families and communities as a basis for designing culturally sensitive interventions.
2. Identify facilitators to increase participation in workplace programs.
3. Identify factors that promote successful health-promoting behaviors in schools.
4. Test community partnership strategies that optimize community change.
5. Design valid and reliable community-level health outcome indicators.

Evidence suggests that successful community partnerships make a difference in promoting change in the health of the community. Additional research is needed to determine factors that facilitate and inhibit the sustainability of community partnerships, particularly in impoverished communities.

Summary

The development and maintenance of healthy lifestyles and healthy communities are critical components of a healthy population. Families, schools, workplaces, and the community all play a role in promoting health. Community-based programs that are designed, implemented, and evaluated in collaboration with community members increase buy-in and the likelihood of success. Community partnerships create a network of community members who can offer quality health promotion and prevention services.

Learning Activities

1. Identify a community-based health promotion program in a community of interest to you and assess its effectiveness by interviewing two persons who live in the community and have participated in the program.
2. Visit an elementary school and assess its health promotion activities for children. Make realistic, cost-effective recommendations, based on your assessment.
3. Identify a workplace health promotion program in your community. Assess its strengths and limitations from the perspectives of the employer and employee. How would you evaluate its effectiveness?
4. Develop three questions about the role and effectiveness of an advanced practice nurse in a community-based nurse-led practice. Interview a nurse practitioner and a client using your questions as a guide.

References

Bernstein, R., Schneider, R., Welch, W., Dressell, A., DeNomie, M., Kusch, J., & Sosa, M. (2017). Biking for health: Results of a pilot randomized controlled trial examining the impact of a bicycling intervention on lower-income adults. *Wisconsin Medical Journal, 116*(3), 154–160.

Bloemraad, I., & Terriquez, V. (2016). Cultures of engagement: The organizational foundation of advancing health in immigrant and low-income communities of color. *Social Science & Medicine, 165,* 214–222.

Bradley, B., & Green, A. (2013). Do health and education agencies in the United States share responsibility for academic achievement and health? A review of 25 years of evidence about the relationship of adolescents' academic achievement and health behaviors. *Journal of Adolescent Health, 52*(5), 523–532. doi:10.1016/j.jadohealth.2013.01.008

Bureau of Labor Statistics. (2017). *Employment Situation Summary Table A. Household data, seasonally adjusted.* Retrieved from https://www.bls.gov/news.release/empsit.a.htm

Carlin, A., Murphy, M., & Gallagher, A. (2016). Do intervention to increase walking work? A systematic review of interventions in children and adolescents. *Sports Medicine, 46*(4), 515–530. doi:10.1007/s40279-015-0432-6

Centers for Disease Control and Prevention. (2005). *National health education standards.* Retrieved from http://www.cdc.gov/healthyschools/sher/standards/index.htm

Centers for Disease Control and Prevention. (2011). School health guidelines to promote healthy eating and physical activity. *MMWR, 60*(5), 1–76.

Centers for Disease Control and Prevention. (2014a). *Healthy places, healthy people: A progress review on nutrition and weight status, & physical activity.* Retrieved from https://www.cdc.gov/nchs/ppt/hp2020/hp2020_nws-and_hp_progress_review_presentation.pdf

Centers for Disease Control and Prevention. (2014b). *Whole school, whole community, whole child model: A collaborative approach to learning and health.* Alexandria, VA: Author.

Centers for Disease Control and Prevention, Division of Tuberculosis Elimination. (2007). *Forging partnerships to eliminate tuberculosis. A guide and toolkit.* Publication No. 00-6552. Atlanta, GA: Author.

Centers for Disease Control and Prevention Foundation. (2015). *Worker illness and injury costs U.S. employers $225.8 billion annually.* Retrieved from https://www.cdcfoundation.org/pr/2015/worker-illness-and-injury-costs-us-employers-225-billion-annually

Chuang, R., Sharma, S., Perry, C., & Diamond, P. (2017). Does the CATCH early childhood program increase physical activity among low-income preschoolers? Results from a pilot study. *American Journal of Health Promotion,* 1–5.

Fabius, R., Loeppke, R., Hohn, T., Fabius, D., Eisenberg, B., Konicki, D., & Larson, P. (2016). Tracking the market performance of companies that integrate a culture of health and safety. *Journal of Occupational and Environmental Medicine, 58*(1), 3. doi:10.1097/JOM.0000000000000638

Grieco, L., Jowers, E., Errisuriz, V., & Bartholomew, J. (2016). Physically active vs. sedentary academic lessons: A dose response study for elementary student time on task. *Preventive Medicine, 89,* 98–103.

Grossmeier, J., Fabius, R., Flynn, J., Noeldner, S., Fabius, D., Goetzel, R., & Anderson, D. (2016). Linking workplace health promotion best practices and organizational financial performance. *Journal of Occupational and Environmental Medicine, 58*(1), 16–22. doi:10.1097/JOM.0000000000000631

Harris, J., Hannon, P., Beresford, S., Linnan, L., & McLellan, D. L. (2014). Health promotion in smaller workplaces in the United States. *Annual Review of Public Health, 35,* 327–342. doi:10.1146/annurev-publhealth-032013-182416

Harris, M. (2016). *The business case for employee health and wellness programs.* White paper prepared for the Society of Industrial and Organizational Psychology. Bowling Green, OH: Society of Industrial and Organizational Psychology.

Jorgensen, M., Villadsen, E., Burr, H., Punnett, L., & Holtermann, A. (2016). Does employee participation in workplace health promotion depend on the work environment? A cross-sectional study of Danish workers. *BMJ Open, 6,* e01516. doi:10.1136/bmjopen-2015-010516

Kolbe, L., Allensworth, D., Potts-Datema, W., & White, D. (2015). What have we learned from collaborative partnerships to concomitantly improve both education and health? *Journal of School Health, 85*(11), 766–774. doi:10.1111/josh.12312

Lang, J. (2017). Using employer case studies to highlight best practices and tailored strategies to build comprehensive workplace health programs. *American Journal of Health Promotion, 31*(1), 79–88.

Lang, J., Cluff, L., Payne, J., Matson-Koffman, D., & Hampton, J. (2017). The Centers for Disease Control and Prevention: Findings from the National Healthy Worksite Survey. *Journal of Occupational and Environmental Medicine, 59*(7), 631–641. doi:10.1097/JOM.0000000000001045

Langford, R., Bonell, C., Komro, K., Murphy, S., Magnus, D., Waters, E., . . . Campbell, R. (2017). The health promoting schools framework: Known unknowns and an agenda for future research. *Health Education & Behavior, 44*(3), 463–475.

Lewallen, T., Hunt, H., Potts-Datema, W., Zaza, S., & Giles, W. (2015). The whole school, whole community, whole child model: A new approach for improving educational attainment and healthy development of students. *Journal of School Health, 85*(11), 729–739. doi:10.1111/josh.12310

Marzec, M. (2017). The foundational influence of a workplace culture of health. *American Journal of Health Promotion, 31*(1), 77–79.

Matthew, R. (2017). Community engagement: Behavioral strategies to enhance the quality of participatory partnerships. *Journal of Community Psychology, 45*(1), 117–127. doi:10.1002/jcop.21830

Mattke, S., Liu, H., Caloyeras, J., Huang, C., van Busum, K., Khodyakov, D., & Shier, V. (2013). *Workplace Wellness Programs Study: Final Report.* RR-254-DOL. Santa Monica, CA: RAND Corporation. Retrieved from www.RAND.org/t/RR254

McCleary, K., Goetzel, R., Roemer, E., Berko, J., Kent, K., & de la Torre, H. (2017). Employer and employee opinions about workplace health promotion (wellness) programs: Results of the 2015 Harris Poll Nielsen Survey. *Journal of Occupational and Environmental Medicine, 59*(3), 256–263. doi:10.1097/JOM.0000000000000946

McLellan, R. (2017). Work, health, and worker wellbeing: Roles and opportunities for employers. *Health Affairs, 36*(2), 206–213. doi:10.1377/hlthaff.2016.1150

Minkler, M. (2012). *Community organizing and community building for health and welfare.* New Brunswick, NJ: Rutgers University Press.

National Academies of Science, Engineering, & Medicine. (2016). *A framework for educating health professionals to address the social determinants of health.* Washington, D.C.: National Academies Press.

Naylor, P., Nettlefold, L., Race, D., Hoy, C., Ashe, M., Higgins, J., & McKay, H. (2015). Implementation of school based physical activity interventions: A systematic review. *Preventive Medicine, 72*, 95–115.

O'Donnell, M. (2015). What is the ROI for workplace health promotion? It really does depend, and that's the point. *American Journal of Health Promotion, 29*(3), v–viii. doi:10.4278/ajhp.29.3v

Ostbye, T., Stroo, M., Eisenstein, E., & Dement, J. (2016). The effects of two workplace weight management programs and weight loss on health care utilization and costs. *Journal of Occupational and Environmental Medicine, 58*(2), 162–169.

Patton, G., Sawyer, S., Santelli, J., Ross, D., Afifi, R., Allen, N., . . . Azzpoardi, P. (2016). Our future: A

Lancet commission on adolescent health and wellbeing. *The Lancet, 387*(10036), 2423–2478.

Peek, M. (2017). Can mHealth interventions reduce health disparities among vulnerable populations? *Diversity and Equity in Health and Care, 14*(2), 44–45.

Penny, T., McIsaac, J., Storey, K., Kontak, J., Ata, N., Kuhle, S., & Kirk, S. (2017). A translational approach to characterization and measurement of health-promoting school ethos. *Health Promotion International*, 1–10. doi:10.1093/heapro/dax039

Perry, H., Zulliger, R., & Rogers, M. (2014). Community health workers in low-, middle-, and high-income countries: An overview of their history, recent evolution, and current effectiveness. *Annual Review of Public Health, 35*, 399–421. doi:10.1146/annurev-publhealth-032013-182354

Pohling, R., Buruck, G., Jungbauer, K., & Leiter, M. (2016). Work-related factors of presenteeism: The mediating role of mental and physical health. *Journal of Occupational Health Psychology, 21*(2), 220–234. doi:10.1037/a0039670

Randall, S., Crawford, T., Currie, J., River, J., & Betihavas, V. (2017). Impact of community based nurse-led clinics on patient outcomes, patient satisfaction, patient access and cost effectiveness: A systematic review. *International Journal of Nursing Studies, 73*, 24–33. doi:10.1016/j.ijnurstu.2017.05.008

Rasberry, C., Slade, S., Lohrmann, D., & Valois, R. (2015). Lessons learned from the whole child and coordinated school health approaches. *Journal of School Health, 85*(11), 759–765. doi:10.1111/josh.12307

Sato, P., Steeves, E., Carnell, S., Cheskin, L., Trude, A., Shipley, C., . . . Gittelsohn, J. (2016). A youth mentor-led nutritional intervention in urban recreation centers: A promising strategy for childhood obesity prevention in low-income neighborhoods. *Health Education Research, 3*(2), 195–206.

Schneider, P., Bassett, D., Rider, B., & Sanders, S. (2016). Physical activity and motivating factors of participants in a financially incentivized worksite wellness program. *International Journal of Health Promotion and Education, 54*(6), 295–303. doi:10.1080/14635240.2016.1174951

Smith, L., Norgate, S., Cherrett, T., Davies, N., Winstanley, C., & Harding, M. (2015). Walking school buses as a form of active transportation for children—A review of the evidence. *Journal of School Health, 85*(3), 197–210. doi:10.1111/josh.12239

Stephenson, A., McDonough, S., Murphy, M., Nugent, C., & Mair, J. (2017). Using computer, mobile and wearable technology enhanced interventions to reduce sedentary behavior: A systematic review and meta-analysis. *International Journal of Behavioral Nutrition and Physical Activity, 14*, 105. doi:10.1186/s12966-017-0561-4

Stylianou, M., Kulinna, P., van der Mars, H., Mahar, M., Adams, M., & Amazeen, E. (2016). Before-school running/walking club: Effects on student on-task behavior. *Preventive Medicine Reports, 3,* 196–202.

Terric, L., & Winslow, C. (2015). Workplace stress management interventions and health promotion. *Annual Review of Organizational Psychology and Organizational Behavior, 2,* 583–603. doi:10.1146/annurev-orgpsych-032414-111341

Terry, P. (2017). The art of health promotion ideas for improving health outcomes. *American Journal of Health Promotion, 30*(6), 475–488. doi:10.1177/0890117116658726

Turunen, H., Sormunen, M., Jourdan, D., von Seelen, J., & Buijs, G. (2017). Health promoting schools—A complex approach and a major means to health improvement. *Health Promotion International, 32*(2), 177–184.

Vedanthan, R., Bansilal, S., Soto, A., Kovacic, J., Latina, J., Jaslow, R., . . . Fuster, V. (2016). Family-based approaches to cardiovascular health promotion. *Journal of the American College of Cardiology, 67*(14), 1725–1737. doi:10.1016/j.jacc.2016.01.036

Wallace, D., & Daroszewski, E. (2015). Convenient care clinic nurse practitioner impact analysis. *Journal of Nursing Education and Practice, 5*(9), 1–10. doi:10.5430/jnep.v5n9p1

Wollesen, B., Menzel, J., Drogemuller, R., Hartwig, C., & Mattes, K. (2017). The effects of a workplace health promotion program in small and middle-sized companies: A pre-posttest analysis. *Journal of Public Health, 25*(1), 37–47.

World Health Organization. (2017). *Health promoting schools. An effective approach to early action on non-communicable disease risk factors.* WHO/NMH/PND/17.3. Geneva, Switzerland: Author.

Wright, L. M., & Leahey, M. (2012). *Nurses and families: A guide to family assessment and intervention.* Philadelphia, PA: F. A. Davis Company.

Xu, H., Wen, L., & Rissel, C. (2015). Associations of parental influences with physical activity and screen time among young children: A systematic review. *Journal of Obesity.* doi:10.1155/2015/546925

Xue, Y., & Intrator, O. (2016). Cultivating the role of nurse practitioners in providing primary care to vulnerable populations in an era of health-care reform. *Policy, Politics, & Nursing Practice, 17*(1), 24–31. doi:10/1177/1527154416645539

CHAPTER 14

Promoting Health through Social and Environmental Change

OBJECTIVES

This chapter will enable the reader to:

1. Justify the rationale for describing health as a social goal.
2. Describe the role of public policy in promoting social and environmental change.
3. Discuss common health-damaging factors in the physical environment and their etiologies.
4. Describe the role of digital technology in promoting social and environmental change.
5. Discuss the relationship between access to health care and health equity.

Recognition that health is influenced by the social and physical environments in which people live has resulted in new approaches to achieve behavior change. As mentioned throughout previous chapters, large-scale change is best accomplished by altering social and environmental structures that influence health. To effectively promote a healthy society, the dynamic relationships among individuals, families, and their social and environmental context must be addressed. Health and social policies that fail to alleviate inequitable living conditions, such as poverty, violence, hunger, and unemployment; environmental threats, such as pollutants in worksites and communities; and inequities in access to care will perpetuate continuing high rates of morbidity and mortality in groups affected by these conditions. Individual and family efforts to adopt healthy behaviors also are likely to be ineffective in the presence of environmental constraints and policies that do not promote healthy living. The need for a social and environmental focus is not new, as the idea goes back in history as far as Hippocrates. Florence Nightingale also stressed the importance of paying attention to the environment to promote health.

HEALTH AS A SOCIAL GOAL

The health of societies, communities, families, and individuals is integrated and insepa-rable, reinforcing the need to address health as both an individual and a social goal. Health is shaped by individual, cultural, socioeconomic, and environmental circum-stances as shown in Figure 14–1. Publication of the social determinants of health by the World Health Organization (WHO) was a significant milestone, as it documented the social, cultural, economic, political, biological, and psychological factors that influence health (World Health Organization, Commission on Social Determinants of Health, 2008). Successful health promotion results when communities, health care profession-als, and policy makers work together to eliminate conditions that contribute to poor health, including inadequate housing, an unsafe water supply, poor nutrition or insuf-ficient food supply, chemical pollutants, poor or absent recreational facilities, inade-quate access to care, and lack of economic opportunity. Globally, governments acknowledge that behavior change strategies must be directed beyond the individual to include community- and policy-level factors.

Health as a social goal requires the integration of theories that address com-munity change (see Chapter 3) with theories that address individual behavior change (see Chapter 2), and health care policy. The three perspectives are comple-mentary. When nurses think only in terms of one-to-one relationships, the success of health promotion and prevention is severely limited.

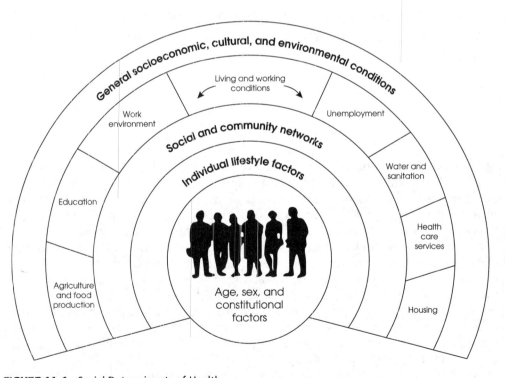

FIGURE 14–1   Social Determinants of Health

Source: Dahlgren and Whitehead (1993), accessible in Dahlgren and Whitehead (2007).

Health behavior change has been successful when the social context in which the individual lives is also targeted. For example, smoking cessation programs have succeeded, in part, due to addressing the individual addictive properties of smoking as well as the social context in which smoking occurs, including the advertising and sale of cigarettes. Tobacco public policy interventions have changed smoking behaviors through laws that reduce exposure to secondhand smoke in public facilities, excise taxes that increase the costs of cigarettes, and regulations to limit advertising and promotion of tobacco products.

The pursuit of health as a social goal requires that all community members (individuals, health professionals, organizations, policy makers) collaboratively engage in the process of change to address the social, political, and economic issues within their neighborhoods and communities. As discussed in earlier chapters, *empowerment* is a social action process through which individuals, groups, and communities work together to gain control over their lives and environments to improve their health through building healthy communities. The empowerment process begins with individuals. Empowered individuals form groups of individuals with similar concerns who work with community organizations and leaders to take actions to address their issues. *Community competence*, a concept related to empowerment, is a community's ability to come together to solve problems and obtain resources. Members of competent communities learn to

- Work collaboratively to identify their needs
- Achieve a working consensus on goals and priorities
- Agree on ways to implement goals
- Collaborate effectively to take action to accomplish goals

Health care professionals assist in the development of community competence by identifying natural community leaders who will facilitate community assessments and actions necessary to strengthen the community. Leadership development is a critical component in building community competence. As a community gains competence in negotiating for resources to address a particular problem, the community becomes empowered. This empowerment enhances problem-solving ability and capacity to address other problems that may arise. In addition, community members gain a sense of ownership through their participation in initiating and promoting change.

When health is considered a social goal as well as an individual one, the health promotion focus includes the community and public policy context. Priority decisions and strategies for social change to address lifestyle issues can best be made when community members work with local and state governments. Socioeconomic and environmental issues are addressed, as health is considered vital to the health and well-being of all individuals and the economic security of the community.

HEALTH IN A CHANGING DIGITAL SOCIAL ENVIRONMENT

Information and communication technology (ICT) has transformed our society to an information- and knowledge-based one in which we are connected globally. ICT is now playing a role in promoting health and reducing health inequities through the delivery of education and access to information resources. Individuals can connect to the Internet almost anywhere anytime of the day or night. Vast amounts of information can be shared to promote behavior change. Personal tracking devices enable consumers to monitor personal physiological data, such as heart rate, body weight, and physical activity. Tracking sensors can also be used in communities to track traffic and air quality. The uses of ICT continue to expand into all areas of life for individuals and communities.

Healthy People 2020 emphasizes equitable access to health information and improved health communication. The WHO Shanghai Conference on Health Promotion in 2016 emphasized the potential of digital technology to promote health by reaching greater numbers of people. Conference recommendations served as a resource in the development of the *Healthy People 2030* framework (Kickbusch & Nutbeam, 2017; Secretary's Advisory Committee on National Health Promotion and Disease Prevention Objectives for 2030, 2017). These initiatives are based on evidence that shows improved health communication and access to information is associated with healthier lifestyle choices, improved client–provider communication, greater participation in health decisions, and greater treatment adherence.

Mobile technologies have rapidly expanded into health promotion as noted throughout the chapters in this book. Short messaging service, or text messaging, is used to educate and answer questions about sexual health for teens, send reminders to take medications, enter health data, deliver health alerts, and offer health promotion programs to address nutrition, weight loss, and physical activity. An advantage of this technology is the widespread ownership of cell phones by diverse racial and ethnic groups throughout the world (Patrick et al., 2016). Cell phones have opened the door to new methods to empower individuals by delivering health information and health-promoting interventions in developed as well as developing nations.

Social media technologies provide an interactive environment for individuals to receive and share online information. Social media sites include social sharing sites, such as YouTube and Flickr; social networking sites, such as Facebook and MySpace; microblogs, including Twitter; virtual worlds, such as Second Life; and text messaging discussion forums or wikis. These technologies reach a broad audience and can be empowering for individuals, as they are able to obtain and share health information, solve problems, and gain diverse insights and perspectives through interactions with others who may or may not have expertise. Because multiple opportunities exist for employing this technology, federal agencies now use social media for government purposes. For example, electronic input was solicited to comment on the *Health People 2030* goals and the proposed revised federal nutrition guidelines.

Comprehensive, computerized health assessments are used to tailor health promotion programs to the knowledge, beliefs, motivations, and prior health behaviors of diverse individuals and families. Personal computers in the home and public libraries offer informational resources to answer questions and provide access to support and discussion groups.

Clients and their health care professionals now link electronically as well. The electronic personal health record (PHR; see Chapter 4) enables individuals to communicate with health care providers. An electronic PHR enables clients to have access to their personal data, act as stewards of their information, and take an active role in their own health. The PHR is a tool to help maintain health and wellness through access to credible information and data, as well as a means to help manage risk factors or promote health. Technological challenges, organizational barriers, economic and market forces, and individual obstacles have limited the nationwide adoption of PHR. However, adoption is a national priority and is ongoing in the government and private sectors.

The information era has also brought about changes that can empower families. Interactive computer technology enables parents to work at home. They can also obtain health information without visiting a health care provider. The Internet revolution is reshaping health promotion, as individuals now conduct health information searches, share information with their families, and ask informed questions of their health care providers.

The information revolution continues to challenge health professionals to think creatively about the delivery of health promotion programs and the potential consequences of this technology on society. Application of these technologies in culturally diverse, low-income communities remains a major challenge due to factors such as varying degrees of computer skills, Internet access, health literacy, and financial stability. Computer skills need to be taught using strategies that account for health literacy levels. Sites to access computers should be available in diverse communities. Although the digital divide has narrowed, rural communities continue to face technology challenges, including the unavailability of broadband services. Public education should be designed for underserved groups to learn how to find and use health information for healthy lifestyle changes.

The digital revolution has its limitations as well. Poverty and illiteracy, costs, security, privacy, and lack of standards continue to challenge the application of ICT. The information provided on social media sites may not be scientifically accurate or credible. In addition, the digital divide further marginalizes socially disadvantaged groups. Another limitation is the pitfall of self-diagnosis, using websites and apps that may not be credible, resulting in inaccurate diagnoses and possible delays in seeking medical care with fatal consequences (Ortega-Navas, 2017).

A critical concern of the use of digital technologies in health promotion is the emphasis on individual responsibility for health, which may divert attention away from the social determinants of health, where greater emphasis is needed (Lupton, 2014). The ethical implications of collecting large amounts of information from individuals have not received adequate attention. Nurses and all health care providers must be at the forefront in assisting clients to understand the privacy and security issues and teaching them how to find and evaluate reliable information. In addition, strategies are needed to apply digital technologies to address the social determinants of health in communities and to assist in the development of public policy.

PROMOTING HEALTH WITH PUBLIC POLICY

Shaping health policies in the public and private sectors to improve health for populations is widely advocated. Policies set goals and limits and define choices. Personal, social, and political factors all influence the development and implementation of health policy. For example, at the personal level, changes in public sentiment have influenced the development of health policy related to smoking in public places in the United States. At the political level, lobbyists have been successful in maintaining the economic interests of the food industries to prevent changes in food content, such as sugar or salt. On a more positive note, public policy has resulted in removal of cigarette commercials from television.

The idea of developing policies for healthier communities is not new. Historically, local governments provided environmental safeguards against infectious diseases. Social, economic, and environmental factors also need attention. Policy formulation to promote health begins at the local level, through identification of problems and development of local ordinances to implement change.

The U.S. government plays a major role in regulating health behavior. State and federal policies regulate a range of health behaviors, including alcohol, tobacco, seat belt use, food safety, and drug use. In addition, the federal government plays a major role in payment for health care services, through Medicaid and Medicare.

The *Healthy People 2020* and *Healthy People 2030* federal initiative's overarching goals are to achieve health equity and eliminate health disparities, and to create social and physical environments that promote good health for all. These goals challenge local, state, and federal governments, as well as policy makers, to promote policies that affect entire populations to address social determinants. Policies should focus on both downstream and upstream factors to promote health. For example, local governments can limit youth access to tobacco in neighborhood markets and vending machines. In addition, local and state policies can be developed to target economic development in communities with high unemployment or promote safe housing in poor neighborhoods. Long-term changes result from modifying upstream factors, or the conditions under which people live.

Local and national policy making can be beneficial for health promotion. Policy making at the local level eliminates the trickle-down time for a policy to have an influence in the community. Community and political leaders, along with local and state health departments, can advise and advocate large-scale changes to promote health. At the national level, the government's role in health promotion includes such things as writing guidelines for healthy eating and physical activity; eliminating environmental contaminants; facilitating access to safe housing, nutritious food, and green space; and facilitating access to quality health care (Whitsel, 2017).

Policy making is value driven, dynamic, often chaotic, and is about social influence, as it involves persuasion, attitude change, decision-making, and compromise. Facts, or science-based information, are usually used in the early phases of policy development to identify problems and solutions, including the economic costs. However, non-science-based, or less verifiable information from stakeholders who offer their informed judgments and personal experiences also is used to promote the legitimacy of a proposed policy. Both types of information are needed to gain support for successful policy making. Although scientific knowledge is critical, stakeholders also need to be informed about the political costs, as well as the resources needed to implement the policy. This additional information aids consensus development. Evidence indicates that collaborative decision-making, effective leadership, maintaining trust, and availability of resources are necessary at both the local and the national level to facilitate policy development (Weiss, Lillefjell, & Magnus, 2016).

Barriers to public health policy formulation are numerous.

- Policy makers may not be committed to the proposed change.
- Scientific evidence substantiating the issue has not been translated into user-friendly language.
- A dominant commercial market, such as the food industry, may hinder policy formulation.

- Timely, relevant information about the issue has not been consistently and personally communicated to policy makers.

These barriers substantiate the need for political champions, or knowledge brokers—respected persons who are articulate proponents of a particular policy and know how to work with policy makers to develop policy. Nurses and other health care professionals are often in positions to be knowledge brokers.

Addressing Obesity with Public Policy

The complex factors that promote obesity reinforce the need for policy interventions to target social and environmental conditions that influence individual lifestyle choices. Lessons learned from successful tobacco control, seat belt use, and the recycling movements have been incorporated in the obesity prevention movement to promote social change (see Graff, Kappagoda, Wooten, McGowan, & Ashe [2012] for a history of the obesity prevention movement). In addition to public policy, organizations play a role in efforts to combat obesity. For example, the Institute of Medicine, the Robert Wood Johnson Foundation, and the National Alliance for Nutrition and Activity Coalition have developed recommendations and programs to combat obesity. Former First Lady Michelle Obama drew attention to obesity in 2010 by launching the Let's Move! campaign. Examples of policies and actions that have occurred are the Healthy, Hunger-Free Kids Act of 2010, which instituted healthy lunches and healthy snacks in school vending machines and snack bars; legal action against food markets making misleading claims and promoting sugary food to young children; and the Safe Routes to School Program to promote walking. In 2014, sugary beverages were removed from all schools as a result of this act.

Local and state governments are key players in obesity prevention, as these entities have control over the social and built environments, including schools, food retailers, restaurants, and the transportation system. Examples of state policies and initiatives enacted in cities are banning sugary beverages in schools, limiting fast-food chains in poverty areas, designing transportation with everyone in mind, and attracting healthy retailers to low-income areas, which often have been saturated with alcohol retail shops and fast-food chains.

A national momentum to decrease sugary beverages in communities through either taxation or warning labels is underway in this country (Falbe & Madsen, 2017). Although there is evidence of the contributing role of sugar in obesity and type 2 diabetes, the beverage associations and juice companies continue to file lawsuits to prohibit warning labels on sugary beverages (Schillinger & Jacobson, 2016). Research evidence is limited; however, information to date indicates that a sugar tax generates revenue that can be used to promote healthy eating and decreases sugar consumption. The implementation of a sugar tax in several cities has demonstrated the feasibility of implementing widespread policy change to combat obesity.

Policies need to be legally feasible and financially viable. Financial viability focuses on the associated costs to implement the policy. If costs are prohibitive, governments may partner with private entities to implement the policy, such as building a recreational facility to increase physical programs, or they may redirect dollars from other programs to implement a policy if it is a priority. Last, policies can be enacted to generate revenues that can be directed to pay for new programs that promote health. For example, a tax on sugary beverages could generate revenue for programs to promote healthy eating.

Local and state health departments are positioned to serve as catalysts for institutional and community changes needed to target obesity. Local and state health policies can support healthy lifestyle programs in schools, communities, and worksites. Health policies that place a higher value on health and provide the resources to implement are a priority for all levels of government. Individuals, communities, and local and state governments, as well as the national government, are all active partners in the effort to prevent obesity.

Policies change behaviors by creating environments that promote healthy behaviors and change social norms. Changing social norms means indirectly influencing behaviors by creating a social climate where the unhealthy behavior becomes less desirable and acceptable. For example, when mandatory seat belt policies were enacted, many people rebelled and refused to wear them in spite of the consequences. However, over time, wearing seat belts is acceptable for almost everyone and probably would continue without a seat belt policy based on the lives saved. A shift in social norms related to eating unhealthy foods has started to occur as well. The momentum to tax sugary beverages is an example. Other examples include the addition of healthy choices at fast-food restaurants and the reduction of sugar in products targeted to children by food companies (Schwartz, Just, Chriqui, & Ammerman, 2017). Policies are necessary to shift social norms, as laws and regulations facilitate environmental changes that promote unhealthy behaviors.

Promoting Health in All Policies

The Helsinki Statement on Health in All Policies (HiAP) calls on governments around the world to ensure that health is considered in all policy making (World Health Organization, 2014). HiAP is a collaborative policy approach that considers the *health* implications of policy decisions and avoids making policies with harmful outcomes in order to improve health and eliminate health inequities. Attention to the health consequences of public policy making is expected to increase the accountability of policy makers. The Helsinki statement is considered a major step toward addressing the social determinants of health and builds on the public health tradition of collaboration to improve health (Rudolph, Caplan, Ben-Moshe, & Dillon, 2013).

Finland's broad approach to policy making to address the health problems of the Finnish people paved the way for the HiAP initiative (Kilpelainen et al., 2016). Policies targeting nutrition, such as dietary consumption of butter, fat content of milk, maximal salt content of some foods, salt labeling, and changing food subsidies, have led to substantial reductions in blood cholesterol levels and cardiovascular disease mortality rates in the population. The success of the Finnish policies is considered to be due to basing policy on sound evidence and promoting ethical policies and activities with and by the stakeholders (individuals and communities) to promote the political decision process.

Obesity is an example of the need for health in all policies, as both individual behaviors and the social and physical environments need to be addressed. Health professionals, in collaboration with schools, the food industry, multiple government sectors, and private organizations and businesses, can develop a comprehensive approach to begin to solve this complex problem. Health in all policies enables all stakeholders to work with policy makers to address problems more efficiently, as resources can be shared and redundancies are avoided.

PROMOTING HEALTH BY CHANGING THE PHYSICAL ENVIRONMENT

The quality of the physical environment in which people live is critical to the health of populations. Traditionally, environmental health practices have concentrated on controlling factors that are beyond the power of most people. However, individuals and communities have control over many external factors that promote healthy environments. Environmental factors that are health damaging are increasing, such as lead in water from aging plumbing in older homes and toxic runoff from shale gas extraction by hydraulic fracturing.

Addressing Health-Damaging Features of Environments

LEAD. The harmful effects of lead in the environment continue to be evident in communities. The sources of this pollutant include lead-based paint, contaminated water from old or soldered lead plumbing, and industry (Laidlaw et al., 2016). In addition, lead has been found in the surface soil and dust following years of accumulation from prior use of leaded gasoline. Younger children who ingest lead absorb greater amounts in their intestines than adults. Elevated lead levels lead to a lower intelligence quotient (IQ), behavior problems, and learning disorders due to its interference in the child's developing nervous system. Exposure and uptake is age dependent; children under 6 years of age are especially vulnerable (Laidlaw et al., 2016).

Although the number of children with elevated lead levels has been reduced, lead paint in older houses remains a childhood environmental disease hazard in the United States (Robert Wood Johnson & Pew Charitable Trusts, 2017). Windows have the highest level of lead paint and lead dust compared to other housing components. Contaminated lead dust settles on floors and windowsills and is ingested through normal hand-to-mouth contact. Exposure to high levels of lead can be fatal, but even low exposures can be toxic to the central nervous system, resulting in delayed learning, behavior problems, impaired hearing, and growth deficits.

The public health crisis in Flint, Michigan, in 2016, refocused attention on lead exposure in children and pregnant women. Drinking water was contaminated as it flowed through old lead pipes (Hanna-Attisha, LaChance, Sadler, & Schnepp, 2016). Lead exposure results from drinking the contaminated water and cooking foods with that water. Aging lead water pipes are found in older homes and more frequently in neighborhoods of poverty where resources are scarce. The federal government has a major role to play in solving this issue through the provision of financial and technical resources to eliminate lead sources and updating and enforcing protocols for lead removal. Priorities should focus on plumbing in houses built before 1986, paint in homes built before 1960, and cleaning contaminated soil (Robert Wood Johnsons Foundation & Pew Charitable Trusts, 2017). The detrimental neurological effects documented in children, which last into adulthood, make lead removal a priority, especially in communities of poverty, where the problem of lead-based paint, old plumbing systems, and lead in the soil due to gasoline has been found to be greater.

TOBACCO SMOKE. Many thousands of people are exposed each year to tobacco smoke and radon, the two leading indoor air hazards. Environmental tobacco smoke may cause lung cancer in nonsmokers. Children of parents who smoke are more likely to develop lower respiratory tract infections and middle ear infections than are children of parents who do not smoke. Asthma and other respiratory diseases are triggered or worsened by tobacco smoke and other substances in the air.

The most common forms of tobacco use among youth are electronic or e-cigarettes and hookah/water pipes. Adolescents in middle and high school are smoking e-cigarettes, and more than 25% have tried them (U.S. Department of Health and Human Services, 2016). E-cigarettes are battery-powered devices that heat a liquid containing nicotine, flavorings, and other additives into an aerosol that is inhaled. They are also called "e-cigs," "vape pens," and "tank systems." The amount of nicotine varies and the amount of nicotine in the vials used may be fatal if ingested orally or transdermally (Gilreath et al., 2016). The aerosol created by e-cigarettes contains chemical flavorings that have been linked with lung disease; organic compounds such as benzene, which is also found in car exhaust; and metals, including nickel, tin, and lead (U.S. Department of Health and Human Services, 2016).

The use of products containing nicotine is addictive, and the effects of nicotine exposure during adolescence can have long-lasting effects on the brain. Brain development continues until the early to mid-20s, so effects may be seen on attention, learning, and susceptibility to addiction.

In 2016, the Food and Drug Administration (FDA) started regulating the manufacturing, importing, packaging, labeling, advertising, and sale of e-cigarettes. Additional policies are needed to prevent access to e-cigarettes by youth. Adolescent users are more likely to subsequently use combustible tobacco products (Barrington-Trimis et al., 2016). In addition, e-cigarettes should be added to smoke-free policies, as they are currently permitted in public areas. Unfortunately, e-cigarettes are becoming a socially acceptable product and have the potential to renormalize tobacco use. Nurses should work with schools to educate adolescents and parents of the dangers of e-cigarettes and discourage their use.

RADON.   The second leading cause of lung cancer, after cigarette smoking, is exposure to radon, a well-known carcinogen that is a by-product of the breakdown of naturally occurring uranium in soil and rocks. When uranium decays in soil and rocks, it can seep into groundwater and diffuse into the air. It has a tendency to collect in mines and basements or other low places in homes, offices, and schools as it seeps through foundation cracks and plumbing gaps and drains or diffuses through construction materials (U.S. Environmental Protection Agency, 2009). Radon can dissolve in water and is found in homes that have their own wells. When radon is inhaled, it is deposited in the lungs and damages surrounding lung tissues, laying the foundation for lung cancer.

The best way to reduce radon is to educate the public to promote radon testing in homes and buildings to measure its concentration in the air. Since 1996, the Environmental Protection Agency (EPA) has led a campaign recommending that people test their homes and take action when radon concentrations exceed normal, safe levels. Do-it-yourself kits are available in retail stores, or the test can be done by a licensed contractor. Based on the strong evidence between radon exposure and lung cancer, programs to test and reduce radon in homes should be priorities to decrease the public health burden.

In 2013, U.S. Department of Housing and Urban Development (HUD) unveiled "Advancing Healthy Housing—A Strategy for Action," a plan that aims to make homes healthier. The plan encourages federal agencies to take actions to reduce the number of homes with high levels of radon, damaged paint, water leaks and roofing problems, and pests. This policy is a positive step in federal housing efforts to promote healthy housing and reduce health inequities for diverse populations. The EPA also issued guidelines for testing and mitigating radon levels in schools, and in 2015 a national radon action plan was released. These guidelines are available on the EPA website (www.epa.gov).

OUTDOOR AIR.   Outdoor air quality continues to be a global environmental problem, contributing to premature morbidity and mortality (Brook, Newby, & Rajagopalan, 2017). The effects are noted in cancer and respiratory and cardiovascular diseases. Motor vehicles account for one-fourth of emissions that produce ground-level ozone, the largest problem in air pollution. Although emission controls that were implemented in Europe and North America have decreased ozone precursors to a small degree, concerns remain due to the increased emission of these precursors in rapidly developing areas of the world. Agricultural emissions are the major sources of pollution in the eastern United States, Europe, Russia, and Asia, surpassing traffic and power generation pollution. Air pollutants other than traffic-related pollution include coal-fired power plants, emissions from domestic fires, and burning biomass fuels in less-developed countries. Emissions from heating and cooking in China and India have been found to have the greatest effect on premature mortality in these countries (Lelieveld, Evans, Fnais, Giannadaki, & Pozzer, 2015).

Worldwide, employers encourage and reward individuals to walk or use public transportation rather than drive their cars. Local and regional governments are designing public transportation systems that are available to outlying communities and streets that facilitate bicyclists and pedestrians. The increasing popularity of hybrid automobiles, which use alternative fuels, and battery-operated vehicles is a positive development. Nationally, support must be increased for alternative fuels, such as ethanol, by commercial and private vehicles and construction of clean energy mass transit systems. Air pollution from traffic is a preventable cause of disease. All health professionals should support campaigns to increase public awareness and advocate for community-level polices and resources needed to reduce the health effects of traffic pollution and smoke.

WATER.   Water quality is a major health concern because of protozoa and chemical contaminants, in addition to toxic metals, such as lead, discussed earlier. Industry and agricultural runoff is a known contaminant of water. For example, the development of intensive animal feeding operations has resulted in the discharge of improperly treated animal wastes into recreational and drinking water. Animal waste runoff may also contaminate the soil. Heavy metals, such as mercury, have been found in water contaminated by mining. Mercury has been found in the breast milk of mothers who live near gold-mining areas and consume fish from contaminated runoff water from mines. Mercury is used to extract the gold from the ore. Mercury is neurotoxic and a hazard to infant development.

HERBICIDES.   Concerns about the toxicity and health risks of glyphosate-based herbicides, commonly marketed under the trade name Roundup have recently been raised. Glyphosates are the most widely used agricultural herbicides in the world for killing weeds; its use has increased 100-fold since being introduced in 1974. Early research on glyphosate toxicity was conducted over 30 years ago and is outdated and insufficient, based on newer, more accurate research methods (Vandenberg et al., 2017). Glyphosates remain in the soil, posing multiple threats to the environment. It has been found in water from runoff and treatment of aquatic weeds. The World Health Organization's International Agency for Research on Cancer has reclassified it as probably carcinogenic in humans. Residues of glyphosates have been found in the food supply consumed by humans and animals (Bai & Ogbourne, 2016).

A consensus statement of concern about the use of glyphosate-based herbicides was published in 2016 to document health issues, based on published research, and offer recommendations for further research and monitoring (Myers et al., 2016). In addition to calling attention to water contamination due to surface runoff and leaching into groundwater and its probable carcinogenic effects, the statement stresses that current safe levels for humans are based on outdated science. Since Roundup is also a commonly used household weed killer, nurses need to be aware of the use of this herbicide and implement educational efforts to teach appropriate use of herbicides and the precautions needed when using glyphosate-based products.

SHALE GAS EXTRACTION.   Technological advances in the production of natural gas have resulted in a boom in an unconventional drilling method to extract natural gas from large underground shale deposits throughout the northeastern and southwestern United States, Europe, China, Argentina, and Australia. The method, which includes horizontal drilling and hydraulic fracturing or "fracking," uses a high-volume, high-pressure technique to drill thousands of feet into the earth to reach and fracture hard rocks (shale) to release natural gas. Large volumes of water, sand, and chemicals are used throughout the process to create fractures in the shale. Although the fracking process has been used for over 60 years, horizontal drilling is a recent advance that enables large amounts of natural gas to be extracted. As much as 5.5 million gallons of water can be used to fracture a gas well one time, and wells may be repeatedly fractured multiple times over the life of the well. Chemicals are also used throughout the operation to reach and release the gas. When the natural gas is released, anywhere from 30 to 70% of the fracturing solution is returned as backwater, which contains additional chemicals and radioactive material released during the process (Estrada & Bhamidimarri, 2016).

The disposal and storage of the backwater, a potential contaminant of soil and water, and air pollution emissions have become significant public health issues (Hays & Shonkoff, 2016). The natural gas industry is not required to disclose the chemicals used in the process, based on their exemption from the Toxic Release Inventory of the National Environmental Policy. The lack of disclosure presents a challenge to study the potential health effects. In addition, the federal government has exempted the industry from the Clean Water Act, the Clean Air Act, and the National Environmental Act. These actions have left a void in environmental regulation of the industry, leaving responsibility to the states, which traditionally have not required accountability for wastewater handling and disposal.

Research has documented health risks for humans and animals from contaminated drinking water, contaminated soil, and air pollution. In a review of papers published between 2009 and 2015, 84% of the studies reported public health hazards or adverse outcomes (Hays & Shonkoff, 2016). Almost three-fourths found water contamination

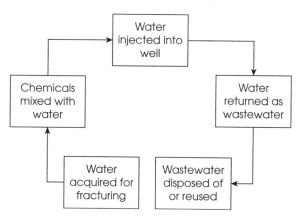

FIGURE 14–2   Hydraulic Fracturing Water Cycle: Potential Sources of Impact on Drinking Water Resources

Source: Adapted from U.S. Environmental Protection Agency (2016).

and almost all (87%) found elevated air pollution emissions. Aquifers have been found to be contaminated with chemicals, such as methane and boron, from the production process and seepage of wastewater. Toxic chemicals exceeding health standards have been measured in shale gas regions.

In 2016, the Environmental Protection Agency issued a final report on the impact of fracturing on drinking water (U.S. Environmental Protection Agency, 2016). Scientific evidence was found for contamination of drinking water due to water withdrawn for fracturing in areas of low water availability, spills and chemicals reaching groundwater, leakage from poorly constructed wells where backwater is stored, injection of poorly treated backwater into groundwater resources, discharge of poorly treated wastewater to surface water, and disposal of wastewater in unlined or poorly lined pits. Figure 14–2 highlights the hydraulic fracturing water cycle and potential sources of water contamination. The information was compiled to inform federal, state, and local agencies to take actions to protect the drinking water. However, no new regulations have been reported to date.

The backwater produced is one of the major concerns due to large volumes of contaminated water (Annevelink, Meesters, & Hendriks, 2016). The contaminated water is either stored in large open reservoirs, recycled on site, treated and discharged by wastewater treatment plants or reinjected in the ground. Reinjecting the water into the ground, or deep well injection, is known to significantly contribute to seismic activity with the potential to produce earthquakes (Estrada & Bhamidimarri, 2016). Open reservoirs have linings that fail, allowing seepage of polluted water. Disposal of water to public wastewater plants also results in poorly treated water, resulting in polluted drinking water and rivers. The main source of water pollution is sealing failures of abandoned wells, resulting in cracks, gaps, and pores that allow seepage into groundwater.

The potential multiple and serious health and environmental issues should be of concern for all health professionals. Rigorous regulations are needed to set standards and monitor the treatment of backwater. Nurses need to be advocates for transparency and careful monitoring of water, air, and chemicals as well as the effects of human and animal exposure to chemicals used in extracting the gas. Clients living in areas of gas extraction need education and ongoing monitoring to prevent or reduce exposure to contaminated water and air to the extent possible, until regulations can be implemented to improve safety standards.

The best available scientific knowledge about the relative risks of various pollutants to health is needed to understand the environmental risks of fracturing, rather than basing policies and regulations on what is emotionally appealing or politically or economically attractive. Many major environmental risks require intensive, multifaceted, and often long-term interventions to change attitudes and reallocate resources for their control. Nurses and other health professionals should play a proactive role by focusing on the local community and its worksites. All health professionals need to advocate for policies that will eliminate or reduce environmental pollutants; ensure safe waste disposal; and require ongoing monitoring and surveillance to verify good-quality air and water, and worker protection from toxic substances.

Promoting Healthy Social and Built Environments

Where people live makes a difference in their health. The social, cultural, socioeconomic, and physical characteristics of neighborhoods play a critical role in early child development. The physical activity behaviors of older adults, the fast growing and least physically active group, are influenced by their neighborhood characteristics. In addition, characteristics of "obesogenic" environments contribute to obesity levels in children and adults.

Components of the neighborhood social environment include socioeconomic composition, crime, disorder, community support, collective efficacy, social capital, neighborhood cohesion, and social connectedness (Gomez et al., 2015; Lin et al., 2017). *Social capital* focuses on supportive networks within the community. *Collective efficacy*, the perception of mutual trust and willingness to help each other, is a measure of neighborhood social capital that has been associated with healthy neighborhoods. *Neighborhood cohesion*, another measure of social capital, refers to neighborhood residents' sense of shared norms, values, and feelings of belonging within their community. *Social connectedness* is the degree of closeness between adults and children in a neighborhood. Questions to assess these characteristics might include

"How do neighbors help each other?"

"How much do you trust your neighbors?"

"Do you feel you are a part of the neighborhood?"

"Do you and your neighbors agree on similar things such as child rearing?"

"How often do you talk with your neighbors?"

"How safe do you feel in your neighborhood?"

"Is there graffiti in your neighborhood?"

The *built environment*, defined as the way in which communities and neighborhoods are designed, includes buildings, spaces, public transportation systems, homes, schools, workplaces, parks, and recreation facilities (Sarkar & Webster, 2017). Table 14–1 provides examples of the components of the built environment associated with health

TABLE 14–1 **Components of the Built Environment Associated with Health Outcomes**

Built Environment Components	Physical and Mental Health Outcomes
• Air, water quality	• Physical activity, walking
• Population density	• Well-being
• Housing density, quality	• Diet quality
• Land use mix, zoning	• Asthma, pulmonary diseases
• Distance to stores, schools, etc.	• Cardiovascular diseases
• Food access, quality	• Type 2 diabetes
• Street patterns, lighting	• Restricted elderly mobility
• Sidewalks	• Body mass index
• Noise	• Obesity
• Safety (crime, traffic)	• Depression
• Public parks, green space	• Stress
• Recreational facilities	• Alcohol abuse

outcomes. These include traffic flow, cleanliness, maintenance of public spaces, zoning and land use mix, presence and conditions of sidewalks, and population density. The physical characteristics of neighborhoods have been linked to physical activity, obesity, cardiovascular risk factors, mental health, collective efficacy, and neighborhood cohesiveness.

Built environments are consistently associated with physical activity. Factors that support walkability and other physical activity include the presence and conditions of sidewalks and trails, availability of recreational facilities, lighting, land use mix, and perceived safety within the neighborhood. Built environments can be configured to promote social interactions and physical activity, such as the addition of benches on walking paths for the elderly (Ottoni, Sims-Gould, Winters, Heijnen, & McKay, 2016). Children who live in neighborhoods that enable them to play, walk, or cycle through their neighborhood are more physically active compared to children in less walkable communities (Villanueva et al., 2016). Physical activity benefits children's physical development as well as their social, emotional, and cognitive development.

Obesity has been linked to factors in the social and built environments, especially for children (Townshend & Lake, 2017). Physical inactivity is more common in neighborhoods with sidewalks in need of repair and absent or poorly maintained recreation centers and parks. Children who live in unsafe neighborhoods are less likely to walk to school and more likely to stay inside and watch television more than 2 hours a day compared to children in safe neighborhoods. The increased availability of fast-food outlets is also associated with obesity. In neighborhoods with limited local food stores and higher numbers of fast-food restaurants, the risk for obesity is increased. The neighborhood social environment also plays a role in obesity, as high poverty neighborhoods are less safe for children, have greater rates of crime, and have lower social connectedness and trust of neighbors (Suglia et al., 2016). Obesogenic environments are more likely to be found in impoverished neighborhoods with crime and traffic safety issues and lack of green space to promote physical activity. Low-income neighborhoods have fewer factors that promote health. However, all of the adverse conditions are amenable to change through the creation of programs and policies that can change environments to promote healthy behaviors.

Health care professionals play a pivotal role in promoting healthy social and built environments. Nurses can help communities define and prioritize issues that need to be addressed and empower its members to advocate with community leaders and policy makers to obtain needed resources for community infrastructure. Nurses also can engage sectors in the community, nonprofit organizations, and local policy makers to provide resources needed to repair or build safe sidewalks, obtain streetlights, and create parks or walking spaces; collaborate with schools to develop health promotion programs that facilitate physical activity; and work with families to promote social interactions that develop connectedness in their neighborhoods.

PROMOTING HEALTH THROUGH LEGISLATION

In a democratic society, it is widely assumed that matters of risk critical to survival and security are subject to regulatory decisions, whereas risks not clearly essential for general health and welfare are issues for personal decision and action. Even essential risks may be left to individual decisions, provided that they do not infringe on the rights of others. Controversy over the role of government continues in relation to legislating environmental and behavioral changes that promote good health and increase longevity. If the government uses the means at its disposal to regulate changes in behavior, it may be faced with ethical problems. However, voluntary, individual approaches may fall short of achieving widespread change in self-damaging behaviors. Public health policy plays a major role in the regulation of advertising and taxation of harmful products as well as communicable disease control, such as quarantine and surveillance. For example, pandemic influenza preparedness requires health policy. Public policy and laws are easier for large-scale health threats.

The balance between public good and individual rights is a difficult dilemma. If the state has a moral obligation to protect the right of its citizens, can health measures that benefit the population as a whole be subverted by minority beliefs? The appropriate balance between public good and individual rights is a challenging one. Many individuals view health promotion legislation as unethical or undue intrusion on their individual freedom. Ethical issues, including individual autonomy, must be thoughtfully considered in matters of health policy.

Personal Choice versus Paternalism

There are two philosophical views about the role of government in health: individualism, or personal choice, and paternalism (Wiley, Berman, & Blanke, 2013). *Individualism* or *personal choice* is based on the "American ideal," in which individuals are given maximum freedom to make their own decisions about their health. Health habits are considered personal choices, so outside interventions by governmental policy are not thought to be warranted. Poor health is attributed to individual behaviors; thus, society's responsibility is minimized. *Paternalism*, the counterpoint, holds that experts (professionals and policy makers) have a moral responsibility to solve health problems because individuals lack the ability to do so. Therefore, laws and public policies are justified for the health of society. The role of individuals in this model is to adhere to policies. Individuals are not blamed for their health problems, as they are viewed as victims of circumstance. Both views have strengths. In the *personal control* or individualism model, control is in the hands of the individuals, promoting a sense of efficacy and empowerment. Second, diversity of opinions is respected in the individualistic view. The strength of the paternalistic view is that it has the potential to reduce health inequities. Health policies are socially responsible as they apply to all segments of the population. In addition, problems over which individuals have no control, such as environmental issues, are recognized and addressed.

Both approaches have limitations as well. An emphasis on personal responsibility for health promotes victim blaming, which becomes problematic, as social and environmental factors also are major determinants of health. However, overemphasis on paternalism or social responsibility may discount individual and group differences and the contributions of individuals to lifestyle behaviors. Public health approaches include individuals and communities, the collective voice, to work together to solve problems.

Deciding whether social changes to enhance health should be voluntary or mandatory is a continuing debate. Questions that have been raised include the following:

- Are government regulations appropriate? If so, how and to what extent?
- Is it coercive to increase cigarette taxes to help defray the cost of smoking-induced disease?
- Should highly refined sugar products also be taxed more heavily to pay for the costs of health problems due to obesity?
- Should taxes on large, high-speed automobiles be proportionately higher than taxes on smaller cars with limited speed and greater fuel economy?
- Which social changes should be voluntary and which should be mandated through legislation?

A balance of voluntary and mandatory action is needed, while continuing to pay close attention to the ethical dimensions of such health-related decisions.

Local, state, and federal governments have been criticized for implementing regulations to change the nutritional content of foods, including sugary beverages, trans fats, and salt, to address national health problems (Brownell et al., 2010). Attacks by the food industry have included derogatory labels, such as "nanny state" or "big brother." The attacks are seen as subversive attempts to divert the focus to government paternalism, rather than the need to address the health problems. Proponents of healthy food legislation are accused of interfering with the market economy and restricting personal choices. Similar criticisms were voiced by the tobacco industry prior to the passing of smoking restriction legislation. Paternalistic government regulations have been common throughout history to protect and improve the health and safety of the public. Current actions are targeted to decrease obesity and its long-term health burden. Laws and regulations that promote personal choice and responsibility are possible when authority is used judiciously to address public health problems that are beyond individual control.

In 2016, the beverage industry lost the battle against tax on sugary beverages (Gostin, 2017). Local governments in cities from Philadelphia to San Francisco have levied taxes on sugary beverages, the main source of added sugar, to begin to address obesity and type 2 diabetes. Momentum for the tax was a result of decreased consumption of sugary beverages in Mexico and Berkeley, California, following a tax, and the recommendation of WHO, which called on governments to tax sugary drinks and other unhealthy foods. The beverage companies have criticized the tax as unfairly targeting small businesses and the poor, and indicated the tax was an example of the "nanny state." The American Beverage Association is continuing to oppose the tax as well as proposals to place warning labels in advertisements of sugary drinks in the federal courts. The cities plan to use the tax revenues for health and wellness programs to prevent obesity.

Health Care Access and Health Equity

The U.S. health care system is considered one of the most expensive in the industrialized world (Dickman, Himmelstein, & Woolhandler, 2017). However, it is the only one without universal health coverage. Income-related disparities in access to care are also greater in the United States than other high-income countries. In the United States, the income gap widened between 1980 and 2015; the top 0.1% of the population now controls as much wealth as the bottom 90%. In contrast, incomes remained stagnant for poor and middle-class Americans during this period (Bor, Cohen, & Galea, 2017). Increases in inequities in health and longevity have occurred with the widening income gap. The life expectancy gap between the wealthiest and poorest is now almost 15 years for men and 10 years for women. Evidence also indicates that the United States has one of the lowest projected future life expectancies of 35 industrialized countries (Kontis et al., 2017). Countries with lower projected life expectancies have higher levels of social inequalities, while gains in countries with higher projected life expectancies are attributed to improvements in socioeconomic status and social capital, expanded access to high-quality health care, and low body mass index and blood pressure. The United States has the highest child and maternal mortality, the highest homicide rate, and the highest body mass index of any high-income country (Kontis et al., 2017). Access to quality health care for all is considered critical to reversing the current downward trajectory of health.

The uninsured or underinsured are less likely to seek needed medical attention due to costs. Many who receive care are not able to pay for prescriptions. Employed persons with insurance coverage are paying higher premiums and greater deductibles and copayments, causing many to cut back on seeking care. Postponing or neglecting care results in health problems that may have been prevented with early diagnosis and treatment. Persons in rural areas experience barriers to finding adequate care. Women who need reproductive care are disadvantaged due to high costs and regulations related to family planning. Many Americans continue to face high medical bills, depleting their saving, accruing debt, and declaring bankruptcy. Unequal access to care and unjust financing have been described as similar to the period in the 1950s and 1960s before the passage of Medicare and Medicaid. During this era, one-fourth of all Americans were not insured and over half of older adults and minorities did not have health insurance (Dickman et al., 2017). Health inequities have increased while resources for wealthy Americans have risen. Policy decisions that promote income inequities as well as inequities in opportunity increase disparities in health, resulting in increases in chronic diseases and decreased life expectancy.

The widening health inequities and need to modify the health care system have placed the debate on universal health care at the forefront. Historically, a universal health care system was suggested by two former presidents: President Franklin Roosevelt in his 1944 State of the Union address and President Harry Truman in a message to Congress that proposed a federally supported universal health care plan. Currently, the government provides health coverage for selected segments of the population, including the military, the disabled, and the elderly. Covering only segments of society reinforces health care as a privilege (Berdion, 2007). In other words, health care is only available for those who can pay or have insurance coverage.

When health care is considered a right rather than a privilege, universal care becomes an ethical issue, not an economic or market-driven one (O'Rourke, 2017). Health care as a right means that the government is responsible for providing medically necessary care, regardless of one's ability to pay. It means equality of access to health care resources provided to everyone. Health care as a right shifts the debate from how to pay for health care and who should qualify to how to provide high-quality care for all (Berdion, 2007).

The need for transformation of the health care system has never been greater. All evidence to date has shown that, without health care reform to make health care accessible and affordable for all, the United States will continue to face accelerating costs, and inequities in life expectancy and health outcomes will continue to increase. Health inequities can begin to be addressed through access to health care, the first step in enabling individuals to learn how to prevent diseases and promote a healthy lifestyle. Health inequities will be eliminated when health care is considered a human right, not a privilege.

CONSIDERATIONS FOR PRACTICE TO PROMOTE SOCIAL AND ENVIRONMENTAL CHANGE

As mentioned throughout the book, health promotion and prevention interventions can no longer focus exclusively on the individual to achieve large-scale behavior change. The comprehensive view of health promotion emphasizes the need for collaboration and partnerships with other health professionals, community leaders, health care organizations, and policy makers at the local, state, and national levels. Advanced practice nurses are in positions to provide leadership to build healthy communities by designing and implementing programs to develop community competence and empowerment, and to participate with community members to identify resources and solve problems. Community members should be involved in all aspects of change. Community-based nurses can teach leadership skills to empower community leaders to play influential roles in changing their communities.

Nurses can also become advocates for policies to decrease social and environmental risks and increase access to health care. Promoting health in all policies should be a priority. This can be accomplished by working with local health departments and state legislatures to make change and participating in lobbying efforts to increase resources and services. Health promotion in the 21st century brings many changes and challenges due to technological advances, increasing population diversity and rising social and health inequities. However, these challenges bring new opportunities for nurses, who, with other health professionals, can create innovative health programs and advocate for policies to improve the health of individuals and their communities.

OPPORTUNITIES FOR RESEARCH IN SOCIAL AND ENVIRONMENTAL CHANGE

Social and environmental approaches to promote health offer many opportunities for research. New programs and innovative interprofessional models need to be developed and evaluated. Diverse racial/ethnic and cultural groups should be included in all research. Culturally appropriate programs should be implemented and tested in low-income and racial/ethnically diverse populations. Community-based participatory research to promote partnerships with communities should be emphasized. The study of individual and environmental factors in health and disease is complex and requires research collaboration, multilevel models, and sophisticated statistical techniques to address the many gaps in knowledge that exist. Additional directions for nursing and interdisciplinary research efforts include the following:

1. Evaluate the effects of community physical activity programs on changing health-related social norms among children and adolescents.
2. Design observational studies to describe the effects of chemicals used in hydraulic fracturing on humans and animals, as well as the air and water supply in affected areas.
3. Design studies to evaluate both short-term and long-term effects of policy change to build safe communities on the health of individuals in low-income communities.
4. Evaluate community programs designed to address health inequities, such as unsafe housing, neighborhood crime, or lack of recreational and walking facilities.
5. Identify factors in the social and/or built environment that facilitate physical activity in adolescents and the elderly; design and test the effects of eliminating the barriers on physical activity, both short-term for the elderly and long-term for adolescents.
6. Evaluate the effectiveness of policy changes that eliminate neighborhood environmental barriers to healthy food choices and active lifestyles on obesity.

Summary

This chapter focuses on the impact of social and physical environments and public policy on the health status of individuals, and communities. Attempting to promote healthy lifestyles without changing environments in which people live results in frustration and failure of health promotion efforts. A balanced approach to disease prevention and health promotion requires attention to (1) individual behaviors, (2) quality of the social and physical environments, (3) inequities in health-promoting options available in communities, and (4) changes in health policy to create access to health care for all who need it. Because health is no longer viewed as an aim in itself, but as a resource for personal and social development, as well as a product of social conditions, changes in public policies should become part of any effort to promote health.

Learning Activities

1. Conduct a home or worksite assessment to identify a health-damaging environmental factor. Describe the history of the problem, its effects on the health of the family or workers, barriers to solving the problem, resources needed to solve the problem, and strategies to obtain resources, if they are not available to solve the problem.

2. Develop three strategies to solve the problem identified in Learning Activity 1, and outline an evaluation plan for your possible solutions.

3. Write a letter to your state legislators voicing your concerns about a health inequity you have identified in a rural or urban community, suggest possible solutions, and ask for a response to your concerns.

4. Describe the strategies you would implement to empower and mobilize individuals in a community who have expressed concerns about possible contamination of their water supply from shale gas extraction.

5. Visit your local or state legislature and observe a session, if possible, that involves passing legislation. Summarize your experience. What did you learn that might increase nurses' involvement in influencing policy?

References

Annevelink, M., Meesters, J., & Hendriks, A. (2016). Environmental contamination due to shale gas development. *Science of the Total Environment, 550,* 431–438. doi:10.1016/j.scitotenv.2016.01.131

Bai, S., & Ogbourne, S. (2016). Glyphosate: Environmental contamination, toxicity and potential risks to human health via food contamination. *Environmental Science and Pollution Research,* 23(19), 18988–19001. doi:10.1007/s11356-016-7425-3

Barrington-Trimis, J., Urman, R., Berhane, K., Unger, J., Cruz, T., Pentz, M., . . . McConnell, R. (2016). E-cigarettes and future cigarette use. *Pediatrics,* 138(1), e2016039. doi:10.1542/peds.2016-0379

Berdion, M. (2007). The right to health care in the United States: Local answers to global responsibilities. *SMU Law Review,* 60(4), 1633–1666.

Bor, J., Cohen, G., & Galea, S. (2017). Population health in an era of rising income inequality: USA, 1980–2015. *Lancet,* 389(10077), 1475–1490. doi:10.1016/S0140-6736(17)30571-8

Brook, R., Newby, D., & Rajagopalan, S. (2017). The global threat of outdoor ambient air pollution to cardiovascular health: Time for intervention. *JAMA Cardiology,* 2(4), 353–354. doi:10.1001/jamacardio.2017.0032

Brownell, K. D., Kersh, R., Ludwig, D. S., Post, R. C., Puhl, R. M., Schwartz, M. B., & Willett, W. C. (2010). Personal responsibility and obesity: A constructive approach to a controversial issue. *Health Affairs,* 29(3), 379–387. doi:10.1377/hlthaff.2009.0739

Dahlgren, G., & Whitehead, M. (1993). *Tackling inequalities in health: What can we learn from what has been tried?* Working paper prepared for the King's Fund International Seminar on Tackling Inequalities in Health, The King's Fund, Ditchley Park, Oxfordshire, London, September 1993.

Dahlgren, G., & Whitehead, M. (2007). *European strategies for tackling social inequities in health: Levelling up Part 2.* Copenhagen, Denmark: WHO Regional Office for Europe. Retrieved from http://www.euro.who.int/__data/assets/pdf_file/0018/103824/E89384.pdf

Dickman, S., Himmelstein, D., & Woolhandler, S. (2017). Inequity and the healthcare system in the USA. *Lancet,* 389(10077), 1431–1441. doi:10.1016/S0140-6736(17)30398-7

Estrada, J., & Bhamidimarri, R. (2016). A review of the issues and treatment options for wastewater from shale gas extraction by hydraulic fracturing. *Fuel,* 182, 292–303. doi:10.1016/j.fuel.2016.05.051

Falbe, J., & Madsen, K. (2017). Growing momentum for sugar-sweetened beverage campaigns and policies: Costs and considerations. *American Journal of Public Health,* 107(6), 835–838. doi:10.2105/AJPH.2017.303805

Gilreath, T., Leventhal, A., Barrington-Trimis, J., Unger, J., Cruz, T., Berhane, K., McConnell, R. (2016). Patterns of alternative tobacco product use: Emergence of hookah and E-cigarettes as preferred products amongst youth. *Journal of Adolescent Health,* 58(2), 181–185. doi:10.1016/j.jadohealth.2015.10.001

Gomez, S., Shariff-Marco, S., De Rouen, M., Keegan, T., Yen, I., Mujahid, M., . . . Glaser, S. L. (2015). The impact of neighborhood social and built environment factors across the cancer continuum: Current research, methodological considerations, and future directions. *Cancer, 121*(14), 2314–2330. doi:10.1002/cncr.29345

Gostin, L. (2017). 2016: The year of the soda tax. *The Milbank Quarterly, 95*, 1–3.

Graff, S. K., Kappagoda, M., Wooten, H. M., McGowan, A. K., & Ashe, M. (2012). Policies for healthier communities: Historical, legal, and practical elements of the obesity prevention movement. *Annual Review of Public Health, 33*, 307–324. doi:10.1146/annurev-publhealth-031811-124608

Hanna-Attisha, M., LaChance, J., Sadler, R., & Schnepp, A. (2016). Elevated blood lead levels in children associated with the Flint drinking water crisis: A spatial analysis of risk and public health response. *American Journal of Public Health, 106*(2), 283–290. doi:10.2105/AJPH.2015.303003

Hays, J., & Shonkoff, S. (2016). Toward an understanding of the environmental and public health impacts of unconventional natural gas development: A categorical assessment of the peer-reviewed scientific literature, 2009–2015. *PLoS ONE, 11*(4), e0154164. doi:10.1371/journal.pone.0154164

Kickbusch, I., & Nutbeam, D. (2017). A watershed for health promotion: The Shanghai Conference 2016. *Health Promotion International, 32*(1), 2–6. doi:10.1093/heapro/daw112

Kilpelainen, K., Parikka, S., Koponen, P., Koskinen, S., Rotko, T., Koskela, T., & Gissler, M. (2016). Finnish experiences of health monitoring: Local, regional, and national data sources for policy evaluation. *Global Health Action, 9*, 28824. doi:10.3402/gha.v9.28824

Kontis, V., Bennett, J., Mathers, C., Li, G., Foreman, K., & Ezzati, M. (2017). Future life expectancy in 35 industrialized countries: Projections with a Bayesian model ensemble. *Lancet, 389*(10076), 1323–1335. doi:10.1016/S0140-6736(16)32381-9

Laidlaw, M., Filippelli, G., Sadler, R., Gonzales, C., Ball, A., & Mielke, H. (2016). Children's blood level seasonality in Flint, Michigan (USA) and soil-sourced lead hazard risks. *International Journal of Environmental Research and Public Health, 13*(4), 358.

Lelieveld, J., Evans, J., Fnais, M., Giannadaki, D., & Pozzer, A. (2015). The contribution of outdoor air pollution sources to premature mortality on a global scale. *Nature, 525*(7569), 367–371. doi:10.1038/nature15371

Lin, E., Witten, K., Oliver, M., Carroll, P., Asiasiga, L., Badland, H., & Parker, K. (2017). Social and built-environment factors related to children's independent mobility: The importance of neighborhood cohesion and connectedness. *Health & Place, 46*, 107–113. doi:10.1016/j.healthplace.2017.05.002

Lupton, D. (2014). Health promotion in the digital era: A critical commentary. *Health Promotion International, 30*(1), 174–183. doi:10.1093/heapro/dau091

Myers, J., Antoniou, M., Blumberg, B., Carroll, L., Colborn, T., Everett, L., & Benbrook, C. (2016). Concerns over use of glyphosate-based herbicides and risks associated with exposures: A consensus statement. *Environmental Health, 15*, 19. doi:10.1186/s12940-016-0117-0

O'Rourke, T. (2017). Lost in the health care reform discussion: Health care as a right or privilege. *American Journal of Health Education, 48*(3), 138–141.

Ortega-Navas, M. (2017). The use of new technologies as a tool for the promotion of health education. *Procedia—Social and Behavioral Sciences, 237*, 23–29. doi:10.1016/j.sbspro.2017.02.006

Ottoni, C., Sims-Gould, J., Winters, M., Heijnen, M., & McKay, H. (2016). "Benches become porches": Built and social environment influences on older adults' experiences of mobility and well-being. *Social Science & Medicine, 169*, 33–41.

Patrick, K., Hekler, E., Estrin, D., Mohr, D., Riper, H., Crane, D., . . . Riley, W. (2016). The pace of technologic change: Implications for digital health behavior intervention research. *American Journal of Preventive Medicine, 51*(5), 816–824. doi:10.1016/j.amepre.2016.05.001

Robert Wood Johnson Foundation & Pew Charitable Trusts. (2017). *10 policies to prevent and respond to childhood lead exposure: An assessment of the risks communities face and key federal, state, and local solutions.* Health Impact Project. Retrieved from http://www.pewtrusts.org/~/media/assets/2017/08/hip_childhood_lead_poisoning_report.pdf

Rudolph, L., Caplan, J., Ben-Moshe, K., & Dillon, L. (2013). *Health in all policies: A guide for state and local governments.* Washington, DC/Oakland, CA: American Public Health Association/Public Health Institute.

Sarkar, C., & Webster, C. (2017). Urban environments and human health: Current trends and future directions. *Current Opinion in Environmental Sustainability, 25*, 33–44. doi:10.1016/j.cosust.2017.06.001

Schillinger, D., & Jacobson, M. (2016). Science and public health on trial: Warning notices on advertisements for sugary drinks. *JAMA, 316*(15), 1545–1546. doi:10.1001/jama.2016.10516

Schwartz, M., Just, D., Chriqui, J., & Ammerman, A. (2017). Appetite self-regulation: Environmental and policy influences on eating behaviors. *Obesity, 25*(Suppl 1), s26–s37. doi:10.1002/oby.21770

Secretary's Advisory Committee on National Health Promotion and Disease Prevention Objectives for 2030. (2017). *Recommendations for an approach to Healthy People 2030.* Retrieved on September 14, 2017, from http://www.healthypeople.gov

Suglia, S., Shelton, R., Hsiao, A., Wang, Y., Rundle, A., & Link, B. (2016). Why the neighborhood social environment is critical in obesity prevention. *Journal of Urban Health, 93*(1), 206–212. doi:10.1007/s11524-015-0017-6

Townshend, T., & Lake, A. (2017). Obesogenic environments: Current evidence of the build and food environments. *Perspectives in Public Health, 137*(1), 38–44.

U.S. Department of Health and Human Services. (2016). *E-cigarette use among youth and young adults: A report of the Surgeon General—Executive summary.* Atlanta, GA: U.S. Department of Health and Human Services, Centers for Disease Control and Prevention, National Center for Chronic Disease Prevention and Health Promotion, Office on Smoking and Health.

U.S. Environmental Protection Agency. (2009). *Radon.* Retrieved from https://www.epa.gov/radon

U.S. Environmental Protection Agency. (2016). *Hydraulic fracturing for oil and gas: Impacts from the hydraulic fracturing water cycle on drinking water resources in the United States.* Washington, DC: Office of Research and Development.

Vandenberg, L., Blumberg, B., Antoniou, M., Benbrook, C., Carroll, L., Colborn, T., . . . Myers, J. (2017). Is it time to reassess current safety standards for glyphosate-based herbicides? *Journal of Epidemiology & Community Health, 71*(6), 613–618. doi:10.1136/jech-2016-208463

Villanueva, K., Badland, H., Kvalsvig, A., O'Connor, M., Christian, H., Woolcock, G., . . . Goldfeld, S. (2016). Can the neighborhood built environment make a difference in children's development? Building the research agenda to create evidence for place-based children's policy. *Academic Pediatrics, 16*(1), 10–19. doi:10.1016/j.acap.2015.09.006

Weiss, D., Lillefjell, M., & Magnus, E. (2016). Facilitators for the development and implementation of health promoting policy and programs—A scoping review at the local community level. *BMC Public Health, 16*(1), 1–15. doi:10.1186/s12889-016-2811-9

Whitsel, L. (2017). Government's role in promoting healthy living. *Progress in Cardiovascular Diseases, 59,* 492–497. doi:10.1016/j.pcad.2017.01.003

Wiley, L., Berman, M., & Blanke, D. (2013). Who's your nanny? Choice, paternalism and public health in the age of personal responsibility. *The Journal of Law, Medicine, & Ethics, 41*(1), 88–91. doi:10.1111/jlme.12048

World Health Organization. (2014). *Health in all policies: Helsinki statement. Framework for country action.* Geneva, Switzerland: Author.

World Health Organization, Commission on Social Determinants of Health. (2008). *Closing the gap in a generation: Health equity through action on the social determinants of health.* Geneva, Switzerland: Author.

INDEX